Instructor's Guide

Guide to Good Food

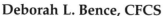

Deborah L. Bence, CFCS
Family and Consumer Science
Author and Editor
Homewood, Illinois

Guide to Good Food Text
by Velda L. Largen
and Deborah L. Bence, CFCS

Publisher
The Goodheart-Willcox Company, Inc.
Tinley Park, Illinois

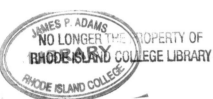
Copyright 1996
by

The Goodheart-Willcox Company, Inc.

Previous editions copyright 1992, 1989

Contents

	Instructor's Guide	Text	Activity Guide

Part 4   Foods of the World

Introduction

Guide to Good Food is a comprehensive text concerned with the nutrient value, appetite appeal, social significance, and cultural aspects of food. Besides the student text, the *Guide to Good Food* learning package includes the *Student Activity Guide, Teacher's Annotated Edition, Instructor's Guide, Transparency Packet, Teacher's Resource Binder,* and *Test Creation Software.* Using these products can help you develop an effective food and nutrition program tailored to your students' unique needs.

Using the Text

The text, *Guide to Good Food,* is designed to help your students learn about food preparation and management. They will learn how to select, store, prepare, and serve foods while preserving nutrients, flavors, textures, and colors.

The text is divided into 4 parts with a total of 31 chapters. The material is organized and presented in a logical sequence of topics for the study of foods and nutrition. The book is directed primarily toward students, but it is also suitable for use as a reference by anyone interested in the management and preparation of food. Although the text was written to be studied in its entirety, individual chapters and sections are complete enough to be studied independently.

The text is straightforward and easy to read. Hundreds of full-color photographs and charts attract student interest and emphasize key concepts. The copy includes references to the illustrations to help students associate the visual images with the written material. This helps reinforce learning.

The text includes an expanded table of contents to give students an overview of the wide variety of topics they will be studying. The glossary at the back of the book helps students learn terms related to foods and nutrition. A complete index helps them find information they want quickly and easily. A separate recipe index helps them locate instructions for preparing specific food products.

Each chapter includes several features designed to help students study effectively and review what they have learned.

A "Taste" of the World of Work. Job titles and descriptions from the *Dictionary of Occupational Titles* are listed at the beginning of each chapter. This helps show students the wide range of careers available in the food industry.

Terms to Know. A list of vocabulary terms appears at the beginning of each chapter. Terms are listed in the order in which they appear in the chapter. These terms are in bold italic type throughout the text so students can recognize them while reading. Discussing these words with students will help them learn concepts to which they are being introduced. To help students become familiar with these terms, you may want to ask them to

- look up, define, and explain each term.
- relate each term to the topic being studied.
- match terms with their definitions.
- find examples of how the terms are used in current newspapers and magazines, cookbooks, and other related materials.

Objectives. A set of behavioral objectives is also found at the beginning of each chapter. These are performance goals that students should be able to achieve after studying the chapter. Review the objectives in each chapter with students to help make them aware of the skills they will be building as they read the chapter material.

Health, consumer, safety, business etiquette, and environmental tips. Throughout the book, students will find color-keyed boxes containing interesting, educational tips. Following these tips will help students apply text information in their daily lives.

Summary. A chapter summary, located at the end of each chapter, provides a review of major concepts.

Review What You Have Read. Review questions at the end of each chapter are included to cover the basic information presented. This section consists of a variety of true/false, completion, multiple choice, and short essay questions. It is designed to help students recall, organize, and use the information presented in the text. Answers to these questions appear in the front section of the *Teacher's Annotated Edition* as well as in the *Instructor's Guide* and the *Teacher's Resource Binder.*

Build Your Basic Skills. Suggested activities at the end of each chapter offer students opportunities to develop verbal, reading, writing, math, and science skills.

Build Your Thinking Skills. This set of end-of-chapter activities promotes the development of such higher-order thinking skills as analysis, synthesis, and evaluation in problem-solving situations.

Both groups of activities encourage students to apply many of the concepts learned in the chapter to real-life situations. Suggestions for both individual and group work are provided in varying degrees of difficulty. Therefore, you may choose and assign activities according to students' interests and abilities.

Using the *Student Activity Guide*

The *Student Activity Guide* designed for use with *Guide to Good Food* helps students recall and review material presented in the text. It also helps them apply what they have learned as they buy, prepare, and store foods.

The activities in the guide are divided into chapters that correspond to the chapters in the text. The text provides the information students will need to complete many of the activities. Other activities will require creative thinking and research beyond the textbook.

You may want to use the exercises in the *Student Activity Guide* that are directly related to textual material as introductory, review, or evaluation tools. Ask students to do the exercises without looking in the book. Then they can use the text to check their answers and to answer questions they could not complete. The pages of the *Student Activity Guide* are perforated so students can easily turn completed activities in to you for evaluation.

The *Student Activity Guide* includes different types of activities. Some have specific answers related to text material. Students can use these activities to review as they study for tests and quizzes. Answers to these activities appear in the *Instructor's Guide* and *Teacher's Resource Binder*.

Other activities, such as case studies and surveys, ask for students' thoughts or opinions. Answers to these activities cannot be judged as right or wrong. These activities allow students to form ideas by considering alternatives and evaluating situations thoughtfully. You can use these thought-provoking exercises as a basis for classroom discussion by asking students to justify their answers and conclusions.

The use of each activity in the *Student Activity Guide* is described in the *Instructor's Guide* and *Teacher's Resource Binder* as a teaching strategy under the related instructional concept. Activities are identified by name and letter.

Using the *Teacher's Annotated Edition*

The *Teacher's Annotated Edition* for *Guide to Good Food* is a special edition of the student text. It is designed to help you more effectively coordinate materials in the *Student Activity Guide* and *Teacher's Resource Binder* with text concepts. It also provides you with additional suggestions to help you add variety to your classroom teaching.

Annotations are located throughout the text. Numbers are placed in the right and left side margins that correspond with annotations located at the bottom of each page. The chart on the next page details the annotations used in the annotated edition.

Along with annotations placed throughout the student text, the *Teacher's Annotated Edition* includes a special front section on colored paper. It begins with a detailed introduction explaining how to use the various components in the teaching package for *Guide to Good Food*. This section also contains several features designed to help you prepare meaningful lessons for your students.

Teaching Suggestions

A number of suggestions are given to help you increase the effectiveness of your classroom teaching. This information includes suggestions for teaching students of varying abilities, evaluating students, communicating with students, and promoting your program.

Scope and Sequence Chart

A "Scope and Sequence Chart," located at the end of the introduction, identifies the major concepts presented in each chapter of the text. This special resource is provided to help you select for study those topics that meet your curriculum needs.

Teaching Aids

The last item in the front section of the annotated text is a chapter-by-chapter teaching aids resource. It

Annotation Term	Annotation Description
Vocabulary	These annotations are placed alongside the list of chapter terms and elsewhere within the chapter. They suggest vocabulary reinforcement activities, such as defining terms, using terms in sentences, looking up terms in the glossary, or comparing important new terms. They may also provide interesting and meaningful information about the origins of words.
Discuss	These annotations provide discussion questions to reteach or reinforce learning. Questions may also relate to charts in the chapter.
Reflect	These annotations provide questions to ask students to think about regarding the concepts presented, often by applying the content to their lives. These questions are often more personal than are the discussion questions.
Activity	These annotations suggest activities that would reteach and reinforce text concepts. (Math or science activities are designated as either *Math Activity* or *Science Activity*.)
Note	These annotations provide additional points the instructor might want to make regarding the topic, or to spark student interest in the topic discussion. Points might include statistics, interesting facts, or historical notes. These may also be notes to the instructor regarding the subject matter.
Example	These annotations provide one or more examples to use in illustrating an important point in the chapter material.
Enrich	These annotations suggest activities that demonstrate the concept, but are more involved and challenging for students. Examples include role-playing, research topics, debates, surveys, bulletin boards, field trips, or guest speakers.
Resource	These annotations refer to activities in the *Student Activity Guide* and reproducible masters in the *Teacher's Resource Binder* that relate to chapter material.
Answers	These annotations indicate where answers to questions may be found.

is designed to assist you in developing lesson plans and evaluating student learning. Each chapter of the text includes the following aids:

Chapter Outline. An outline of the chapter's main points is provided to give you an overview of the content and organization of chapter material.

Answer Key. Answers for the "Review What You Have Read" questions at the end of each chapter are supplied to assist you in clarifying student understanding of chapter concepts.

Using the *Instructor's Guide*

The *Instructor's Guide* for *Guide to Good Food* suggests many methods of presenting the concepts in the text to students. It begins with some of the same helpful information found in the *Teacher's Annotated Edition,* including teaching suggestions and a "Scope and Sequence Chart."

Basic Skills Chart

Another feature of the *Instructor's Guide* is a "Basic Skills Chart." This chart has been included to identify those activities that encourage the development of the following basic skills: verbal, reading, writing, mathematical, scientific, and analytical. (Analytical skills involve the higher-order thinking skills of analysis, synthesis, and evaluation in problem-solving situations.) The chart includes activities from the *Student Activity Guide* and strategies from the *Instructor's Guide* and *Teacher's Resource Binder.* Incorporating a variety of these activities into your daily lesson plans will provide your students with vital practice in the development of basic skills. Also, if you find that students in your classes are weak in a specific basic skill, you can select activities to strengthen that particular skill area.

Chapter-by-Chapter Resources

Like the *Student Activity Guide,* the *Instructor's Guide* is divided into chapters that match the chapters in the text. Each chapter contains the following features:

Objectives. These are the objectives that students will be able to accomplish after reading the chapter and completing the suggested activities.

Bulletin Boards. Bulletin board ideas are described for each chapter. Many of these ideas are illustrated for you. Putting up bulletin board displays can often be a stimulating student activity.

Teaching Materials. A list of materials available to supplement each chapter in the text is provided. The list includes the names of all the activities contained in the *Student Activity Guide* and all the masters contained in the *Teacher's Resource Binder.*

Introductory Activities. These motivational exercises are designed to stimulate your students' interest in the chapter they will be studying. The activities help create a sense of curiosity that students will want to satisfy by reading the chapter.

Strategies to Reteach, Reinforce, Enrich, and Extend Text Concepts. A variety of student learning strategies is described for teaching each of the major concepts discussed in the text. Each major concept appears in the guide in bold type. The student learning experiences for each concept follow. Activities from the *Student Activity Guide* are identified for your convenience in planning daily lessons. They are identified with the letters *SAG* following the title and letter of the activity. (*What's Behind the Dietary Guidelines?* Activity A, SAG.)

The number of each learning strategy is followed by a code in bold type. These codes identify the teaching goals each strategy is designed to accomplish. The following codes have been used:

RT identifies activities designed to help you *reteach* concepts. These strategies present the chapter concepts in a different way to allow students additional learning opportunities.

RF identifies activities designed to *reinforce* concepts to students. These strategies present techniques and activities to help clarify facts, terms, principles, and concepts, making it easier for students to understand.

ER identifies activities designed to *enrich* learning. These strategies help students learn more about the concepts presented by involving them more fully in the material. Enrichment strategies include diverse experiences, such as demonstrations, field trips, guest speakers, panels, and surveys.

EX identifies activities designed to *extend* learning. These strategies promote thinking skills, such as critical thinking, creative thinking, problem solving, and decision making. Students must analyze, synthesize, and evaluate to complete these activities.

Chapter Review. These review activities are designed to help students summarize key information from the chapter. You can use these activities to help students check their learning and prepare for chapter tests.

Above and Beyond. This section gives suggestions for enrichment activities that require work beyond the average class assignments. Although these activities could enhance the learning of any student, they are recommended for gifted or above average students.

Answer Key. This section provides answers for review questions at the end of each chapter in the text, for activities in the *Student Activity Guide,* and for the chapter tests.

Chapter Test Masters. Individual tests with clear, specific questions that cover all the chapter topics are provided. True/false, multiple choice, and matching questions are used to measure student learning about facts and definitions. Essay questions are also provided in the chapter tests. Some of these require students to list information, while others encourage students to express their opinions and creativity. You may wish to modify the tests and tailor the questions to your classroom needs.

Using the Transparency Packet

Color transparencies for *Guide to Good Food* are available to add variety to your classroom lecture as you discuss topics included in the text with your students. You will find some transparencies useful in illustrating and reinforcing information presented in the text. Others will provide you with an opportunity to extend learning beyond the scope of the text. Attractive colors are visually appealing and hold students' attention. Suggestions for how you can use the transparencies in the classroom are included in the packet.

Using the *Teacher's Resource Binder*

The *Teacher's Resource Binder* for *Guide to Good Food* combines the *Instructor's Guide* with the transparency packet. A convenient three-ring binder holds all the materials from both products, allowing you to remove materials for easy copying. You can also insert additional resource materials of your own. Handy dividers organize pages into parts corresponding with the textbook so you can easily find the items you need.

Besides the transparencies and the items found in the *Instructor's Guide,* the *Teacher's Resource Binder* includes the following materials:

Comprehensive Tests. A comprehensive test covering each of the four parts of the text is provided in the back of the *Teacher's Resource Binder.* These tests consist of true/false, multiple choice, matching, and essay questions. The answer key for each test identifies the chapter to which each question relates. This will assist you if you wish to modify the tests to meet your individual classroom needs.

Foods Lab Resources. The front of the *Teacher's Resource Binder* includes suggestions for managing the foods lab. Ideas are given for lab preparation, lab policies, and working with exceptional students. Information is included for using food science masters. Reproducible masters are also provided for making market orders, planning lab time, and evaluating food products and lab experiences.

Reproducible Masters. Each chapter includes several reproducible masters. These masters are designed to enhance the presentation of concepts in the text. Some of the masters are designated as *transparency masters* for use with an overhead projector. These are often charts or graphs that can serve as a basis for class discussion of important concepts. You can also use them as student handouts.

Some of the masters are designed as *reproducible masters.* You can copy these masters to use as student handouts. Many of them include activities that encourage creative and critical thinking. You may wish to use these activities as a basis for class discussion. Some masters provide material not contained in the text that you may want students to know.

Each chapter also includes a reproducible master for a study sheet. Study sheets are designed to be completed by students as they read the chapter and focus on key concepts. Students can then use the completed study sheets as chapter summaries to review for tests. The chapter answer keys include any answers needed for the reproducible masters.

In chapters focusing on food preparation, many of the masters are designated as *recipe masters.* These masters include all the recipes used in the text, plus a number of additional recipes. You can copy these masters for students to use in the foods lab as they gain hands-on experience in various food preparation techniques. This eliminates the need to carry textbooks into the lab. It also provides students with copies of the recipes they can take home with them.

Chapters 13 through 25 include *food science masters.* These masters are intended to heighten students' awareness of the scientific principles used in food preparation. Each one describes a procedure for students to follow. Space is also included for students to record their observations and formulate conclusions.

Using the *Test Creation Software*

Besides the printed supplements designed to support *Guide to Good Food, Test Creation Software* is available. The database for this software package includes all the test master questions from the *Instructor's Guide/Teacher's Resource Binder* plus an additional 25 percent new questions prepared just for this product. You can choose the EasyTest option to have the computer generate a test for you with randomly selected questions. You can also opt to choose specific questions from the database and, if you wish, add questions to create customized tests to meet your classroom needs. You may want to make different versions of the same test to use during different class periods. Answer keys are generated automatically to simplify grading.

Using the Computer Review Games

Software designed for student use is available to accompany *Guide to Good Food.* It uses five game formats as challenging, fun methods of reviewing text information. One game is provided for each chapter. Each game contains questions that help students review key facts, concepts, and vocabulary terms. Randomized questions make each game different every time students play it. Immediate feedback and an explanation of the correct answer are given for each question.

You may incorporate the review games into your program in a variety of ways. Since the programs are self-guiding, you can have students work at their pace with minimum supervision. You might allow students to use the software outside class time as a review for a chapter test. You may find the software useful in reinforcing concepts for lower level or difficult-to-motivate students. You may also use the games as a thought-provoking preview to the chapter.

Teaching Techniques

You can make the study of foods and nutrition exciting and relevant by using a variety of teaching techniques. Below are some principles that will help you choose and use different teaching techniques in your classroom.

- Make learning stimulating. One way to do this is to involve students in lesson planning. When possible, allow them to select the modes of learning that they enjoy most. For example, some students will do well with oral reports; others prefer written assignments. Some learn well through group projects; others do better working independently. You can also make courses more interesting by presenting a variety of learning activities and projects from which students may choose to fulfill their work requirement.
- Make learning realistic. You can do this by relating the subject matter to issues that concern young people. Students gain the most from learning when they can apply it to real-life situations. Case studies, role-playing, and drawing on personal experiences all make learning more realistic and relevant.
- Make learning varied. Try using several different techniques to teach the same concept. Make use of outside resources and current events as they apply to material being presented in class. Students learn through their senses of sight, hearing, touch, taste, and smell. The more senses they use, the easier it will be for them to retain information. Bulletin boards, films, tapes, and transparencies all appeal to the senses.
- Make learning success-oriented. Experiencing success increases self-esteem and confidence. Guarantee success for your students by presenting a variety of learning activities. Key these activities to different ability levels so that each student can enjoy both success and challenge. You also will want to allow for individual learning styles and talents. For instance, creative students may excel at designing projects, while analytical students may be more proficient at organizing details. Build in opportunities for individual students to work in ways that let them succeed and shine.
- Make learning personal. Young people become more personally involved in learning if you establish a comfortable rapport with them. Work toward a relaxed classroom atmosphere in which students can feel at ease when sharing their feelings and ideas in group discussions and activities.

Following are descriptions of various teaching techniques you may want to try. Keep in mind that not all methods work equally well in all classrooms. A technique that works beautifully with one group of students may not be successful with another. The techniques you choose will depend on the topic, your teaching goals, and the needs of your students.

One final consideration concerns students' right to privacy. Some activities, such as autobiographies, diaries, and opinion papers, may invade students' privacy. You can maintain a level of confidentiality by letting students turn in unsigned papers in these situations. You may also encourage students to pursue some of these activities at home for personal enlightenment without fear of evaluation or judgment.

Helping Students Gain Basic Information

Many teaching techniques can be grouped according to different goals you may have for your students. One group of techniques is designed to convey information to students. Two of the most common techniques in this group are reading and lecture. Using a number of variations can make these techniques seem less common and more interesting. For instance, students may enjoy taking turns to read aloud as a change of pace from silent reading. You can energize lectures with flip charts, overhead transparencies, and other visual materials. Classroom discussions of different aspects of the material being presented get students involved and help impart information.

Other ways to present basic information include the use of outside resources. Guest speakers, whether speaking individually or as part of a panel, can bring a new outlook to classroom material. You can videotape guest lectures to show again to other classes or to use for review. Besides videotapes, students also enjoy films and filmstrips related to material being studied.

Helping Students Question and Evaluate

A second group of teaching techniques helps students develop analytic and judgmental skills. These techniques help your students go beyond what they see on the surface. As you employ these techniques, encourage students to think about points raised by others. Ask them to evaluate how new ideas relate to their attitudes about various subjects.

Discussion is an excellent technique for helping students consider an issue from a new point of view. To be effective, discussion sessions require a great deal of planning and preparation. Consider the size of the discussion group and the physical arrangement. Since many students are reluctant to contribute in a large group, you may want to divide the class into smaller groups for discussion sessions. You can also enhance participation by arranging the room so students can see each other.

Discussion can take a number of forms. Generally it is a good idea to reserve group discussions involving the entire class for smaller classes. Buzz groups consisting of two to six students offer a way to get willing participation from students who are not naturally outgoing. They discuss an issue among themselves and then appoint a spokesperson to report back to the entire class.

Debate is an excellent way to explore opposite sides of an issue. You may want to divide the class into two groups, each to take an opposing side of the issue. You can also ask students to work in smaller groups and explore opposing sides of different issues. Each group can select students from the group to present the points for their side.

Helping Students Participate

Another group of teaching techniques is designed to promote student participation in classroom activities and discussion. There are many ways to involve students and encourage them to interact. Case studies, surveys, opinionnaires, stories, and pictures can all be used to boost classroom participation. These techniques allow students to react to or evaluate situations in which they are not directly involved. Open-ended sentences often stimulate discussion. However, it is wise to steer away from overly personal or confidential matters when selecting sentences for completion. Students may be reluctant to deal with confidential issues in front of classmates.

The *fishbowl* can be a good way to stimulate class discussion. A larger observation group encircles an interactive group of five to eight students. The encircled students discuss a given topic while the others listen. Observers are not permitted to talk or interrupt. Positions can be reversed at the end of a fishbowl session to allow some of the observers to become the participants.

One of the most effective techniques for encouraging participation is the *cooperative learning group*. The teacher has a particular goal or task in mind. Small groups of learners are matched to complete the task or goal, and each person in the group is assigned a role. The success of the group is measured not only in terms of outcome, but in the successful performance of each member in his or her role.

In cooperative learning groups, students learn to work together toward a group goal. Each member is dependent upon others for the outcome. This interdependence is a basic component of any cooperative learning group. The value of each group member is affirmed as learners work toward their goal.

The success of the group depends on individual performance. Mix groups in terms of abilities and talents so that there are opportunities for the students to learn from one another. Also, as groups work together over time, rotate the roles so that everyone has an opportunity to practice and develop different skills. Possible roles include leader, timer, recorder, and reporter.

The interaction of students in a cooperative learning group creates a tutoring relationship. While cooperative learning groups may involve more than just group discussion, discussion is always part of the process by which cooperative learning groups function.

Helping Students Apply Learning

Some techniques are particularly good for helping students use what they have learned. Simulation games and role-playing allow students to practice solving problems and making decisions under nonthreatening circumstances. Role-playing allows students to examine others' feelings as well as their own. It can help them learn effective ways to react or cope when confronted with similar situations in real life.

Role-plays can be structured, with the actors following written scripts, or they may be improvised in response to a classroom discussion. Students may act out a role as they see it being played, or they may act out the role as they presume a person in that position would behave. Roles are not rehearsed and lines are composed on the spot. The follow-up discussion should focus on the feelings and emotions felt by the participants and the manner in which the problem was resolved. Role-playing helps students consider how they would behave in similar situations in their lives.

Helping Students Develop Creativity

You can use some techniques to help students generate new ideas. For example, brainstorming encourages students to exchange and pool their ideas and to come up with new thoughts and solutions to problems. No evaluation or criticism of ideas is allowed. The format of spontaneously expressing any opinions or reactions that come to mind lets students be creative without fear of judgment.

You also can promote creativity by letting students choose from a variety of assignments related to the same material. For example, suppose you wanted students to know how to control spending when making food purchases. You might have students compare prices of various sizes and brands of particular food items. You could give them the choice of seeing how much money they could save if they used coupons. Having students interview an experienced meal manager about budgeting techniques he or she has found helpful would be an option, too. Any teaching techniques you use to encourage students to develop ideas will foster their creativity.

Helping Students Review Information

Certain techniques aid students in recalling and retaining knowledge. Games can be effective for drills on vocabulary and information. Crossword puzzles and mazes can make the review of vocabulary terms more interesting. Structured outlines of subject matter can also be effective review tools. Open-book quizzes, bulletin board displays, and problem-solving sessions all offer ways to review and apply material presented in the classroom.

Teaching Students of Varying Abilities

The students in your classroom represent a wide range of ability levels. Special needs students who are mainstreamed require unique teaching strategies. You must not overlook gifted students. You need to challenge them up to their potential. All the students in between will have individual needs to consider, too. Often you will have to meet the needs of all of these students in the same classroom setting. It is a challenge to adapt daily lessons to meet the demands of all your students.

To tailor your teaching to mainstreamed and lower-ability students, consider the following strategies:

- Before assigning a chapter in the text, discuss and define the key words that appear at the beginning of each chapter. These terms are defined in the glossary at the back of the text. Ask students to write out the definitions and interpret what they think the terms mean. You might want to invite students to guess what they think words mean before they look up the definitions. You can also ask them to use new words in sentences and to find the sentences in the text where the new terms are used.
- When introducing a new chapter, review previously learned information students need to know before they can understand the new material. Review previously learned vocabulary terms they will encounter again.
- Use the "Introductory Activities" section in the *Instructor's Guide* or *Teacher's Resource Binder* for each chapter. Students who have difficulty reading need a compelling reason to read the material. These introductory activities can provide the necessary motivation. Students will want to read the text to satisfy their curiosity.
- Break the chapters into smaller parts, and assign only one section at a time. Define the terms, answer the "Review What You Have Read" questions, and discuss the concepts presented in each section before proceeding to the next. It often helps to rephrase questions and problems in simple language and to

repeat important concepts in different ways. Assign activities in the *Student Activity Guide* that relate to each section in the book. These reinforce the concepts presented. In addition, many of these activities are designed to improve reading comprehension.

- Ask students, individually or in pairs, to answer the "Review What You Have Read" questions at the end of each chapter in the text. This will help them focus on the essential information contained in the chapter.
- Use the buddy system. Pair nonreaders with those who read well. Ask students who have mastered the material to work with those who need assistance. It also may be possible to find a parent volunteer who can provide individual attention where needed.
- Select a variety of educational experiences to reinforce the learning of each concept. Look for activities that will help reluctant learners relate information to real-life situations. It helps to draw on the experiences of students at home, in school, and in the community.
- Give directions orally as well as in writing. You will need to explain assignments as thoroughly and simply as possible. Ask questions to be certain students understand what they are to do. Encourage them to ask for help if they need it. You will also want to follow up as assignments proceed to be sure no one is falling behind on required work.
- Use the overhead projector and the transparency masters included in the *Teacher's Resource Binder.* A visual presentation of concepts will increase students' ability to comprehend the material. You may want to develop other transparencies to use in reviewing key points covered in each chapter.

If you have advanced or gifted students in your class, you will need to find ways to challenge them. These students require assignments that involve critical thinking and problem solving. Because advanced students are more capable of independent work, they can use the library and outside resources to research topics in depth. Learning experiences listed in the "Basic Skills Chart" that involve analytical skills are appropriate for gifted students. You may be able to draw on the talents of advanced students in developing case studies and learning activities to use with the entire class.

Evaluation Techniques

You can use a variety of evaluation tools to assess student achievement. Try using the reproducible forms, "Evaluating Individual Participation," "Evaluating Individual Reports," and "Evaluating Group Participation," included with the introductory material in the front of the *Teacher's Resource Binder.* These rating scales allow you to observe a student's performance and rank it along a continuum. This lets students see what levels they have surpassed and what levels they can still strive to reach.

In some situations, it is worthwhile to allow students to evaluate themselves. When evaluating an independent study project, for example, students may be the best judge of whether they met the objectives they set for themselves. Students can think about what they have learned and see how they have improved. They can analyze their strengths and weaknesses.

You may ask students to evaluate their peers from time to time. This gives the student performing the evaluation an opportunity to practice giving constructive criticism. It also gives the student being evaluated the opportunity to accept criticism from his or her peers.

Tests and quizzes are also effective evaluation tools. You may give these in either written or oral form. In either case, however, you should use both objective and subjective questions to help you adequately assess student knowledge and understanding of class material.

Communicating with Students

Communicating with students involves not only sending clear messages, but also receiving and interpreting feedback. Following are some suggestions for productive communication with your students:

- Recognize the importance of body language and nonverbal communication, both in presenting material and interpreting student responses. Eye contact, relaxed but attentive body position, natural gestures, and alert facial expression all make for a presentation of material that will command attention. The same positive nonverbal cues from students indicate their response and reactions. Voice is also an important nonverbal communicator. Cultivating a warm, lively, enthusiastic speaking voice will make classroom presentations more interesting. By your tone, you can convey a sense of acceptance and expectation to which your students will respond.

- Use humor whenever possible. Humor is not only good medicine, it opens doors and teaches lasting lessons. Laughter and amusement will reduce tension, make points in a nonthreatening and memorable way, increase the fun and pleasure in classroom learning, and break down stubborn barriers. Relevant cartoons, quotations, jokes, and amusing stories all bring a light touch to the classroom.
- Ask questions that promote recall, discussion, and thought. Good questions are tools that open the door to communication. Open-ended inquiries that ask what, where, why, when, and how will stimulate thoughtful answers. You can draw out students by asking for their opinions and conclusions. Questions with yes or no answers tend to discourage rather than promote further communication. Avoid inquiries that are too personal or that might put students on the spot.
- Rephrase students' responses to be sure both you and they understand what has been said. Paraphrasing information students give is a great way to clarify, refine, and reinforce material and ideas under discussion. For example, you might say, "This is what I hear you saying. . .correct me if I'm wrong." Positive acknowledgment of student contributions, insights, and successes encourages more active participation and open communication. Comments such as, "That's a very good point. I hadn't thought of it that way before." or, "What a great idea." will encourage youngsters to express themselves.
- Listen for what students say, what they mean, and what they do not say. Really

listening may be the single most important step you can take to promote open communication. As students answer questions and express their ideas and concerns, try not only to hear what they say, but to understand what they mean. What is not said can also be important. Make room for silence and time to think and reflect during discussion sessions.

- Share your feelings and experiences. The measure of what students communicate to you will depend in part on what you are willing to share with them. Express your personal experiences, ideas, and feelings when they are relevant. Do not forget to tell students about a few of your mistakes. Sharing will give students a sense of exchange and relationship.
- Lead discussion sessions to rational conclusions. Whether with an entire class or with individual students, it is important to identify and resolve conflicting thoughts and contradictions. This will help students think clearly and logically. For example, in a discussion of weight management, students may want the physical benefits of maintaining a healthy weight without giving any thought to their food choices. Pointing out and discussing the inconsistency in these two positions will lead students to more logically consider both health and food choices.
- Create a nonjudgmental atmosphere. Students will only communicate freely and openly in a comfortable environment. You can make them comfortable by respecting their ideas, by accepting them for who they are, and by honoring their confidences. It is also important to avoid criticizing a student or discussing personal matters in front of others.
- Use written communication to advantage. The more ways you approach students, the more likely you are to reach them on different levels. The written word can often be an excellent way to connect. Written messages can take different forms—a notice on the chalkboard, a note attached to homework, a memo to parents (with good news as well as bad), or a letter exchange involving class members.

- Be open and available for private discussions of personal or disciplinary problems. It is important to let students know they can come to you with personal concerns as well as questions regarding course material. Be careful not to violate students' trust by discussing confidential matters outside a professional setting.

Promoting Your Program

Your class is likely to be the first foods class some of your students have taken. Many students and their parents may have preconceived ideas about what foods and nutrition curriculum includes. You need to identify these preconceptions and, if necessary, gently alter them to give students and their parents a more accurate idea of what your class entails. You may need to make them aware of the value foods classes hold for students at a variety of levels.

Your public relations campaign can begin by using the reproducible master, "Daily Diet," found in the introductory materials of the *Teacher's Resource Binder.* Add your name and the name of your school underneath the masthead. Then send copies of the page home as a newsletter to inform parents about what their children will be studying in your class. You can also use copies promotionally to encourage students to enroll in your class.

Students and their parents are not likely to be the only ones who are not totally aware of the importance of family and consumer science classes. You can make people more aware through good public relations. It pays to make the student body and faculty aware of your program. With good public relations, you can increase your enrollment, gain support from administrators and other teachers, and achieve recognition in the community. Following are some ways to promote your program:

- Create visibility. It is important to let people know what is going on in family and consumer science classes. Ways to do this include announcements of projects and activities at faculty meetings and in school bulletins or newspapers, displays in school showcases or on bulletin boards, and articles and press releases in school and community newspapers. "Hungry to Learn?" is a reproducible

flyer describing the importance of foods classes. It is included with the introductory materials of the *Teacher's Resource Binder.* Add the title of your class and your name and room number to the flyer. Then post copies of it around your school or pass them out to students. Ask your students what they feel they have gained by taking your class. Add some of their ideas to your flyer. (If you decide to use direct quotations, be sure to get permission from your students.)

- Interact within the school. Foods and nutrition information is related to many fields of learning. You can strengthen your program and contribute to other disciplines by cooperating with other teachers. For example, you can work with a science teacher to present information on the scientific principles involved in cooking food, a social studies teacher to cover the cultural aspects of food, or a business teacher to discuss food budgeting. Invite administrators and other teachers to visit your classes. The more interaction you can generate, the more you promote your foods and nutrition class.

- Contribute to the educational objectives of the school. If your school follows stated educational objectives and strives to strengthen specific skills, include these overall goals in your teaching. For example, if students need special help in developing verbal or writing skills, select projects and assignments that will help them in these areas. The "Basic Skills Chart" in the *Instructor's Guide* and *Teacher's Resource Binder* will give you ideas for activities that strengthen specific skills. Show administrators examples of work that indicate student improvement in needed skills.

- Serve as a resource center. Foods and nutrition information is of practical use and interest to almost everyone. You can sell your program by making your department a resource center of foods and nutrition materials related to weight management, healthy food choices, appliance selection, food preparation, and consumer skills. Invite faculty members, students, and parents to tap into the wealth of foods and nutrition information available in your classroom.

- Generate involvement and activity in the community. You are teaching concepts students can apply in their everyday lives. You can involve students in community life and bring the community into your classroom through field trips, interviews with businesspeople and community leaders, surveys, and presentations from guest speakers. You may be able to set up cooperative projects between the school and community organizations around a variety of topics.

- Connect with parents. If you can get them involved, parents may be your best allies in teaching foods and nutrition. Let parents know when their children have done good work. Moms and dads have had experiences related to many of the issues you discuss in class. They have purchased foods and appliances, planned menus,

and prepared meals. Call on them to share individually or as part of a panel addressing a specific topic. Parents can be a rich source of real-life experience. Keep them informed about classroom activities and invite them to participate as they are able.

- Establish a student sales staff. Enthusiastic students will be your best salespeople. Encourage them to tell their parents and friends what they are learning in your classes. You might create bulletin boards or write letters to parents that focus on what students are learning in your classes. Ask students to put together a newsletter highlighting their experiences in your foods and nutrition class. Students could write a column from your department for the school paper.

We appreciate the contributions of the following Goodheart-Willcox authors to this introduction: "Teaching Techniques" from *Changes and Choices,* by Ruth E. Bragg; and "Evaluation Techniques" from *Contemporary Living,* by Verdene Ryder.

Scope and Sequence

In planning your program, you may want to use the "Scope and Sequence Chart" below. This chart identifies the major concepts presented in each chapter of the text. Refer to the chart to find the material that meets your curriculum needs. Bold numbers indicate chapters in which concepts are found.

Part 1
The Importance of Food

Social/Cultural Aspects

1: The history of food; cultural influences; social influences; psychological influences

4: Childhood obesity; acne; adolescent obesity; vegetarian diet; factors that contribute to overeating; identifying eating habits; underweight; eating disorders

6: Choosing a career; finding a job

Nutrition and Health

2: Nutrients—carbohydrates, fats, proteins, vitamins, minerals, trace elements, water; total energy value of food

3: Recommended Dietary Allowances; Dietary Guidelines for Americans; Food Guide Pyramid

4: Nutrition during pregnancy, lactation, infancy, early childhood, the elementary school years, the teen years, adulthood, old age; nutrition for athletes; exercise and fitness; nutrition during illness; weight management

5: Food-borne illnesses

6: Careers in dietetics and nutrition

Safety and Sanitation

5: Personal and kitchen cleanliness; sanitation in food preparation and storage; eating safely when eating out; safety in the kitchen; preventing chemical poisonings, cuts, burns and fires, falls, electric shock, and choking

6: Careers in food handling industry; careers in food service-sanitation

Career Options

1: Food historian; demographer; advertising production manager

2: Research dietitian; dietetic technician; teaching dietitian

3: Nutrition consultant; food columnist; family and consumer science professional

4: School cafeteria head cook; dietary aide; reducing salon attendant

5: Scullion; sanitarian; safety inspector

6: Employment agency manager; personnel psychologist; career placement services counselor; preparing for a career; skills for success; careers in food service; catering; food-related careers in education and business; entrepreneurship

Consumer Skills

3: Choosing wisely when shopping for food; choosing wisely when eating out

6: Careers in customer service; food professionals in communications, business, and consumer affairs

Meal Management

3: Choosing wisely when preparing food

4: Feeding infants; meals for preschoolers; planning meals for school-age children, teens, adults

6: Choosing a career in foods; careers in management

Food Preparation Skills

3: Healthful preparation tips

6: Careers in food preparation

Food Science and Technology

1: Social influences; mass media; current trends

2: Functions of nutrients; digestion and absorption; metabolism; energy needs

6: The food service industry; careers in research

Part 2
The Management of Food

Social/Cultural Aspects

7: Design needs of people with physical disabilities

Nutrition and Health

10: Provide good nutrition

11: Organic foods; food additives

Safety and Sanitation

7: Lighting; ventilation; electrical wiring

8: Safety seals; use and care of kitchen appliances; general use and care for portable appliances

9: Use and care of cooking and baking utensils

Career Options

7: Interior designer; tableware salesperson; formal waiter

8: Appliance line assembler; wholesale appliance sales representative; household appliance inspector

9: Housewares designer; wholesale housewares demonstrator; cutlery grinder

10: Domestic cook; caterer; head banquet waiter

11: Comparison shopper; retail food demonstrator; nutrition aide

12: Sandwich maker; time-study engineer; food technologist

Foods Lab Equipment

7: Kitchen and dining area design; dinnerware; flatware; beverageware; table linens

8: Styles and features of major kitchen appliances; portable kitchen appliances

9: Small equipment; cooking and baking utensils

Consumer Skills

7: Selecting wall coverings, floor coverings, countertops, and cabinets; low-cost redecorating; choosing and caring for table appointments

8: Warranties; service contracts; purchase considerations for portable appliances

9: Choosing small equipment; choosing cooking and baking utensils

10: Use planned spending; factors affecting food purchases; food budgeting; reducing food expenses

11: Types of stores; shopping tips; comparing costs; food labeling; universal product code; open dating; unit pricing; generic products; sources of consumer information

Meal Management

7: Planning kitchen work centers; kitchen floor plans; planning the dining area; meal service; setting the table; waiting on the table; clearing and serving

10: Preparing satisfying meals; planning a meal; controlling use of time and energy to plan meals

12: Using a time-work schedule; cooperation in the kitchen

Food Preparation Skills

10: Work simplification

12: Choosing a recipe; using microwave recipes; measuring ingredients; adjusting recipes; converting recipes for microwave use; preparing simple recipes

Food Science and Technology

8: Energy Guide labels; trends in major kitchen appliances; convection ovens; induction cooktops; trends in portable kitchen appliances; bread machines

10: Convenience foods

11: Food additives

12: Microwave cooking; microwaving sandwiches

Part 3
The Preparation of Food

Nutrition and Health

13: Nutritional value of meat

14: Nutritional value of poultry

15: Nutritional value of fish and shellfish

16: Nutritional value of eggs; using raw eggs

17: Nutritional value of dairy products; making the lowfat choice

18: Nutritional value of fruit

19: Nutritional value of vegetables

21: Nutritional value of cereals

22: Ingredient adjustment in baked products

Safety and Sanitation

13: Inspection and grading of meat; storing meat; cooking meat safely

14: Inspection and grading of poultry; storing poultry; storing fish and shellfish

16: Egg grades; storing eggs

17: Storing dairy products

18: Storing fresh fruit

19: Storing fresh vegetables; storing canned, frozen, and dried vegetables

20: Storing herbs and spices

21: Storing cereal products

22: Storing baked products

23: Storing cookies

24: Barbecue safety; transporting and serving food outdoors; cleaning up

25: Food spoilage; preparing jars and closures; pressure canning; checking for spoilage; freezing foods; thawing

Career Options

13: Barbecue cook; meat cutter; livestock sales representative

14: Poultry farmer; poultry boner; wholesale poultry feed product sales representative

15: Raw shellfish preparer; fish hatchery attendant; net fisher

16: Egg candler; egg breaker; egg-producing farm farmworker

17: Cheese blender; ice cream chef; dairy farm supervisor

18: Extractor-machine operator; produce broker; grove supervisor

19: Vegetable harvest worker; vegetable sorter; botanist

20: Salad maker; soup cook; spice sales representative

21: Cash grain farmer; cereal popper; miller

22: Oven tender; baker; dividing-machine operator

23: Cake decorator; pastry chef; candy maker

24: Social director; coffee roaster; food and beverage analyst

25: Pickler; freezer tunnel operator; dehydrator tender

Foods Lab Equipment

23: Baking utensils

24: Barbecue tools; coffeemakers

25: Canning jars and closures; freezers and suitable containers

Consumer Skills

13: Selecting meat; meat labeling; cost of meat per serving

14: Buying poultry

15: Selecting and purchasing fish and shellfish

16: Selecting eggs

17: Types of milk; cost of dairy products

18: Selecting fresh fruit; choosing canned, frozen, and dried fruit

19: Cost of fresh vegetables; selecting fresh vegetables; choosing canned, frozen, and dried vegetables

21: Types of cereal products; cost of cereal products

22: Cost of baked products

24: Dining out; restaurant basics; types of restaurants

Meal Management

13: Deciding how much meat to buy

18: Serving raw fruits

19: Serving vegetables

20: Gourmet cooking

24: Planning a party; outdoor entertaining

Food Preparation Skills

13: Methods of meat cookery

14: Methods of cooking poultry

15: Methods of cooking finfish

16: Eggs as ingredients; methods of cooking eggs

17: Cooking with milk and cream; preparing whipped cream; preparing common milk-based foods; preparing frozen desserts; cooking with cheese; preparing cheese dishes

18: Preparing fruits; methods of cooking fruit; preparing preserved fruits

19: Preparing vegetables; methods of cooking vegetables; preparing canned, frozen, and dried vegetables

20: Preparing salad ingredients; salad dressings; preparing casseroles; preparing stock soups

21: Cooking starches; cooking cereal products

22: Mixing methods for baked products; mixing methods for yeast breads

23: Mixing methods for cakes; preparing shortened, unshortened, and chiffon cakes' mixing methods for cookies; preparing pastry

24: Preparing food for parties; preparing beverages

25: Pressure canning; making jellied products; packing fruits; freezing vegetables; freezing meat, poultry, and fish; freezing prepared foods; procedures for drying foods

Food Science and Technology

13: Food science principles of cooking meat; microwaving meats

14: Food science principles of cooking poultry; microwaving poultry

15: Food science principles of cooking finfish; principles and methods of cooking shellfish

16: Food science principles of cooking eggs; egg substitutes; microwaving eggs

17: Food science principles of cooking with milk; microwaving milk products; food science principles of cooking puddings and gelatin creams; food science principles of preparing frozen desserts; food science principles of cooking with cheese; microwaving cheese

18: Food science principles of cooking fruit; microwaving fruit

19: Food science principles of cooking vegetables; microwaving vegetables

20: Microwaving casseroles and soups

21: Food science principles of cooking starches; food science principles of cooking cereal products; microwaving cereal products

22: Food science principles of preparing quick breads; microwaving quick breads; food science principles of preparing yeast breads; microwaving yeast breads

23: Functions of cake ingredients; food science principles of preparing cakes; microwaving cakes; microwaving cookies; food science principles of preparing pastry; microwaving pie; food science principles of candy making; microwaving candy

24: Microwaving appetizers

25: Functions of jelly ingredients; freeze-drying; aseptic packaging; retort packaging; irradiation

Part 4
Foods of the World

Social/Cultural Aspects

26: Historical overview of Native Americans, first colonists, and immigrants; development of regional cuisines

27: Climate, geography, and culture of Latin America; Mexican culture; Mexican regional cuisine; South American culture and influences

28: Climate, geography, and culture of European countries; development of the cuisines; foundations of French cooking; regional differences

29: Climate, geography, and culture of Mediterranean countries; development of cuisines; regional differences

30: Climate, geography, and culture of Middle East and Africa; Jewish dietary laws; development of cuisines; regional differences

31: Climate, geography, and culture of Russia, India, China, and Japan; development of cuisines; regional differences; British rule; Indian social order; Japanese tea ceremony and eating customs

Nutrition and Health

26: Nutritional value of various cultural foods

27: Nutritional value of Latin American foods

Safety and Sanitation

26: Traditional preservation techniques

Career Options

26: Restaurant critic; tourist-information assistant; travel writer

27: Spanish interpreter; Mexican-food-machine tender; Mexican food cook

28: Tea taster; sommelier; tour guide

29: International airplane flight attendant; press tender; Italian chef

30: Foreign correspondent; travel clerk; moshgiach

31: Travel agent; Japanese translator; Chinese-style food cook

Foods Lab Equipment

26: Traditional food preparation tools

27: Latin American food preparation tools

28: European food preparation tools

29: Mediterranean food preparation tools

30: Traditional food preparation tools

31: Asian food preparation tools; Chinese cooking utensils; the use of chopsticks; basic Japanese ingredients

Consumer Skills

27: Mexican economy

31: Russian economy; Indian economy; Japanese industry

Meal Management

Food Preparation Skills

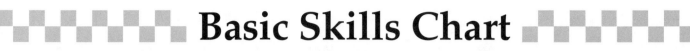

Basic Skills Chart

The chart below has been designed to identify those activities in the *Guide to Good Food Student Activity Guide* and *Instructor's Guide/Teacher's Resource Binder* that specifically encourage the development of basic skills. The following abbreviations are used in the chart:

SAG...Activities in the *Student Activity Guide* (designated by letter).

IG/TRB...Strategies described in the *Instructor's Guide/Teacher's Resource Binder* (referred to by number).

Activities listed as "Verbal" include the following types: role-playing, conducting interviews, oral reports, and debates.

Activities listed as "Reading" may involve actual reading in and out of the classroom. However, many of these activities are designed to improve reading comprehension of the concepts presented in each chapter. Some are designed to improve understanding of vocabulary terms.

Activities that involve writing are listed under "Writing." The list includes activities that allow students to practice composition skills, such as letter writing, informative writing, and creative writing.

The "Math" list includes activities that require students to use computation skills in solving typical problems they may come across in their everyday experiences with foods.

Activities listed as "Science" will enhance student understanding of scientific knowledge. Activities that involve scientific experimentation are included in this category. Also included are activities dealing with the scientific study of nutrients and the chemical properties of foods.

The final category, "Analytical," lists those activities that involve the higher order thinking skills of analysis, synthesis, and evaluation. Activities that involve decision making, problem solving, and critical thinking are included in this section.

	Verbal	Reading	Writing	Math	Science	Analytical
Chapter 1	IG/TRB: 1, 3, 5, 6, 7, 9, 10, 12, 14, 15, 16, 17, 18, 23, 24, 26, 27	IG/TRB: 4, 11, 13, 20, 25, 29, 31	SAG: A, B IG/TRB: 1, 2, 8, 19, 21, 28, 30			SAG: B IG/TRB: 22
Chapter 2	IG/TRB: 2, 3, 6, 8, 10, 13, 14, 18, 20, 22, 23, 25, 26, 27, 32, 36	SAG: A IG/TRB: 4, 12, 16, 24, 31, 42	SAG: A, B, C, D IG/TRB: 5, 7, 9, 12, 14, 15, 19, 29, 33, 34, 35, 37, 38, 39, 40, 41	IG/TRB: 11, 26	SAG: A, B, D IG/TRB: 10, 17, 21, 23, 28, 30, 37, 43	IG/TRB: 1, 10, 14, 17, 21, 39
Chapter 3	IG/TRB: 1, 6, 8, 13, 14, 20, 27, 29, 31, 34, 35, 36, 37, 41, 43	IG/TRB: 4, 7, 16, 21, 46	SAG: A, B, C, D IG/TRB: 2, 10, 12, 15, 17, 22, 25, 38, 40, 45, 47	SAG: B IG/TRB: 9, 18, 31	SAG: B IG/TRB: 5, 11, 17, 19, 23, 30	SAG: B, E IG/TRB: 2, 3, 5, 11, 18, 19, 21, 22, 24, 26, 28, 32, 39, 42
Chapter 4	SAG: A IG/TRB: 1, 2, 4, 5, 7, 8, 9, 12, 15, 17, 20, 21, 22, 23, 25, 26, 28, 31, 32, 33, 34, 36, 40, 41, 42, 45, 52, 54	IG/TRB: 6, 24, 46, 47, 49, 58, 59	SAG: A, D IG/TRB: 3, 10, 13, 14, 18, 19, 43, 51, 55, 56, 57	IG/TRB: 29, 44, 48, 50	SAG: B IG/TRB: 9, 16, 19, 37, 50, 60	SAG: C IG/TRB: 11, 16, 22, 27, 30, 35, 38, 39, 46, 48, 53
Chapter 5	IG/TRB: 1, 2, 3, 6, 9, 16, 21, 22, 25, 26, 28, 29, 31, 33, 34, 35, 37, 39, 42, 43	SAG: A IG/TRB: 3, 4, 14, 18, 19, 36, 41, 42	SAG: D IG/TRB: 5, 7, 8, 10, 11, 13, 15, 17, 20, 23, 24, 25, 27, 30, 32, 38, 40, 42	IG/TRB: 12	SAG: A, B IG/TRB: 39	SAG: C

	Verbal	Reading	Writing	Math	Science	Analytical
Chapter 6	IG/TRB: 1, 6, 8, 9, 10, 13, 14, 15, 16, 17, 18, 19, 21, 23, 25, 26, 27, 28, 30, 33, 37	IG/TRB: 3, 24, 35, 36, 38, 39	SAG: B, C, D, E IG/TRB: 2, 4, 5, 7, 11, 12, 19, 20, 22, 29, 30, 32, 34, 38		IG/TRB: 39	SAG: A, E IG/TRB: 31, 39
Chapter 7	SAG: C IG/TRB: 1, 2, 4, 8, 9, 14, 15, 17, 19, 20, 26, 27, 30, 33, 34, 37, 40, 41, 42, 43, 45, 46, 48, 49, 50, 52, 54, 58	SAG: E IG/TRB: 10, 12, 47, 56, 57	SAG: A, B, D IG/TRB: 3, 11, 16, 22, 25, 28, 29, 36, 38, 39, 51, 53, 55	SAG: C IG/TRB: 6, 7, 24, 32, 35		IG/TRB: 5, 13, 18, 21, 23, 31, 32, 35
Chapter 8	SAG: A, B IG/TRB: 1, 2, 3, 4, 5, 6, 7, 11, 12, 14, 15, 17, 18, 22, 24, 25, 28, 31, 35, 40, 41, 44, 45, 47, 50	IG/TRB: 9, 10, 16, 19, 20, 23, 30, 37, 49	SAG: B, C IG/TRB: 8, 13, 36, 38, 48	SAG: A IG/TRB: 26, 27, 34, 47		SAG: A, C, D IG/TRB: 21, 27, 29, 32, 33, 38, 39, 42, 43, 46
Chapter 9	IG/TRB: 1, 2, 3, 4, 5, 6, 7, 8, 9, 11, 12, 14, 16, 19, 20, 21, 22, 25, 29	IG/TRB: 28, 30	SAG: A, C, D IG/TRB: 13, 15, 24, 26, 27, 29	IG/TRB: 5		SAG: B IG/TRB: 10, 17, 18, 23
Chapter 10	IG/TRB: 1, 2, 8, 12, 13, 14, 23, 26, 27, 28, 29, 31, 35, 37, 38, 39, 40, 41, 48	IG/TRB: 30, 42, 46, 48	SAG: A, B IG/TRB: 3, 4, 6, 11, 19, 22, 24, 25, 33, 34, 36, 44, 45, 47	SAG: B IG/TRB: 14, 15, 16, 17, 18, 20, 21	IG/TRB: 9, 10, 11, 13, 15	SAG: C, D IG/TRB: 5, 7, 21, 32, 43
Chapter 11	IG/TRB: 2, 6, 7, 8, 20, 31, 35, 36	IG/TRB: 5, 14, 23, 24, 32, 33, 37, 38, 40	SAG: B, E IG/TRB: 3, 9, 12, 13, 15, 16, 19, 25, 34	SAG: D, E IG/TRB: 7, 8, 10, 11, 17, 27, 28, 39	SAG: D IG/TRB: 18, 20, 21, 22	SAG: A, C IG/TRB: 1, 4, 10, 29, 30
Chapter 12	IG/TRB: 1, 2, 6, 8, 9, 10, 13, 15, 21, 22, 24, 25, 28, 29	SAG: A, B IG/TRB: 3, 5, 12, 27, 31	SAG: B, C, D IG/TRB: 7, 17, 19, 23, 26, 30	SAG: C IG/TRB: 14, 16, 18		IG/TRB: 1, 4, 11, 20, 32
Chapter 13	IG/TRB: 1, 2, 3, 5, 6, 9, 10, 12, 13, 14, 17, 19, 21, 26, 27, 30, 31	SAG: C IG/TRB: 4, 37, 38, 39	SAG: A, B, C, D IG/TRB: 11, 20, 22, 23, 34, 35, 36, 37	IG/TRB: 7, 15, 16, 17, 18, 24, 25	IG/TRB: 7	IG/TRB: 7, 8, 28, 29, 32, 33

	Verbal	Reading	Writing	Math	Science	Analytical
Chapter 14	IG/TRB: 2, 4, 7, 8, 9, 10, 14, 17, 18, 19, 20, 22, 23, 25, 26, 27, 28	IG/TRB: 1, 6, 11, 32, 35	SAG: A, B, C IG/TRB: 4, 15, 16, 29, 30, 31	IG/TRB: 12	SAG: C IG/TRB: 3, 13	IG/TRB: 21, 24, 33, 34
Chapter 15	IG/TRB: 2, 4, 7, 11, 13, 18, 20, 23, 25, 30, 31	SAG: A, B, D IG/TRB: 1, 3, 10, 17, 24, 29	SAG: B, C, D IG/TRB: 6, 12, 14, 21, 22, 28	IG/TRB: 8, 9	SAG: B IG/TRB: 5, 19	SAG: A IG/TRB: 15, 27
Chapter 16	SAG: B IG/TRB: 2, 3, 5, 12, 13, 17, 25, 26, 27, 28, 29, 30, 31, 32, 38	IG/TRB: 4, 7, 8, 10, 37	SAG: A, C, D IG/TRB: 1, 11, 20, 31, 34, 35, 36	IG/TRB: 6	SAG: A, B, C IG/TRB: 32	IG/TRB: 9, 14, 15, 16, 19, 21, 22, 23, 24, 33
Chapter 17	SAG: B IG/TRB: 1, 3, 9, 15, 16, 19, 26, 28, 30, 34, 35, 40	IG/TRB: 7, 44	SAG: A, D, E IG/TRB: 2, 18, 24, 36, 39, 43, 45	IG/TRB: 9, 13, 14, 15, 17	SAG: C IG/TRB: 5, 12, 20, 21, 22, 23, 25, 27, 32, 33, 37	SAG: A, B IG/TRB: 4, 5, 6, 8, 10, 11, 19, 31, 40, 41, 42
Chapter 18	IG/TRB: 1, 2, 3, 4, 5, 8, 9, 14, 18, 20, 21, 22, 27	SAG: B IG/TRB: 10, 19, 27, 28, 30, 31, 32	SAG: A IG/TRB: 11, 29	IG/TRB: 12, 13, 16, 17, 24	IG/TRB: 1, 6, 7, 23, 25, 26	SAG: B IG/TRB: 15
Chapter 19	SAG: C IG/TRB: 1, 2, 3, 5, 6, 8, 11, 13, 19, 20	IG/TRB: 22, 24	SAG: A, B IG/TRB: 4, 9, 10, 16, 17, 21	IG/TRB: 8	SAG: C IG/TRB: 7, 12, 14, 15, 18	SAG: C IG/TRB: 7
Chapter 20	IG/TRB: 1, 2, 5, 6, 10, 13, 14, 15, 18	IG/TRB: 3, 12, 19, 23, 25	SAG: A, B, C, D IG/TRB: 9, 11, 20, 22, 24		SAG: A, C IG/TRB: 8	SAG: B IG/TRB: 2, 4, 7, 17, 19, 21
Chapter 21	IG/TRB: 1, 2, 3, 4, 5, 6, 7, 8, 9, 11, 13, 18, 19, 20	SAG: C IG/TRB: 26, 27	SAG: A, B, C IG/TRB: 12, 17, 19, 21, 23, 24, 25	IG/TRB: 10	SAG: A, B IG/TRB: 3, 15, 16, 20, 22	SAG: B IG/TRB: 4, 5, 14
Chapter 22	IG/TRB: 2, 6, 7, 8, 11, 12, 14, 15, 22, 23, 26, 28, 29, 32	IG/TRB: 1, 31	SAG: B, C, D IG/TRB: 5, 13, 16, 18, 19, 24, 27, 30	IG/TRB: 4, 10	SAG: A, B IG/TRB: 3, 7, 9, 19, 20, 21, 26	SAG: A IG/TRB: 17, 18, 19, 25, 32, 33
Chapter 23	IG/TRB: 3, 4, 6, 8, 11, 15, 16, 17, 18, 19, 21, 35, 37	SAG: F IG/TRB: 28, 38, 46	SAG: A, B, C, D, E, F IG/TRB: 1, 7, 9, 12, 22, 27, 29, 30, 36, 39, 44, 45, 47	IG/TRB: 2	SAG: A, F IG/TRB: 2, 25, 49	SAG: B, D IG/TRB: 5, 8, 9, 10, 13, 14, 20, 23, 24, 26, 31, 33, 34, 40, 41, 42, 43, 48

	Verbal	Reading	Writing	Math	Science	Analytical
Chapter 24	SAG: D IG/TRB: 1, 2, 3, 5, 6, 7, 8, 9, 13, 14, 17, 18, 26, 28, 31, 35, 36, 38, 39, 40	IG/TRB: 15, 23, 32, 45, 47	SAG: A, C, D, E IG/TRB: 4, 9, 10, 11, 12, 16, 24, 25, 27, 29, 30, 33, 34, 44	SAG: E IG/TRB: 28, 37, 41, 43, 46	IG/TRB: 20	SAG: B, C, D, E IG/TRB: 12, 19, 21, 22, 36, 42
Chapter 25	IG/TRB: 1, 2, 6, 7, 8, 9, 15, 22, 24, 28, 29, 30, 34	IG/TRB: 13, 33, 37, 38	SAG: A, B, C, D, E IG/TRB: 4, 10, 12, 16, 17, 18, 21, 27, 32, 35, 39, 40, 41	IG/TRB: 34, 39, 40	SAG: A, B, D, E, F IG/TRB: 3, 5, 36	IG/TRB: 19, 20, 23, 25, 26
Chapter 26	IG/TRB: 1, 2, 3, 4, 5, 7, 8, 9, 10, 13, 16, 19, 20, 25, 27, 28, 40, 41, 48	IG/TRB: 6, 14, 21, 22, 27, 30, 31, 34, 35, 47, 48	SAG: A, B, C IG/TRB: 11, 14, 15, 17, 23, 26, 34, 37, 39, 41, 42, 43, 44, 45, 46			IG/TRB: 18, 24, 29, 33, 38
Chapter 27	IG/TRB: 1, 2, 3, 5, 6, 9, 10, 13, 22	IG/TRB: 4, 7, 14, 15, 21	SAG: A, B, C IG/TRB: 4, 11, 12, 16, 17, 18, 19, 20			SAG: C IG/TRB: 12
Chapter 28	IG/TRB: 1, 2, 3, 4, 7, 11, 15, 16, 19, 20, 22, 24, 25, 26, 27, 28, 29, 34, 35, 36, 37, 38, 42, 43, 44, 45, 46, 47, 48	IG/TRB: 5, 6, 8, 10, 12, 13, 18, 21, 34, 49, 54, 55	SAG: A, B, C, D, E IG/TRB: 14, 23, 32, 33, 39, 40, 41, 50, 51, 52, 53	IG/TRB: 17		SAG: E IG/TRB: 9, 23, 32, 40, 50
Chapter 29	IG/TRB: 1, 2, 3, 4, 5, 9 , 10, 18, 20, 21 , 24, 27, 29, 31, 32	SAG: C IG/TRB: 6, 8, 15, 16, 19, 28, 30, 36	SAG: A, B, C, D, E IG/TRB: 7, 13, 14, 17, 22, 24, 25, 26, 33, 34, 35, 37			SAG: E IG/TRB: 11, 12, 23, 24, 32, 37
Chapter 30	IG/TRB: 1, 2, 3, 4, 7, 9, 10, 11, 13, 19, 20, 21, 24, 26, 27, 29, 31	SAG: C IG/TRB: 5, 6, 8, 12, 16, 18, 23, 28, 30, 32, 33, 35, 37	SAG: A, B, C, D IG/TRB: 14, 25, 36	IG/TRB: 34		SAG: D IG/TRB: 5, 13, 15, 17, 22, 24, 38
Chapter 31	IG/TRB: 1, 2, 3, 5, 8, 9, 11, 14, 16, 17, 18, 19, 21, 22, 24, 25, 26, 28, 29, 30, 31, 33, 36, 39, 40	SAG: B IG/TRB: 4, 12, 13, 22, 24, 27, 34, 37, 44	SAG: A, B, C, D, E IG/TRB: 6, 7, 10, 20, 23, 26, 32, 41, 43, 45			IG/TRB: 9, 15, 19, 31, 40, 42

How Food Affects Life
Chapter **1**

Objectives

After studying this chapter, students will be able to
- explain how the search for food led to the development of civilization.
- discuss factors that influence food habits.

Bulletin Boards

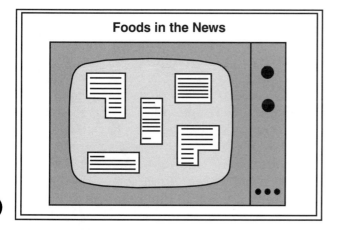

I. Title: "Foods in the News"

Make the bulletin board look like a giant TV. Have students bring in newspaper and magazine articles about foods to post inside the screen.

II. Title: "How Food Affects Life"

Divide the bulletin board into three sections labeled *cultural influences, social influences,* and *psychological influences.* Place pictures of foods clipped from magazines on the bulletin board with tags identifying why each food belongs in a particular section. You may wish to use this bulletin board as an introductory activity, filling in a different section each day to introduce the concepts listed above over a three-day period. You may wish to have students participate in clipping and tagging the food pictures. They can then explain to the class why they have chosen certain pictures to go in a particular section of the bulletin board.

Teaching Materials

Text, pages 13-22

Student Activity Guide, pages 7-8
   A. *Your Food Habits*
   B. *Advertising Analysis*

Teacher's Resource Binder
   The Roles Foods Play, transparency master 1-1
   Food—The Foundation of Civilization, transparency master 1-2
   America's Melting Pot of Foods, transparency master 1-3
   "Light" Product Comparison, reproducible master 1-4
   Chapter 1 Study Sheet, reproducible master 1-5
   Poverty and World Hunger, reproducible master 1-6
   Advertising Techniques, color transparency CT-1
   Chapter 1 Test

Software, diskette for Part One
   Hangman, chapter review game

Introductory Activities

1. Have students make a list of reasons they think food is important. Invite each student to share his or her list with the class. Make a master list on the chalkboard.
2. Ask students to write down the first thing that comes to mind when they hear each of the following words: appetizers, apple pie, bagel, bread, cake, chicken soup, chocolate, fish, hot dogs, meat, milk, orange juice, pancakes, pizza, popcorn, potatoes, rice, spaghetti, tortilla, turkey, vegetables. Invite students to share their responses in small groups to see how various foods call different images to mind for different people.
3. *The Roles Foods Play,* transparency master 1-1, TRB. Use the master as you explain the historical, cultural, social, and psychological significance of foods.

Strategies to Reteach, Reinforce, Enrich, and Extend Text Concepts

The History of Food

4. **EX** Have students research the types of plant and animal foods that prehistoric peoples ate. They should summarize their findings in written reports.

5 **ER** Field trip. Tour a historical museum to view exhibits of early hunting tools and cooking utensils.

6. **ER** Guest speaker. Invite a curator from a historical museum to speak to your class about how people evolved from hunting to herding animals and from gathering to farming plant foods.

7. **RT** *Food—The Foundation of Civilization,* transparency master 1-2, TRB. Use the transparency to illustrate for students the progression from eating food raw, to using fire to cook it, to the domestication of animals and the cultivation of crops. Discuss with students how this progression in the way food was obtained and eaten paralleled the development of civilization.

Cultural Influences

8. **RF** *Your Food Habits,* Activity A, SAG. Students are to answer a series of questions to help them identify their food habits.

9. **RT** *America's Melting Pot of Foods,* transparency master 1-3, TRB. Use the transparency as you briefly explain to students how various factors have influenced cuisine in the United States.

10. **RF** In a large group discussion, have students take turns giving examples of groups of people who strongly influenced food customs in the United States and the foods they introduced.

11. **ER** Have each student select a food of some religious significance. Ask students to research how the food they selected came to have this significance and give a brief oral report to the class.

12. **ER** Panel discussion. Invite a Protestant minister, a Catholic priest, and a Jewish rabbi to speak to your class. Ask each panelist to discuss foods that are significant in his or her religion.

13. **ER** Divide the class into four groups. Have each group research the food customs of one of the following religions: Judaism, Islam, Buddhism, and Hinduism. Each group will share its findings with the class.

14. **ER** Guest speaker. Invite a rabbi to your class to discuss Jewish dietary laws. Ask the rabbi to also discuss special foods that are served on religious holidays such as Passover. In lab, prepare a Passover meal.

Social Influences

15. **EX** Have the class brainstorm to see how many kinds of social situations they can identify that involve food. Write the ideas on the chalkboard.

16. **RF** Ask students to discuss how their family's eating habits have changed in the last ten years.

17. **RF** Lead a class discussion on reasons why family meal traditions are changing.

18. **RT** *Advertising Techniques,* color transparency, CT-1. Use the transparency to introduce students to some of the advertising techniques used to promote food products.

19. **RF** Have students keep a record of all the food advertisements they see during two hours of television viewing. Discuss their findings in class.

20. **RF** *Advertising Analysis,* Activity B, SAG. Students are to clip food ads from newspapers or magazines. Then they are to identify the types of techniques used to persuade people to buy the foods being advertised.

21. **ER** Ask students to write a paragraph about a current trend affecting food products or eating habits. Then have them write a follow-up paragraph describing a specific product or situation as evidence of the trend.

22. **ER** *Light Product Comparison,* reproducible master 1-4, TRB. Have students compare samples of foods in their regular and light versions. (Examples might include pineapple canned in heavy syrup and pineapple canned in juice, tuna packed in oil and tuna packed in water, and green beans canned with salt and green beans canned with no added salt.) Then discuss how the current emphasis on health and fitness has led to an increased number of "light" products. Ask students if they think these products will continue to be popular and to explain why or why not.

Psychological Influences

23. **RF** Invite students to talk about various happy occasions that they associate with particular foods. Ask them to describe how those occasions would differ if those particular foods were not a part of them.

24. **ER** Guest speaker. Invite a psychologist to speak to your class about how a person's perceptions of various foods can trigger certain pleasant or unpleasant sensations. Ask the psychologist to explain how some of these perceptions are formed.

25. **RF** Have students use pictures found in magazines to prepare a collage illustrating

how people associate foods with pleasurable experiences.

26. **ER** Guest speaker. Invite a dietitian to your class to discuss how emotions may cause overeating and undereating.

Chapter Review

27. **RF** On a slip of paper, have each student write a question about one of the concepts in the chapter. Have students write their names on the slips and turn them in to you. Redistribute the questions to the class, making sure that no student gets his or her question. Go around the room and have each student read the question he or she was given out loud. Ask the students to answer the questions they read. If a student is unable to answer the question, call on the author of the question to provide an answer and an explanation.

28. **RT** *Chapter 1 Study Sheet,* reproducible master 1-5, TRB. Have students complete the statements as they read text pages 14-21.

29. **RF** *Hangman,* software, diskette for Part One. Have students play chapter review game according to the instructions that appear on the screen.

Above and Beyond

30. **ER** Have students use at least two resources to prepare a two-page written report on the development of some aspect of cuisine in the United States. You may wish to give students the option of giving an oral presentation instead of writing a report. Students should make visual aids to use in their presentations if they select this option.

31. **EX** *Poverty and World Hunger,* reproducible master 1-6, TRB. After reading the handout, have students plan a world hunger awareness week in your school. They should plan daily activities to inform other students about the problem and ways they can become involved in programs targeted at alleviating the problem.

Answer Key

Text

Review What You Have Read, page 22

1. herding domesticated animals and farming plant foods
2. they were introduced by English explorers
3. (List one:) people of a certain race, citizens of a given country, followers of a specific religion
4. true
5. Moslems and Orthodox Jews cannot eat pork because they consider swine to be unclean.
6. When family members do not eat together, they miss an important opportunity to communicate.
7. true
8. (List one:) Media advertising encourages people to try new food products. Media advertising encourages people to continue buying products that have been available for years. Media news reports and articles inform people about new health findings related to various food products. (Students may justify other responses.)
9. (List two:) smaller living units, spending more time at home, cooking as a leisure activity, increased number of dual-income families, increased emphasis on fitness, eating ethnic foods, grazing (Students may justify other responses.)
10. Babies learn to connect food with warmth and security.

Teacher's Resources

Chapter 1 Test

1. E	10. D	18. T
2. F	11. T	19. F
3. C	12. F	20. T
4. H	13. T	21. B
5. K	14. T	22. D
6. A	15. F	23. A
7. J	16. F	24. B
8. B	17. F	25. D
9. I		

26. (List three:) explorers, Native Americans, European immigrants, Asian immigrants, African slaves
27. Technology has created labor-saving equipment and convenience foods. Rising incomes have made it easier for people to buy these items. Families can also eat more meals away from home.
28. Media introduces people to, reminds them of, and informs them about food products. Advertisements encourage people to buy food products. News reports and articles inform people about health findings.
29. (Student response. See pages 19-20 in the text.)
30. Food appeals to a person's senses of sight, taste, and smell and to the need for social contact.

How Food Affects Life

Name _____

Date _____ Period _____ Score _____

Chapter 1 Test

Matching: Match the following foods and food customs with the associated cultural groups.

_____ 1. Chowders.

_____ 2. Sausages.

_____ 3. Cookies, coleslaw, waffles.

_____ 4. Pastas, rich tomato sauces.

_____ 5. Pierogi, poppyseed cakes.

_____ 6 Stir-fried dishes.

_____ 7. Eat only with the right hand.

_____ 8. Use bread and wine to symbolize Christ's body and blood.

_____ 9. Fast on Yom Kippur, the Day of Atonement.

_____ 10. Buried food with their dead.

A. Chinese
B. Christians
C. Dutch
D. Egyptians
E. French
F. Germans
G. Hindus
H. Italians
I. Jews
J. Moslems
K. Poles

True/False: Circle *T* if the statement is true or *F* if the statement is false.

T   F   11. The domestication of animals and the production of plant foods led to the growth of trade and the development of civilization.

T   F   12. Christopher Columbus was searching for gold when he discovered America.

T   F   13. Many people are part of more than one cultural group.

T   F   14. Groups of immigrants to the United States brought with them foods that were native to their homelands.

T   F   15. Immigrant groups did not settle in any specific areas, so foods from a variety of origins can be found throughout the United States.

T   F   16. Cattle are considered sacred by the Jews and cannot be used for food.

T   F   17. Family has little impact on the foods people eat and how they eat them.

T   F   18. Mass media is used to inform people about health findings related to food.

T   F   19. An increased emphasis on fitness has led to the growing popularity of carry-out foods.

T   F   20. Some people eat food to soothe their feelings of anger or frustration.

Multiple Choice: Choose the best response. Write the letter in the space provided.

_____ 21. The first food probably was eaten _____.
  A. boiled in a clay pot
  B. raw
  C. roasted over an open fire
  D. wrapped in leaves and steamed

(Continued)

Name _____

_____ 22. Which group of explorers introduced cane sugar, wheat, oranges, and sheep to the United States?
  A. Dutch.
  B. English.
  C. Portuguese.
  D. Spanish.

_____ 23. The customs and beliefs of a racial, religious, or social group form the group's _____.
  A. culture
  B. fasting
  C. grazing
  D. melting pot

_____ 24. A decrease in the number of meals family members eat together is often the result of _____.
  A. bad manners
  B. busy schedules
  C. efforts to lose weight
  D. increasing food costs

_____ 25. An increased emphasis on fitness has caused some people to _____.
  A. become more physically active
  B. eat lighter meals
  C. reduce the amount of fats, salt, and sugar in their diets
  D. All of the above.

Essay Questions: Provide complete responses to the following questions or statements.

26. Name three groups that helped form the "melting pot" culture in the United States.
27. How have modern technology and rising incomes affected family food habits?
28. How can mass media affect people's food habits?
29. Describe two current trends that affect what, when, and how people eat.
30. How can food be psychologically satisfying?

Nutritional Needs

Objectives

After studying this chapter, students will be able to
- define good nutrition.
- name the key nutrients, describe their functions, and list important sources of each.
- explain the process of digestion, absorption, and metabolism.

Bulletin Boards

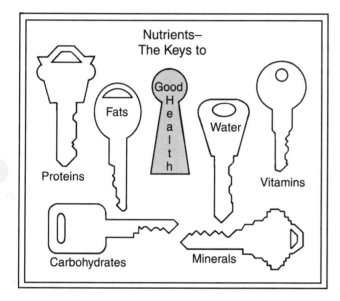

I. Title: "Nutrients—The Keys to Good Health"

Use construction paper or other material to make six large cutouts of keys. Label each with one of the six key nutrients—fats, carbohydrates, proteins, vitamins, minerals, and water. Place the keys around a keyhole labeled "Good Health," as shown.

II. Title: "Is There a Weak Link in Your Nutrient Chain?"

Use construction paper or other material to make six large cutouts of chain links. Label each with one of the six basic nutrient groups—fats, carbohydrates, proteins, vitamins, minerals, and water.

Teaching Materials

Text, pages 23-52
Student Activity Guide, pages 9-14

A. *Nutrient Facts*
B. *Nutrient Deficiencies and Excesses*
C. *Nutrition Maze*
D. *How the Body Uses Food*

Teacher's Resource Binder
Nutrient Sources and Functions, reproducible master 2-1
Carbohydrate Content of Foods, reproducible master 2-2
The Gastrointestinal Tract, transparency master 2-3
Chapter 2 Study Sheet, reproducible master 2-4
Basic Nutrient Groups, color transparency CT-2A
Complementary Proteins, color transparency CT-2B
Chapter 2 Test
Software, diskette for Part One
Tic Tac Toe, chapter review game

Introductory Activities

1. Ask students if they feel they follow well-balanced diets. Have them explain why or why not.
2. Have students complete the statement, "A person can be overweight and yet be malnourished because..." Discuss in class.

Strategies to Reteach, Reinforce, Enrich, and Extend Text Concepts

The Nutrients

3. **RT** *Basic Nutrient Groups,* color transparency CT-2A, TRB. Use the transparency to introduce the six nutrient groups.
4. **RT** *Nutrient Sources and Functions,* reproducible master 2-1, TRB. Encourage students to use the handout as a study guide as they learn about the various nutrients.
5. **RF** On a large piece of paper, list the six nutrient groups. Ask students to tell you as much as they can about each group and note their comments on the paper. Save the paper and refer to it again at the end of the chapter. (See strategy 39.)

6. **RF** *Nutrient Facts*, Activity A, SAG. As you discuss the various nutrients in class, have the students complete the chart by listing the functions and food sources of each nutrient. After completing the chart, have them answer the questions to show their understanding of the importance of nutrients in their diet.

7. **RF** *Nutrient Deficiencies and Excesses*, Activity B, SAG. Have students complete the activity by identifying whether nutrient deficiencies or excesses cause the various conditions. Have them match these conditions with descriptions of their symptoms. Then have them identify the particular nutrient related to each condition.

8. **ER** Guest speaker. Invite a registered dietitian to speak to your class about the nutritional needs of teenagers. Ask the speaker to focus on any problem nutrients and offer suggestions for meeting those needs.

Carbohydrates

9. **ER** Have students design a poster that they could use to study carbohydrates. Have them use pictures to illustrate important carbohydrate sources. Be sure they include a list of the important functions of carbohydrates and the effects of a deficiency or excess of carbohydrates in the diet.

10. **EX** After discussing the differences between the simple carbohydrates and the complex carbohydrates, have students debate the pros and cons of excesses of both groups in the diet. For instance, an excess of simple sugars can cause weight gain, whereas an excess of fiber in the diet is recommended.

11. **RF** *Carbohydrate Content of Foods*, reproducible master 2-2, TRB. Students are to use Appendix B (Nutritive Values of Foods) on pages 617-634 of the text to calculate the percentage of calories from carbohydrates found in various foods.

12. **ER** Have students investigate the effects sugar can have on teeth and summarize their findings in a two-page written report.

13. **ER** Guest speaker. Invite a dentist to speak to your class about the effects too much sugar can have on teeth. Ask the speaker to offer suggestions for preventing dental caries.

14. **ER** Have students test a variety of foods for the presence of starch by dropping a few drops of iodine on each food item. If starch is present, the iodine will change from reddish-brown to a blue-black color. Once students have recorded and discussed their observations, be sure to properly dispose of all tested food items. Iodine is poisonous—instruct students not to eat any tested food items!

Fats

15. **ER** Have students design a poster for fats similar to the poster described in strategy 9.

16. **RF** Provide students with the health sections of newspapers and health-related magazines. Have each student find an article that deals with the topics of saturated fats in the diet, cholesterol, or the relationship between fats and cancer or heart disease. Have each student read his or her article to the class as a basis for a discussion of reducing fats in the diet.

17. **EX** Have students record all the foods they eat for one day. Then have them analyze their lists for sources of visible and invisible fat in their diets.

18. **ER** Guest speaker. Invite a representative from a local affiliate of the American Heart Association to speak to your class about the relationship between heart disease and fat in the diet. Ask the speaker to offer suggestions for following a heart-healthy diet.

Proteins

19. **ER** Have students design a poster for proteins similar to the poster described in strategy 9.

20. **RF** *Complementary Proteins*, color transparency CT-2B, TRB. Use the transparency to show students the complementary relationship of nonmeat protein sources. Have them list foods in each category shown in the diagram. Then have them suggest examples of dishes that take advantage of this relationship to form high quality protein.

21. **EX** Bring examples of meat analogs made of textured vegetable proteins to class and prepare them for students to sample. Have students evaluate the taste, texture, and appearance of the analogs compared to their all-meat equivalents.

Vitamins

22. **ER** Have students describe how foods can lose water-soluble vitamins during cooking. Then have them investigate cooking techniques that can reduce these losses.

23. **RF** Have students read the label of a multivitamin supplement. Ask them to note the percentage of the Daily Values provided for each of the vitamins in the supplement. Use their findings as the basis for a discussion of the effects of excess fat-soluble and water-soluble vitamins in the body.
24. **ER** Have students visit the aisle of a drugstore or grocery store in which vitamin supplements are stocked. Ask them to take inventory of the variety of supplements that are available and report their findings in class.
25. **EX** Have two teams of students debate the statement "Most people need to take vitamin supplements." Instruct the students to conduct research that will give them sufficient information to support their arguments.

Minerals

26. **EX** Discuss with students the importance of having sufficient calcium intake during the formative years as a measure to prevent the development of osteoporosis later in life. Then have students plan a weekly set of menus that provide at least 1,200 mg of calcium each day—the RDA for teens 11 to 18 years of age.
27. **RF** Discuss with students the relationship of minerals that work together in the body, such as calcium and phosphorus and sodium, chlorine, and potassium. Have students identify common functions, food sources, and deficiencies of each of the minerals in these two nutrient teams.
28. **EX** Have students use the nutrition labels from a variety of processed foods, such as cured meats, canned soups, frozen entrees, snack foods, and condiments, to evaluate sodium content. Have them suggest ideas for reducing excess sodium in the diet.
29. **EX** Have students plan menus for two days that provide at least 18 mg of iron each day.

Water

30. **EX** Have students use Appendix B (Nutritive Values of Foods) on pages 617-634 of the text to rank the following foods according to the percentage of water they contain: lettuce, whole milk, white bread, apples, potatoes, sunflower seeds, green beans, butter, saltine crackers, sirloin steak (cooked), watermelon, and ice cream.

31. **ER** Have students investigate the increased water needs of an athlete during competition.

Digestion, Absorption, and Metabolism

32. **RT** *The Gastrointestinal Tract*, transparency master 2-3, TRB. Label the various organs of the gastrointestinal tract as you discuss their roles in digestion and absorption with your class.
33. **RF** Have students explain how worry, hurried meals, and fatigue can affect the process of digestion.
34. **ER** Have students draw diagrams illustrating the metabolic pathways of carbohydrates, fats, and proteins.

Energy Needs

35. **RF** Have students define *energy* and list the various activities for which the body needs energy.
36. **RF** Have students explain how two people who are the same weight and age can have different basal metabolic rates.
37. **EX** Have students list all the foods they have eaten or drunk for the last two days. Have them label each food as a low fuel value food, an intermediate fuel value food, or a high fuel value food.
38. **RF** *How the Body Uses Food*, Activity D, SAG. Students are to write answers to questions about the processes of digestion, absorption, metabolism, and energy needs.

Chapter Review

39. **EX** Review with the class the information they listed about the six nutrient groups on a large sheet of paper in strategy 5. Ask them to evaluate what they have learned about nutrients since starting to study the chapter. Ask them each to write one suggestion of how they might use the information they have learned.
40. **RF** *Nutrition Maze*, Activity C, SAG. Students are to complete statements about nutrition by filling in blanks. Then they are to find terms in a word maze and circle them.
41. **RT** *Chapter 2 Study Sheet*, reproducible master 2-4, TRB. Have students complete the statements as they read text pages 24-50.
42. **RF** *Tic Tac Toe*, Software, diskette for Part One. Have students play chapter review game according to the instructions that appear on the screen.

Above and Beyond

43. **ER** Have students investigate how to assemble a simple calorimeter and use it to measure the calorie content of various food samples. Suggested samples include bread or other food high in carbohydrates, meat or other food high in proteins, vegetable oil or other food high in fats, and celery or other food high in water content. Students should carefully record integral data and observations and summarize their work in a written report. (You may wish to coordinate this learning experience with your school's science department.)

Answer Key

Text

Review What You Have Read, page 52

1. true
2. carbohydrates, fats or lipids, proteins, vitamins, minerals, water
3. E, B, C, D, A
4. saturated fatty acids
5. (List three functions of each:) carbohydrates—furnish the body with energy, provide cellulose needed for bulk, help the body digest fats efficiently, make foods more palatable, spare proteins so they can be used for growth and maintenance
   fats—serve as an energy storage source in the body, protect internal organs from injury, insulate the body from shock and temperature changes, carry the fat-soluble vitamins, serve as a source of essential fatty acids
   proteins—provide amino acids needed for growth, maintenance, and repair of body tissues; aid in formation of enzymes, some hormones, and antibodies; provide energy; regulate bodily processes
6. complete protein
7. Vitamins A, D, E, and K are fat-soluble. They can be stored in the body whereas water-soluble vitamins cannot be stored.
8. (List three functions and four important food sources:) functions—helps in the formation and maintenance of collagen, helps make the walls of blood vessels firm, helps wounds heal, aids in the formation of hemoglobin, helps the body fight infections
   sources—citrus fruits, strawberries, cantaloupe, leafy green vegetables, green peppers, broccoli, cabbage

9. thiamin
10. osmosis
11. peristalsis
12. true

Student Activity Guide

Nutrient Deficiencies and Excesses, Activity B, page 11

1. M; carbohydrate (sugar) excess
2. E; fat (cholesterol) excess
3. I; protein deficiency
4. B; vitamin A deficiency
5. L; vitamin D deficiency
6. G; vitamin C deficiency
7. A; thiamin deficiency
8. F; niacin deficiency
9. J; vitamin B-12 deficiency
10. H; calcium deficiency
11. K; sodium excess
12. D; iron deficiency
13. C; iodine deficiency

Nutrition Maze, Activity C, pages 12-13

1. calcium
2. iron
3. monosaccharides
4. gastric juices
5. metabolism
6. malnutrition
7. calorie
8. minerals
9. trace
10. water
11. fat
12. protein
13. amino acids
14. complete
15. incomplete
16. saturated
17. unsaturated
18. cholesterol
19. carbohydrates
20. nutrients
21. lipids
22. vitamins
23. sunlight
24. clotting
25. bleeding
26. carotene
27. starch
28. hydrogenation

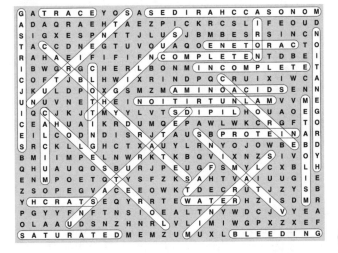

How the Body Uses Food, Activity D, page 14
1. Peristalsis is the process whereby food is pushed through the digestive tract.
2. Digestive enzymes help break down carbohydrates, proteins, and fats into simple substances that can be absorbed and used by the body.
3. proteins—2, fats—3, carbohydrates—1
4. 1-inch cube Cheddar cheese—4 g protein, 6 g fat, Tr carbohydrate
   apple—Tr protein, Tr fat, 21 g carbohydrate
   roasted chicken drumstick—12 g protein, 2 g fat, 0 g carbohydrate
5. The cheese would satisfy hunger longest because it has the highest fat content. Fats stay in the stomach longer than carbohydrates or proteins.
6. in the small intestine
7. Villi are hairlike fingers that line the small intestine and increase its absorptive surface by more than 600 percent.
8. within the cells
9. (List one for each:) Carbohydrates: used for energy, converted to glycogen, stored as fat. Fats: used for fuel. Proteins: used for cell maintenance; used for cell growth; used for the synthesis of enzymes, antibodies, and nonessential amino acids; used as an energy source.
10. A. 6'1" tall person
    B. male
    C. 15-year-old
    D. a person with a body temperature of 101.2°F

Teacher's Resources

Chapter 2 Test

1. J	15. F	28. A
2. E	16. T	29. D
3. H	17. F	30. A
4. A	18. F	31. C
5. B	19. T	32. A
6. G	20. F	33. A
7. D	21. F	34. C
8. C	22. F	35. A
9. K	23. T	36. D
10. F	24. F	37. B
11. T	25. T	38. D
12. T	26. A	39. C
13. T	27. C	40. D
14. T		

41. Poor nutrition over an extended time. The body does not receive the nutrients it needs for energy, growth, repair, and the regulation of body processes.
42. Visible fats are fats you can see. Examples include butter, margarine, and marbling in meat cuts. Invisible fats are those you cannot see. Examples include the fat in eggs, whipped cream, and baked products. (Students may justify other examples.)
43. A protein that lacks a particular amino acid can be supplemented with another protein that contains that amino acid. Together, the two proteins provide a higher quality protein than either would have provided alone.
44. The control of osmosis (the process whereby fluids flow in and out of cells through the cell walls).
45. Body size and composition, age, health, and secretions of the endocrine glands.

Nutritional Needs

Name _____

Date _____ **Period** _____ **Score** _____

Chapter 2 Test

Matching: Match the following terms and identifying phrases.

_____ 1. The study of how the body uses food.

_____ 2. Protein that contains all nine essential amino acids in adequate amounts.

_____ 3. Inorganic substances that become part of the bones, tissues, and body fluids.

_____ 4. The amount of energy the human body needs just to stay alive and carry on vital life processes.

_____ 5. A unit used in nutrition to measure the energy value of food.

_____ 6. The process by which hydrogen is chemically added to an unsaturated fat.

_____ 7. A fatlike substance found in every cell in the body.

_____ 8. The body's chief source of energy.

_____ 9. The process that pushes food through the digestive tract.

_____ 10. An indigestible material in plant foods that provides bulk in the diet.

A. basal metabolism
B. calorie
C. carbohydrate
D. cholesterol
E. complete protein
F. fiber
G. hydrogenation
H. minerals
I. nutrient
J. nutrition
K. peristalsis

True/False: Circle *T* if the statement is true or *F* if the statement is false.

T   F   11. An overweight person may be malnourished.

T   F   12. The foods a teenage girl eats today may affect her pregnancy in later years.

T   F   13. A nutrient is a chemical substance in food that helps maintain the body.

T   F   14. Starch is the most abundant carbohydrate in the body.

T   F   15. Meats are an excellent source of carbohydrates.

T   F   16. Fats are important energy sources.

T   F   17. Cholesterol occurs only in foods of plant origin.

T   F   18. Adults need more protein per pound of body weight than children because they are larger.

T   F   19. If a diet does not supply enough fats and carbohydrates, the body will use proteins for energy before using them to support growth and maintenance.

T   F   20. The body does not store fat-soluble vitamins.

T   F   21. Calcium, phosphorus, and potassium are known as trace elements.

T   F   22. Iron is needed to prevent osteoporosis in old age.

T   F   23. Your body's water intake comes from the liquids you drink, the foods you eat, and metabolism.

(Continued)

Name _____

T   F   24. Food is pushed through the digestive tract by villi.

T   F   25. When the amount of energy you obtain from foods is greater than the amount of energy you expend, your body weight increases.

Multiple Choice: Choose the best response. Write the letter in the space provided.

_____   26. Which of the following is *not* a carbohydrate?
      A. Amino acid.
      B. Cellulose.
      C. Dextrin.
      D. Fructose.

_____   27. A fatty acid that has as many hydrogen atoms as it can hold is called _____.
      A. cholesterol
      B. polyunsaturated fatty acid
      C. saturated fatty acid
      D. unsaturated fatty acid

_____   28. Proteins are made up of small units called _____.
      A. amino acids
      B. disaccharides
      C. lipids
      D. monosaccharides

_____   29. Proteins are provided by _____.
      A. dried beans, peas, and nuts
      B. meat, fish, and poultry
      C. milk and eggs
      D. All of the above.

_____   30. The following vitamins are fat-soluble: _____.
      A. A, D, E, K
      B. C, D, K, riboflavin
      C. Folic acid, biotin, and vitamin C
      D. Niacin, C, E, K

_____   31. A deficiency of which of the following vitamins can cause scurvy?
      A. Niacin.
      B. Thiamin.
      C. Vitamin C.
      D. Vitamin D.

_____   32. Which of the following minerals is found in the greatest amount in the human body?
      A. Calcium.
      B. Magnesium.
      C. Phosphorus.
      D. Sodium.

_____   33. Milk and milk products are the best dietary sources of _____.
      A. calcium
      B. iron
      C. magnesium
      D. sodium

(Continued)

Name _____

_____ 34. Which of the following groups of nutrients work as a team?
 A. Calcium, iron, fluorine.
 B. Calcium, sodium, potassium.
 C. Sodium, potassium, chlorine.
 D. Sodium, potassium, fluorine.

_____ 35. Over half of the iron in the human body is found in the _____.
 A. blood
 B. bones
 C. heart
 D. tissues

_____ 36. In which of the following cases might a person need to increase his or her intake of fluids?
 A. The person is suffering from a severe case of diarrhea.
 B. The person is involved in active sports.
 C. The person lives in a hot climate.
 D. All of the above.

_____ 37. The digestive process begins in the _____.
 A. colon
 B. mouth
 C. small intestine
 D. stomach

_____ 38. The body absorbs nearly all carbohydrates as _____.
 A. amino acids
 B. diglycerides
 C. disaccharides
 D. monosaccharides

_____ 39. After the body absorbs nutrients, the nutrients undergo the chemical processes known as _____.
 A. absorption
 B. digestion
 C. metabolism
 D. peristalsis

_____ 40. An adult's total energy needs depend on _____.
 A. basal metabolism
 B. heat produced by the ingestion of food
 C. physical activity
 D. All of the above.

Essay Questions: Provide complete responses to the following questions or statements.

41. Define malnutrition.
42. Explain what is meant by visible and invisible fats and give two examples of each.
43. How can proteins complement one another?
44. What is the main function performed by sodium, chlorine, and potassium?
45. What factors cause a person's basal metabolism to vary?

Making Healthy Food Choices

Objectives

After studying this chapter, students will be able to
- explain how they can use the Recommended Dietary Allowances.
- list the Dietary Guidelines for Americans.
- identify how many daily servings they need from each group in the Food Guide Pyramid.
- explain how they can use the Dietary Guidelines when shopping for food, preparing food, and eating out.

Bulletin Boards

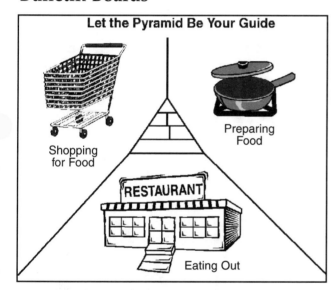

Let the Pyramid Be Your Guide

Shopping for Food

Preparing Food

RESTAURANT

Eating Out

I. Title: "Let the Pyramid Be Your Guide"

Place an illustration of the Food Guide Pyramid in the center of the bulletin board. Divide the bulletin board into three segments along the sides of the Pyramid. Place a cutout of a shopping cart in one segment labeled "shopping for food." Place a cutout of a saucepan in another segment labeled "preparing food." Place a cutout of a restaurant in the third segment labeled "eating out."

II. Title: "Is Your Diet in Balance?"

Draw or cut out a large balance. On either side of the balance, place blocks cut from construction paper labeled with the seven Dietary Guidelines for Americans. Place the blocks labeled "eat a variety of foods;" "balance the food you eat with physical activity—maintain or improve your weight;" and "choose a diet with plenty of grain products, vegetables, and fruits" on one side of the balance. Place the blocks labeled "choose a diet low in fat, saturated fat, and cholesterol;" "choose a diet moderate in sugars;" "choose a diet moderate in salt and sodium;" and "if you drink alcoholic beverages, do so in moderation" on the other side of the balance. Point out to students that the bulletin board illustrates how they should balance a variety of wise food choices with moderate use of some food components.

Teaching Materials

Text, pages 53-67
Student Activity Guide, pages 15-20
   A. *What's Behind the Dietary Guidelines?*
   B. *Do You Follow the Pyramid?*
   C. *Choosing Wisely When Shopping*
   D. *Preparing Healthful Food*
   E. *Dining Habits Survey*

Teacher's Resource Binder
   Dietary Guidelines for Americans—A Framework for Good Nutrition, transparency master 3-1
   Healthy Shopping, transparency master 3-2
   Tips for Making Healthy Food Choices, reproducible master 3-3
   Chapter 3 Study Sheet, reproducible master 3-4
   Calorie Sources in the Diet, color transparency CT-3A
   Food Guide Pyramid, color transparency CT-3B
   Recommended Daily Servings, color transparency CT-3C
   Chapter 3 Test

Software, diskette for Part One
   In Reverse, chapter review game

Introductory Activities

1. Ask students what they consider to be the benefits of healthy eating. Find out if they consider themselves to be healthy eaters. Have them explain the reasons behind their responses.

2. Take a poll of your students to find out how often they shop for food, prepare food, and eat out. Ask them what factors affect their food choices in each of these situations. Explain that in this chapter they will be learning some tips that can help them make healthy food choices.

Strategies to Reteach, Reinforce, Enrich, and Extend Text Concepts

The Recommended Dietary Allowances

3. **EX** Have students use the RDA chart on page 616 of the text to compare the RDA for their sex and age group with the RDA for children ages 7 to 10 and adults ages 19 to 24. Ask students to explain the reasons for the differences in recommendations.

4. **ER** Have students investigate how the RDA are revised. Ask students to find out who reviews the RDA, how often they revise the RDA, and what factors might cause them to recommend changes. Have them report their findings in class

5. **EX** Have students compare the RDA for their age and sex groups with amounts of the various nutrients they actually consume over a three-day period.

Dietary Guidelines for Americans

6. **RF** *What's Behind the Dietary Guidelines?* Activity A, SAG. Students are to explain why each of the Dietary Guidelines for Americans was established.

7. **ER** Have each student find a health article that relates to one of the Dietary Guidelines for Americans and share it with the class.

8. **RT** *Dietary Guidelines for Americans—A Framework for Good Nutrition,* transparency master 3-1, TRB. Discuss with students how the seven guidelines are interrelated and how they work together to support a healthy diet.

9. **EX** Body shape is one indication of healthy weight. Have students divide their waist measurements by their hip measurements. Quotients near or above one indicate an increased risk for weight-related health problems.

10. **ER** Ask groups of students to design posters illustrating foods that are low in fat, cholesterol, sugars, or sodium. Display posters in class.

11. **EX** Refer to the bulletin board "Is Your Diet in Balance?" Have students brainstorm a list of grain products, vegetables, fruits, and other foods that are low in fat, saturated fat, and cholesterol. Then have them brainstorm lists of foods that are high in sodium, sugar, and/or fat. Ask them which types of foods they are more likely to consume and have them evaluate whether their diets are in balance.

12. **RF** Ask students to define *balance, moderation,* and *variety* as they relate to the Dietary Guidelines.

13. **EX** Give students examples of high-fat entrees, high-sodium snacks, and desserts that are high in sugar. Have students suggest other foods they might eat at the same meal or at other times throughout the day to balance each example.

The Food Guide Pyramid

14. **EX** Have students describe how the Food Guide Pyramid could be adapted to fit a two-meal-a-day pattern and a five-meal-a-day pattern.

15. **ER** Have students make a poster illustrating a wide variety of foods from each of the groups in the Food Guide Pyramid.

16. **RF** Have students read the ingredient labels on at least 20 bread and cereal product packages. Ask them to identify which products contain whole grains and which do not.

17. **ER** Have students design a chart that groups vegetables into the following categories: dark green, deep yellow, starchy, legumes, and other. Charts should include brief statements about the specific nutrient contributions of each group.

18. **EX** Have students compare one serving of fresh fruit with one serving of fruit juice in terms of the calories and fiber provided.

19. **EX** Have students use Appendix B (Nutritive Values of Foods) on pages 617-634 of the text to compare the protein and fat content of the following foods: ground beef patty, lamb chops, ham steak, roasted chicken breast, broiled halibut, cooked lentils, scrambled eggs, and peanut butter.

20. **ER** Divide the class into three groups. Assign each group a different one of the following: dried beans, peas, and lentils. Ask each group to prepare a presentation about their assigned food. Presentations should

include pictures of the food, nutritional information, and recipes.

21. **EX** Have students investigate dairy substitutes given to people who are allergic to cow's milk. Ask them to find out how these products compare nutritionally to cow's milk products.

22. **EX** Have students keep a list of all the fats, oils, and sweets they include in their diet for one day. Then ask them to evaluate whether some of these foods are replacing foods from the five basic food groups.

23. **RF** Ask students what fats, oils, and sweets a typical teen might eat in one day. Write their responses on the chalkboard. Then have them use Appendix B (Nutritive Values of Foods) on pages 617-634 of the text to find the calorie, fat, and sodium content of the foods on the list. Use this information as the basis for a discussion of fats, oils, and sweets in the diet.

24. **EX** *Do You Follow the Pyramid?* Activity B, SAG. Students are to record their food and beverage intake for one day. They are to use this information to analyze their diets in comparison to the Food Guide Pyramid.

Choosing Wisely When Shopping for Food

25. **EX** Have students compare the nutritional value of a variety of fresh foods with their processed counterparts. Ask them to write a brief conclusion based on their comparisons.

26. **ER** Have students prepare a simple entree, such as macaroni and cheese or spaghetti, from scratch and from a convenience product. Ask them to compare the time required to make the foods and the nutrient content of the foods.

27. **ER** Have students visit the meat case of a grocery store to compare visible fat and marbling of various meat cuts. Ask them to inquire if select grade meats are available.

28. **EX** Have students compare nutrition labeling on several similar products. Ask them to choose which of the products they would buy based on this comparison and give reasons for their choices.

29. **ER** Have students visit a grocery store and make a list of canned vegetables that are available without added salt and canned fruits that are available without added sugar. Have them share their findings in class.

30. **ER** Have students visit a grocery store and make a list of the variety of reduced-fat products that are available. Have students sample some of these products and compare their taste and nutritional value with their high-fat counterparts.

31. **RF** Have students calculate the percentage of calories from fat that a reduced-fat processed meat product provides. Use their findings as the basis of a discussion of why consumers may need to limit their use of even some reduced-fat products.

32. **RT** Increase student awareness of the types of information found on package labels and encourage students to use label information when shopping. Have students read and evaluate package labels from a variety of the processed foods discussed in the text.

33. **RF** *Choosing Wisely When Shopping,* Activity C, SAG. Students are to determine whether the various statements listed on the worksheet about purchasing foods are true or false.

34. **RT** *Healthy Shopping,* transparency master 3-2, TRB. Use the transparency to highlight some basic guidelines for making healthy choices when shopping for food. Ask students which of these guidelines they already follow. Have them give specific examples of how they might put each guideline into practice.

35. **ER** Guest speaker. Invite a grocery store manager to speak to your class about how the increasing array of health-oriented food products has affected grocery display and advertising. Ask the speaker to also discuss how these products have affected the purchasing habits of consumers.

Choosing Wisely When Preparing Food

36. **RF** Demonstrate for students how to prepare and cook meat, poultry, and fish to reduce fat and calories.

37. **RT** Show students various examples of 3-ounce (84g) portions of lean, cooked meat, poultry, and fish.

38. **RF** Have students use Appendix B (Nutritive Values of Foods) on pages 617-634 of the text and a cookbook to compose a list of interesting, inexpensive, and nutritious main dishes made with legumes and/or grain products to replace or stretch meat, poultry, and fish.

39. **EX** Have students evaluate a variety of recipes to see where ingredients can be reduced, replaced, or omitted to limit fat, sugars, and sodium.
40. **RF** *Preparing Healthful Food*, Activity D, SAG. Students are to provide answers to the questions about how to prepare foods according to the recommendations of the Dietary Guidelines for Americans.

Choosing Wisely When Eating Out

41. **EX** Bring in menus from a variety of restaurants. Have students identify menu terms that might indicate foods that are high in fat, sugars, and sodium. Ask students to make healthful selections from each menu and explain their choices.
42. **ER** *Dining Habits Survey*, Activity E, SAG. Students are to survey five teens about their habits and preferences when dining out. They are to use their survey findings to make a general recommendation for teens regarding their food choices when eating out.
43. **ER** Guest speaker. Invite a restaurant manager to speak to your class about how the menu at his or her establishment meets the demands of consumers looking for healthful food options.

Chapter Review

44. **RT** *Tips for Making Healthy Food Choices*, reproducible master 3-3, TRB. If possible, duplicate this handout on colored paper. Have students fold the handout on the dotted lines to create a brochure. Ask them to use crayons or markers to decorate the brochure. You may wish to have students decorate extra brochures to pass out to other students as part of a nutrition awareness program.
45. **RT** *Chapter 3 Study Sheet*, reproducible master 3-4, TRB. Have students complete the statements as they read text pages 54-65.
46. **RF** Software, diskette for Part One. Have students play chapter review game according to the instructions that appear on the screen.

Above and Beyond

47. **EX** Have students plan a Healthy Food Choices Awareness Week in your school. Have them prepare informational posters about the Dietary Guidelines for Americans and the Food Guide Pyramid. Have them write articles for the school paper about food habits in the United States, current health recommendations, and food product trends. Have them prepare self-tests and brochures about shopping for and preparing foods and eating out. Class members should distribute these materials to other students to increase awareness of current food habits and possible need for change. Have your class prepare samples of lowfat, low-sodium, low-sugar snacks to pass out to other students along with recipes. Have your students present demonstrations of cooking techniques that follow the Dietary Guidelines for Americans. Have them work with the cafeteria manager to introduce a few new healthful and appealing food options into the cafeteria menu.

Answer Key

Text

Review What You Have Read, page 67
1. heredity, environment, and such personal health habits as rest, exercise, smoking, and abusing alcohol and other drugs
2. Eat a variety of foods.
   Balance the food you eat with physical activity. Maintain or improve your weight.
   Choose a diet with plenty of grain products, vegetables, and fruits.
   Choose a diet low in fat, saturated fat, and cholesterol.
   Choose a diet moderate in sugars.
   Choose a diet moderate in salt and sodium.
   If you drink alcoholic beverages, do so in moderation.
3. 30 percent
4. false
5.

	Teenage Girls	Teenage Boys
Breads, cereals, rice, and pasta	9	11
Vegetables	4	5
Fruits	3	4
Milk, yogurt, and cheese	3	3
Meat, poultry, fish, dry beans, eggs, and nuts	6 ounces	7 ounces

6. true
7. In most cases, processing decreases the nutritional value of foods.
8. (List five. Student response. See page 60 in the text.)
9. Read labels to be sure products are 100 percent juice.
10. (Name four:) broiling, roasting, grilling, braising, stewing, stir-frying, microwaving
11. Use a gravy separator or chill drippings and skim fat before making gravies.
12. D

Student Activity Guide

Choosing Wisely When Shopping, Activity C, page 18

1. T	12. T
2. T	13. F
3. F	14. T
4. F	15. T
5. T	16. T
6. F	17. F
7. T	18. T
8. F	19. T
9. T	20. T
10. T	21. T
11. F	22. F

Preparing Healthful Food, Activity D, page 19
1. Preparing foods from scratch gives you more control over the amount of added fat, sugars, and salt.
2. All visible fat should be trimmed from meat. Skin should be removed from poultry.
3. A 3-ounce (84 g) portion of meat, poultry, or fish is about the size of the palm of a woman's hand.
4. (lowfat entree of student's choice)
5. Using only half the amount of butter or margarine suggested on packages will help reduce fat when preparing packaged pasta, rice, stuffing, and sauce mixes.
6. Salad dressings, mayonnaise, sour cream, and cream cheese should be used in moderation. Using reduced-fat versions of these products or replacing them with plain, nonfat yogurt will also help limit the fat they contribute.
7. Vegetables can be flavored with herbs and lemon juice instead of salt and butter.
8. Salt can be omitted from recipes calling for other sodium-containing ingredients, such as cheese or condensed soup.
9. Adding vanilla or spices, such as cinnamon, ginger, or cloves, makes recipes for baked goods seem sweeter when the amount of sugar in the recipes has been reduced.
10. Portions of omelets and scrambled eggs can be stretched by adding extra egg whites in place of whole eggs, which contain high-cholesterol yolks.

Teacher's Resources

Chapter 3 Test

1. C		14. F	
2. A		15. T	
3. A		16. T	
4. E		17. F	
5. D		18. T	
6. B		19. T	
7. F		20. T	
8. D		21. D	
9. F		22. C	
10. C		23. A	
11. T		24. A	
12. F		25. D	
13. F			

26. You can use the RDA to analyze your diet. You can compare the nutrient content of the foods you eat with the RDA for your sex and age group. This comparison can help you determine whether you are getting enough of the various nutrients.
27. Eat a variety of foods. Balance the food you eat with physical activity—maintain or improve your weight. Choose a diet with plenty of grain products, vegetables, and fruits. Choose a diet low in fat, saturated fat, and cholesterol. Choose a diet moderate in sugars. Choose a diet moderate in salt and sodium. If you drink alcoholic beverages, do so in moderation.
28. Teenage girls: 2,200 calories, bread group—9 servings, vegetable group—4 servings, fruit group—3 servings, milk group—3 servings, meat group—6 ounces (168g), 73 grams of fat, 12 teaspoons of added sugars.
Teenage guys: 2,800 calories, bread group—11 servings, vegetable group—5 servings, fruit group—4 servings, milk group—3 servings, meat group—7 ounces (196g), 93 grams of fat, 18 teaspoons of added sugars.
29. (Student response. See pages 60-62 in the text.)
30. (Student response. See pages 62 and 64 in the text.)

Making Healthy Food Choices

Name _____

Date _____ Period _____ Score _____

Chapter 3 Test

Matching: Match each of the following foods with the group from the Food Guide Pyramid to which it belongs. (You may use some food groups more than once.)

_____ 1. Cherries.

_____ 2. Tortillas.

_____ 3. Bagels.

_____ 4. Swiss cheese.

_____ 5. Eggs.

_____ 6. Spinach.

_____ 7. Shortening.

_____ 8. Tofu.

_____ 9. Honey.

_____ 10. Raisins.

A. breads, cereals, rice, and pasta
B. vegetables
C. fruits
D. meat, poultry, fish, dry beans, eggs, and nuts
E. milk, yogurt, and cheese
F. fats, oils, and sweets

True/False: Circle *T* if the statement is true or *F* If the statement is false.

T   F   11. The RDA is not a useful guide for people who are sick or convalescing.

T   F   12. Following the Dietary Guidelines for Americans means giving up all high-fat foods.

T   F   13. People with low incomes cannot use the Food Guide Pyramid.

T   F   14. The Food Guide Pyramid recommends two to three servings from the fats, oils, and sweets group each day.

T   F   15. Canned peaches, frozen corn, and vitamin fortified cereal are examples of processed foods.

T   F   16. Nutrition labeling can help shoppers see how their food choices fit with the Dietary Guidelines for Americans.

T   F   17. Meal managers cannot control the amount of fat, salt, and sugar in foods prepared from scratch.

T   F   18. Broiling, grilling, and microwaving are lowfat cooking methods recommended for preparing meat, poultry, and fish.

T   F   19. A high-fat, high-sodium meal eaten in a restaurant can be balanced with other meals that are lower in fat and sodium.

T   F   20. The more varied a restaurant menu is, the easier it is to find healthful food options.

Multiple Choice: Choose the best response. Write the letter in the space provided.

_____ 21. The RDA is used to _____.
A. calculate the approximate nutritional needs of a large group of people
B. evaluate the diets of individuals
C. formulate regulations for the composition of foods, dietary supplements, and drugs
D. All of the above.

(Continued)

Name _____

_____22.   The Dietary Guidelines for Americans recommend moderation in the use of _____.
    A. fruits
    B. grain products
    C. sugars
    D. vegetables

_____   23. Which of the following counts as one serving of chopped, cooked, or canned fruit?
    A. ½ cup.
    B. ¾ cup.
    C. 1 cup.
    D. 2 to 3 ounces.

_____   24. Which of the following preparation tips will *not* help reduce fat, sugars, or sodium?
    A. Use mayonnaise instead of yogurt when making dressings and dips.
    B. Flavor vegetables with herbs and lemon juice instead of salt and butter.
    C. Dust cakes with powdered sugar instead of spreading them with frosting.
    D. Use evaporated milk instead of cream.

_____   25. Which of the following menu terms indicates that a food may be high in sodium?
    A. Breaded.
    B. Fried.
    C. Served with gravy.
    D. Smoked.

Essay Questions: Provide complete responses to the following questions or statements.

26. How can you use the Recommended Dietary Allowances?
27. List the Dietary Guidelines for Americans.
28. Give the level of daily calorie intake that is generally appropriate for someone of your age and sex. Then identify the number of daily servings from each food group and limits for fat and sugar that correspond to this calorie level.
29. Give three tips for making healthy food choices when shopping for food.
30. Give three tips for healthful food preparation.

Nutrition Through the Life Cycle

Objectives

After studying this chapter, students will be able to
- plan a well-balanced diet for themselves and for other people in different stages of the life cycle.
- discuss the importance of exercise in maintaining a suitable level of fitness.
- identify factors that contribute to weight problems and eating disorders.
- explain the philosophy behind weight management.

Bulletin Boards

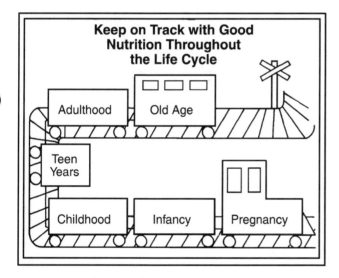

I. Title: "Keep on Track with Good Nutrition Throughout the Life Cycle"

Use colorful construction paper to cut out the cars of a train. Place the train on a track that you've drawn on the bulletin board. Label each car with one of the stages of the life cycle.

II. Title: "Nutrition Is Important at Every Age"

Cut photos from magazines showing pregnant women, infants, preschoolers, school-age children, teenagers, adults, and senior citizens. Group the photos according to the age of the subjects and place the groups around the bulletin board. Under each group, place a card identifying problem nutrients for people in that age group.

Teaching Materials

Text, pages 69-92

Student Activity Guide, pages 21-26
    A. *Baby Food*
    B. *Making a Weight Management Plan*
    C. *Diets in the Life Cycle*
    D. *Nutrition Advice*

Teacher's Resource Binder

    How Do Nutritional Needs Change Throughout Life? transparency master 4-1

    Burning Calories, reproducible master 4-2

    Why Don't Fad Diets Ever Go Out of Fashion? reproducible master 4-3

    Sweet Impostors, reproducible master 4-4

    Progression of Eating Disorders, transparency master 4-5

    Chapter 4 Study Sheet, reproducible master 4-6

    Eat to Compete, color transparency CT-4

    Chapter 4 Test

Software, diskette for Part One
    Reverse Thinking, chapter review game

Introductory Activity

1. *How Do Nutritional Needs Change Throughout Life?* transparency master 4-1, TRB. For each stage of the life cycle, have students suggest reasons why nutritional needs might differ from the stage before.
2. Ask students if they have younger children or older adults in their family who eat different foods or different amounts of food than the students. Discuss why these family members have different food needs.

Strategies to Reteach, Reinforce, Enrich, and Extend Text Concepts

Nutrition During Pregnancy and Lactation

3. Have students plan sample daily menus for a pregnant woman of a given income level for one week. Identify for students foods that the woman does and does not like. Instruct students that their menus should include

foods that are rich in protein, calcium, and iron; foods that the woman likes; and foods that the woman can afford.

4. **ER** Discuss with students how drugs, tobacco, alcohol, and over-the-counter medications, other than those prescribed by a physician, can be harmful for pregnant and lactating women and their infants. Have students design a brochure warning expectant mothers about these dangers.

5. **ER** Guest speaker. Invite an obstetrician to your class to discuss the importance of diet during pregnancy.

Nutrition During Infancy and Early Childhood

6. **ER** Have students research the advantages of breast-feeding over formula-feeding. Ask them to summarize their findings in a written report.

7. **ER** Panel discussion. Invite several new mothers to speak to your class about infant feeding and the advantages and disadvantages of various feeding methods.

8. **ER** *Baby Food*, Activity A, SAG. Students are to interview the mother of an infant and record her responses to the questions on the worksheet.

9. **ER** Field trip. Visit a supermarket and investigate different kinds of baby foods. Record average costs of strained fruits, vegetables, main dishes, and desserts. Prepare similar products using a blender. Compare appearance, texture, and cost of home-prepared foods and commercially-prepared foods.

10. **EX** Have students plan meals for a preschool child for two days. They should design menus for one of the days for a preschool child who does not like to drink milk.

11. **EX** Have students look at the label of a multivitamin/mineral supplement designed for young children. Have them evaluate how the amount of each nutrient provided by the supplement compares with the RDA for this age group.

12. **ER** Field trip. Arrange your students to take a lunch or nutritious snack that they have planned and prepared to a nursery school. Have your students note the children's reactions to the foods served. Afterward, discuss with your students what changes might be desirable if they were to repeat the field trip.

Nutrition in the Elementary School Years

13. **ER** Have students plan one day's menus for a school-age child. Have them show how snacks can fit into the daily food plan.

14. **ER** Have students plan two nutritious breakfasts. They should build one breakfast around traditional breakfast foods. The other breakfast should contain foods that are not usually considered to be breakfast foods. Invite students to share their menus and state which one they think school-age children would prefer.

15. **RF** Discuss with students factors that might contribute to childhood obesity. Ask students what types of physical activity and snack foods might be appropriate for a child who has a weight problem.

Nutrition in the Teen Years

16. **RF** Have students divide a sheet of paper into four sections. Have them label the sections "busy schedules," "skipped meals," "reducing diets," and "junk foods." In each section, have them write suggestions appropriate for the heading that teens could use to avoid or make up for that particular cause of nutrient deficiencies in their diet.

17. **RT** Discuss with students possible variations that could be made in a family meal pattern to allow for the increased nutritional needs of teenage family members.

18. **ER** Have students design a poster illustrating nutritious snacks for teens.

19. **EX** Have students use cookbooks to find recipes that call for milk as a primary ingredient. Ask them to write menus for one day using these recipes in place of fluid milk to meet the recommended number of servings for a teenager.

20. **EX** Have students brainstorm a list of foods that would help obese adolescents meet their nutritional needs without exceeding their calorie goals.

21. **ER** Guest speaker. Invite a registered dietitian to speak to your class about teenage weight problems, dieting, and exercise.

22. **RT** Take a poll of students who are involved in athletics to find out what kinds of diets they follow. Use your findings as the basis for a discussion of nutrition for athletes.

23. **RT** *Eat to Compete*, color transparency CT-4, TRB. Use the transparency to highlight nutri-

tion recommendations for athletes. Explain the reason behind each recommendation.

24. **ER** Have students investigate the dangers of rapid weight loss and weight gain that some athletes practice to make certain weight classes for competition. Ask them to suggest safe alternatives to these practices.

25. **ER** Guest speaker. Invite the coach of one of the school teams to speak to your class about nutrition concerns of teenage athletes. Ask the coach to share the diet advice he or she gives to team members.

Nutrition in Adulthood

26. **RF** Discuss with students why adults may have nutritional deficiencies. Ask students to suggest ways that adults can avoid diet-related deficiencies.

27. **ER** Have students develop a survey about adult eating habits. Have them each to use the survey to interview three adults. Then have them compile their findings in an article for the school paper.

Nutrition in Old Age

28. **RF** Discuss with students the special problems that may need to be considered when planning meals for the elderly. Then ask students to suggest menu ideas for a luncheon for an older adult and write their suggestions on the chalkboard. Ask students to consider the physical as well as the nutritive characteristics of the food. Menu items should be easy to chew and digest while still being flavorful and attractive.

29. **EX** Have students plan low-cost menus that meet the nutritional needs and financial constraints of older adults that older adults could prepare with a minimum of effort.

30. **ER** Have students investigate community programs that provide food service for older adults.

31. **ER** Field trip. Visit a geriatric center. Talk to the staff dietitian about diets suitable for elderly adults.

32. **ER** Guest audience or field trip. Invite a group of senior citizens to your class or visit a senior citizen center. Have your students prepare for this group of older adults the luncheon menu they planned in strategy 28.

Exercise and Fitness

33. **RT** Discuss with students the various benefits of exercise.

34. **EX** Have students brainstorm a list of exercise habits they can begin to develop now that will help them stay healthy and active throughout life.

35. **RF** Have each student divide a sheet of paper horizontally into three sections. Have students label the sections "daily tasks," "moderate activities," and "vigorous activities." Ask them to list forms of exercise they enjoy that fit under each heading.

36. **ER** Guest speaker. Invite a physical therapist to speak to your class about injuries that commonly result from inappropriate exercise programs and techniques. Ask the speaker to explain how to avoid such injuries.

Special Diets

37. **EX** Have students use several vegetarian cookbooks to plan vegetarian menus for three days that provide all of the nutrients needed by an adult for each day.

38. **ER** Have students prepare one of the vegetarian meals they planned in strategy 37. Have them evaluate the flavor and appearance of the meal.

39. **EX** Have students compare recipes designed for people on special diets with standard recipes and evaluate the differences.

40. **ER** Guest speaker. Invite a dietitian to speak to your class about how common illnesses can affect appetite and nutrient needs.

Weight Management

41. **RT** Demonstrate how to perform the pinch test.

42. **RT** Discuss with students the hazards of being obese.

43. **RT** Ask students to list factors that contribute to overeating.

44. **EX** *Burning Calories,* reproducible master 4-2, TRB. Have students compute their daily calorie needs. Then have them figure their energy expenditures based on the activity chart. Students should complete the activity by comparing the two figures and writing a brief evaluation.

45. **RT** Discuss with students the dangers of fad reducing diets.

46. **EX** *Why Don't Fad Diets Ever Go Out of Fashion?* reproducible master 4-3, TRB. After reading the article, students are to complete a chart to evaluate some of the fad diets that are currently popular.

47. **RF** *Sweet Impostors,* reproducible master 4-4, TRB. Students are to read an article and then answer questions about high-intensity sweeteners.
48. **EX** *Making a Weight Management Plan,* Activity B, SAG. Students are to complete the activity by analyzing the menus and suggesting substitutions where appropriate to help an adult lose weight. Then they are to answer questions about weight management.
49. **ER** Have students investigate health problems that could lead people to be underweight.
50. **EX** Have students plan menus for one week that would provide an underweight teen with enough calories to gain about 2 pounds (1 kg). Remind students that the foods they add to standard menus should be high in nutrients as well as calories.

Eating Disorders

51. **ER** Have students use articles and pamphlets about eating disorders to write a brief report about the causes and treatment of anorexia nervosa and bulimia.
52. **RT** Discuss with students standards they might use to determine when further weight reduction would not be appropriate.
53. **RF** Ask students to list appropriate and inappropriate uses for laxatives, diuretics, and weight-loss aids.
54. **RT** *Progression of Eating Disorders,* transparency master 4-5, TRB. Use the transparency as you discuss with students the emotional stages through which someone with an eating disorder passes before and after seeking treatment.

Chapter Review

55. **EX** *Diets in the Life Cycle,* Activity C, SAG. Students are to complete the activity by answering questions about how they can amend given menus to meet the various nutritional needs of people at different points in the life cycle.
56. **EX** *Nutrition Advice,* Activity D, SAG. Students are to use chapter information to answer letters written to a nutrition advice columnist.
57. **RT** *Chapter 4 Study Sheet,* reproducible master 4-6, TRB. Have students complete the statements as they read text pages 70-91.

58. **RF** *Reverse Thinking,* Software, diskette for Part One. Have students play the chapter review game according to the instructions that appear on the screen.

Above and Beyond

59. **EX** Divide the class into groups. Have each group research the nutritional value of foods at a different fast-food chain. Each group should prepare a presentation using visual aids to suggest the most nutritious meal options at the chain investigated.
60. **EX** Have students use the data gathered in strategy 59 to compare the nutritional value of similar items at the various fast-food chains.

Answer Key

Text
Review What You Have Read, page 92
1. If the mother's diet does not meet the nutrient needs of the fetus, the needed nutrients are taken from the mother's tissues.
2. Alcohol and other drugs can pass to a baby through breast milk.
3. false
4. (List three:) Serve foods that are mild flavored, soft, and lukewarm. Serve finger foods. Serve brightly colored foods. Serve small portions. Create a pleasant eating atmosphere with child-sized chair, table, and eating utensils.
5. School-age children who have trouble eating large meals can meet their nutritional needs by eating nutritious snacks.
6. A
7. false
8. (List two:) limited income, difficulty shopping, loneliness, dental and digestive problems
9. Stretching exercises improve flexibility. Calisthenics build strength and muscle endurance. Activities that raise the heart rate for more than 20 minutes promote cardiovascular endurance.
10. true
11. (List four:) soothe a sore throat, cool a fever, flush bacteria out of the urinary tract, replace fluids lost through diarrhea and perspiration caused by fever, keep sinus and nasal secretions flowing

12. The weight ranges on height-weight tables are wide to account for varying body composition. Someone who has low muscle mass but falls at the high end of the range may have excess body fat.
13. To lose 1 pound (.45 kg) a week, you would need to increase the difference between energy intake and expenditure by roughly 500 calories a day through a combination of reduced calories and increased physical activity.
14. true
15. Eating disorders are usually triggered by some type of personal stress.

Student Activity Guide

Making a Weight Management Plan, Activity B, pages 22-23
1. (List five:) early death; more likely to suffer from hypertension; more likely to suffer from diabetes; more likely to suffer from heart ailments; more likely to suffer from cancer; higher insurance rates; strain on bones, muscles, heart, and other organs; more effort needed to walk, breathe, and regulate body temperature; social pressures
2. medical problems, overeating (Students may also sight specific social or emotional reasons that people overeat.)
3. (Student response. See pages 87-88 in the text.)
4. sex, age, size, body composition, and level of activity
5. A good weight management plan is part of a lifestyle that involves using food choices and exercise to reach and/or maintain a healthy weight.

Teacher's Resources

Chapter 4 Test

1. F	11. F	21. D
2. C	12. T	22. B
3. D	13. F	23. B
4. B	14. F	24. B
5. E	15. T	25. D
6. T	16. T	26. D
7. T	17. F	27. A
8. F	18. T	28. C
9. F	19. F	29. C
10. T	20. T	30. A

31. Teen mothers need high levels of nutrients to support their own growth. Deficiencies could negatively affect a teenage mother's development as well as the development of her baby.
32. Breast milk is easy for a baby to digest. It contains immune substances that help a baby resist infection. It also helps protect the baby from allergies.
33. Setting good examples. Encouraging their children to try new foods. Refraining from using food as a punishment or a reward.
34. (Student response. See pages 87-88 in the text.)
35. Anorexia nervosa is an eating disorder characterized by self-starvation. Bulimia nervosa is an eating disorder characterized by repeated eating binges followed by purging via vomiting or taking laxatives or diuretics. Treatment of these eating disorders may begin with hospitalization to combat malnutrition. Once the victim's body is renourished, he or she must begin psychological counseling. Therapists often urge family members to take part in therapy.

Nutrition in the Life Cycle

Name _____

Date _____ Period _____ Score _____

Chapter 4 Test

Matching: Match the following terms and identifying phrases.

_____ 1. Using resources like food choices and exercise to reach and/or maintain a healthy weight.

_____ 2. A condition whereby a person exceeds the healthy weight for his or her height and body composition by 20 percent or more.

_____ 3. A condition whereby a person exceeds the healthy weight for his or her height and body composition by 10 percent.

_____ 4. The body's ability to meet physical demands.

_____ 5. A condition whereby a person weighs 10 percent less than the healthy weight for his or her height and body composition.

A. diet
B. fitness
C. obesity
D. overweight
E. underweight
F. weight management

True/False: Circle *T* if the statement is true or *F* if the statement is false.

T   F   6. A pregnant woman should never take any medication except under the advice of her obstetrician.

T   F   7. During lactation a woman has increased energy, protein, mineral, and vitamin needs.

T   F   8. Infants are born with reserves of most of the needed nutrients.

T   F   9. Growth is faster between the ages of two and six than during infancy.

T   F   10. Studies show that children who eat breakfast are more likely to do better in school than children who skip breakfast.

T   F   11. Teenage boys often have more nutritional deficiencies than teenage girls.

T   F   12. Energy needs decrease in adulthood.

T   F   13. As a person grows older, needs for all nutrients decrease.

T   F   14. Stretching exercises promote cardiovascular endurance.

T   F   15. Lacto-ovo vegetarian diets pose no serious health problems because they include enough foods from each of the food groups to supply all the needed nutrients.

T   F   16. Drinking liquids is a recommended treatment for many everyday health problems.

T   F   17. Fat tissue weighs more than muscle and bone tissue.

T   F   18. Efforts to lose weight are most successful when they are part of a lifelong commitment to maintain good health.

T   F   19. To gain weight, underweight people should eat a higher proportion of calories from fat than other people.

T   F   20. Vomiting, excessive exercise, and depression are all symptoms of eating disorders.

(Continued)

Name _____

Multiple Choice: Choose the best response. Write the letter in the space provided.

_____ 21. Poor nutrition in any stage of a person's life cycle can _____.
   A. create health problems
   B. always be corrected during later stages
   C. shorten the life span
   D. Both A and C.

_____ 22. Pregnant women should follow a diet _____.
   A. consisting mainly of dairy products
   B. that is well-balanced, consisting of a variety of foods
   C. that contains no fat
   D. that includes twice the amount of calories she normally consumes since she is "eating for two"

_____ 23. The first solid foods to be introduced into the diet of most babies are _____.
   A. crackers and zwieback
   B. cereals
   C. pureed fruits and vegetables
   D. strained meats, poultry, and simple desserts

_____ 24. Which of the following might encourage good eating in a preschool child?
   A. Large portions.
   B. Bright colored finger foods.
   C. Spicy foods with crunchy textures served piping hot.
   D. Sitting at a "grown-up" table and using "grown-up" eating utensils.

_____ 25. During the adolescent growth spurt, teenagers need _____.
   A. more energy
   B. as much protein as adults
   C. the same amounts of vitamins and minerals as adults
   D. All of the above.

_____ 26. About which of the following nutrients do athletes need to be most concerned?
   A. Calcium.
   B. Protein.
   C. Vitamin C.
   D. Water.

_____ 27. Which of the following is *not* a problem affecting the diet of elderly people?
   A. Busy schedules keep them from having time to eat.
   B. Limited income makes nutritious foods difficult to afford.
   C. Limited mobility makes shopping difficult.
   D. Loneliness makes eating less appealing.

_____ 28. Which of the following is *not* a benefit of exercise?
   A. It keeps skin healthy.
   B. It reduces the risk of heart disease, stroke, and colon disorders.
   C. It slows metabolism.
   D. It tones muscles.

_____ 29. Which of the following does not affect a person's daily calorie need?
   A. Age.
   B. Body composition.
   C. Eating habits.
   D. Sex.

(Continued)

Name _____

_____ 30. When planning a weight management plan, keep in mind that 1 pound (.45 kg) of fat is
equal to about _____.
   A. 3,500 calories
   B. 2,000 calories
   C. 1,600 calories
   D. 1,200 calories

Essay Questions: Provide complete responses to the following questions or statements.

31. Explain why nutrient deficiencies can especially be a problem in the case of teenage pregnancies.
32. Why do many experts recommend that mothers breast-feed their infants?
33. Explain how parents can promote healthy attitudes about good nutrition.
34. List five tips for successfully following a weight management plan to reduce weight.
35. Explain the difference between anorexia nervosa and bulimia nervosa and describe the treatment
used to deal with these disorders.

Safeguarding the the Family's Health

Objectives

After studying this chapter, students will be able to
- discuss causes, symptoms, and treatment of common food-borne illnesses.
- describe important standards of personal and kitchen cleanliness.
- give examples of how following good safety practices can help you prevent kitchen accidents.
- apply basic first aid measures in the home.

Bulletin Board

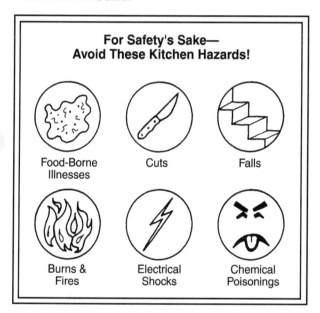

Title: "For Safety's Sake—Avoid These Kitchen Hazards!"

Use drawings or photos from magazines to illustrate the six main sources of danger in the kitchen—food-borne illnesses, cuts, falls, burns and fires, electrical shocks, and chemical poisonings.

Teaching Materials

Text, pages 93-106
Student Activity Guide, pages 27-30
  A. *Kitchen Sanitation*
  B. *Sanitation in Food Preparation and Storage*
  C. *Safety Is No Accident*
  D. *Handling Emergencies*

Teacher's Resource Binder
  Dangers in the Kitchen, transparency master 5-1
  Say No to, transparency master 5-2 (to be used as an overlay with *Dangers in the Kitchen*)
  Poison Treatment, reproducible master 5-3
  Chapter 5 Study Sheet, reproducible master 5-4
  Fire Triangle, color transparency CT-5
  Chapter 5 Test
Software, diskette for Part One
  The Matching Game, chapter review game

Introductory Activities

1. *Dangers in the Kitchen*, transparency master 5-1, TRB. Cover the title of the transparency master. Tell the students to ask you yes-or-no questions to help them identify what the six items pictured have in common. When the students give the correct response, uncover the title. (This master is also used in introductory activity 2.)
2. *Say No to*, transparency master 5-2, TRB. Use this master as an overlay with *Dangers in the Kitchen*. Cover everything except the top two pictures on the transparency. Ask students to identify what each picture is showing and explain why it is a danger in the kitchen. When students give the correct responses, uncover the labels under the pictures. Repeat this process with the other two sets of pictures on the master.

Strategies to Reteach, Reinforce, Enrich, and Extend Text Concepts

Food-Borne Illnesses

3. **ER** Divide the class into groups. Have each group research a different one of the food-borne illnesses mentioned in the text. Have each group design a poster illustrating the cause, food sources, symptoms, and prevention of the illness. Then have the groups use their posters to give presentations to the rest of the class. (Groups of four work well for this learning experience, allowing each student to present a different aspect of the illness.)

4. **RF** Have students read and discuss articles about incidents of food-borne illness.
5. **RF** Have students make a list of foods that have natural poisons.
6. **ER** Guest speaker. Invite a botanist to speak to your class about mushroom identification and natural food poisons.

Kitchen Sanitation

7. **RF** Have students develop a checklist of personal and kitchen cleanliness standards that they can use to evaluate their cooking habits at home.
8. **RF** Have students write to the county health department to obtain a list of the standards established for food service workers.
9. **EX** Have students brainstorm a list of personal hygiene standards that they can practice in the foods laboratory. Write their ideas on the chalkboard. Then discuss with students how they can carry out listed standards in the classroom and at home.
10. **ER** Have students develop slogans that relate to the hygiene standards listed in strategy 9. Have them use decorative writing and/or illustrations to put these slogans on signs that they post around the classroom.
11. **EX** Have the class set up standards for maintaining clean food laboratory units.
12. **ER** Have students measure the temperature of the tap water they will use to wash dishes in the laboratory. Evaluate whether this temperature is sufficient for thorough cleaning.
13. **ER** Have each lab group draw a chart illustrating the order in which dishes should be washed. Laminate the charts and post them near the sink in each lab.
14. **EX** *Kitchen Sanitation,* Activity A, SAG. Students are to read a story and then list 10 guidelines of personal and kitchen cleanliness that the character in the story failed to follow.
15. **RT** Have students list 10 guidelines for maintaining sanitation in food preparation and storage.
16. **ER** Have students demonstrate proper techniques for wrapping foods for refrigerator and freezer storage. Ask them to discuss characteristics of appropriate wrapping materials and storage containers used in their demonstration.
17. **RF** Have students prepare a chart listing

the optimum storage times for a variety of foods.
18. **ER** Have students investigate safe options for thawing foods and report their findings in class.
19. **ER** Have students research one type of insect or rodent that poses a health threat when it infests food. Have them write a two-page report summarizing the type of threat posed, how to prevent infestation, and how to get rid of the pests once infestation occurs.
20. **ER** Have students develop a brochure providing tips for proper sanitation in food preparation and storage when cooking for special occasions, such as picnics, barbecues, and buffets.
21. **ER** Field trip. Visit a school cafeteria, hospital, or hotel kitchen and observe the sanitary standards being followed in quantity food preparation.
22. **ER** Guest speaker. Invite a public health inspector to speak to your class about health codes and inspections for food service establishments. Ask the speaker to discuss how often inspections are conducted. He or she should also mention what the most common violations are and what the penalties are for noncompliance with state health regulations.
23. **RF** *Sanitation in Food Preparation and Storage,* Activity B, SAG. Students are to complete the activity by answering questions related to sanitation in food preparation and storage.

Safety in the Kitchen

24. **RF** Have students make a list of guidelines for preventing chemical poisonings. Encourage students to use these guidelines when using and storing poisonous chemicals in their homes.
25. **RT** *Poison Treatment,* reproducible master 5-3, TRB. Have each student complete the top of the sheet with specified phone numbers to contact if there is a poisoning. Go over the sheet with students. Then encourage them to post it near a phone or inside a medicine cabinet in their home.
26. **RT** Demonstrate the proper use and care of a knife.
27. **RF** Have students list different types of cuts that might occur in the kitchen and give suggestions for preventing each type.
28. **RT** *Fire Triangle,* color transparency CT-5,

TRB. Use the transparency to illustrate the three components necessary for a fire—oxygen, fuel, and heat. Explain how removing any one of these components, such as smothering a fire to remove oxygen, will extinguish the fire.

29. **RF** Show students how to use the fire extinguisher in your classroom. Then ask students to repeat the demonstration back to you.
30. **RF** Have students list three ways burns can be prevented in the kitchen.
31. **ER** Guest speaker. Invite a member of the fire department to speak to your class about fire prevention in the kitchen.
32. **RF** Have students list three common causes of falls in the kitchen. Ask them to explain how they can avoid each cause.
33. **RT** Discuss electrical safety with students. Demonstrate how to correctly unplug an appliance. Show examples of safety covers for outlets and appropriate and inappropriate extension cords for use with appliances.
34. **ER** Guest speaker. Invite a Red Cross instructor or the school nurse to your class to demonstrate basic first aid techniques and the abdominal thrust.
35. **EX** Have students role-play giving basic first aid for minor injuries that occur in the kitchen.
36. **ER** Have each student explore one of the other sources of danger in the kitchen discussed in the chapter. (Some students may suggest a source of danger not discussed in the chapter that they would like to explore.) Have students give brief oral reports about the types of hazards these items may cause and give suggestions for using these items safely.
37. **RF** *Safety Is No Accident,* Activity C, SAG. Students are to play a game as a review of kitchen safety.
38. **EX** *Handling Emergencies,* Activity D, SAG. Students are to provide appropriate responses to the emergency situations described on the worksheet.

Chapter Review

39. **RF** Go around the room and ask each student to give one tip related to sanitation and safety in the kitchen.
40. **RT** *Chapter 5 Study Sheet,* reproducible master 5-4, TRB. Have students complete the statements as they read text pages 94-105.

41. **RF** *The Matching Game,* Software, diskette for Part One. Have students play the chapter review game according to the instructions that appear on the screen.

Above and Beyond

42. **EX** Arrange with school administrators for your class to sponsor a school-wide Food and Kitchen Safety Awareness Week. You may wish to coordinate this project with teachers in other departments. Science classes could gather information about harmful bacteria that cause food-borne illnesses. Health classes could prepare presentations on basic first aid. Art classes could design pamphlets and posters. English classes could write press releases and articles for the school newspaper. Your students should plan to exhibit any of the materials they created as part of the other learning experiences for this chapter. They may also wish to design additional brochures, posters, and handouts to distribute; plan demonstrations and displays about safe practices in the kitchen; and prepare oral presentations, videotapes, and slide shows to inform other teachers and students about kitchen safety and sanitation.
43. **ER** As a service project, have students make puppets and write a puppet show to present information about kitchen safety to young children. Arrange for your students to perform their show at a local preschool or kindergarten.

Answer Key

Review What You Have Read, page 106
1. infants, pregnant women, the elderly, and people with impaired immunity
2. 160°F (71°C)
3. (List six. Student response. See pages 95-96 in the text.)
4. (List five. Student response. See pages 96-97 in the text.)
5. Keep hot foods above 140°F (60°C) and cold foods below 40°F (5°C).
6. Divide food into small, shallow containers.
7. in food service establishments
8. false
9. (List five. Student response. See page 102 in the text.)
10. To pick up broken glass, pick up large pieces

while wearing rubber gloves. Sweep smaller pieces into a disposable dustpan and use damp paper towels to wipe up any remaining fragments.

11. To extinguish a grease fire, pour baking soda or salt on flames or use a fire extinguisher.
12. (List three. Student response. See page 103 in the text.)
13. a nonconducting material, such as rope, a long piece of dry cloth, or a wooden pole
14. (Student response. See pages 103-104 in the text.)
15. People can injure themselves by bumping into open cabinet doors and drawers.

Student Activity Guide

Kitchen Sanitation, Activity A, page 27
(List 10:) Gina did not wash her hands before beginning work. Gina was not wearing clean clothes or a clean apron. Gina did not tie back her hair. Gina did not wash her hands after touching her hair. Gina stored her onions under the kitchen sink. Gina handled food when she had an open cut on her finger. Gina did not wash her hands after handling raw meat. Gina used a dish towel to wipe her hands. Gina did not wash the tomato before cutting it. Gina used the same cutting board for raw meat and fresh tomatoes. Gina fed her dog in the kitchen. Gina did not dust off the can of spaghetti sauce before opening it. Gina did not wipe up her spill and remove dirty utensils from her work area.

Sanitation in Food Preparation and Storage, Activity B, page 28
1. (Students should color in the area between 60° and 126°F.)
2. Temperatures in this zone allow rapid growth of bacteria and production of toxins by some bacteria.
3. two hours
4. Always keep hot foods hot and keep cold foods cold.
5. They should be wrapped in moistureproof and vaporproof wraps.
6. They should be boiled for 10 to 20 minutes before tasting.
7. They should be reheated to at least 165°F (74°C).
8. Raw poultry, meat, and fish should be stuffed just before baking. Stuffing should reach an internal temperature of at least

165°F (74°C). Stuffing should then be removed promptly from the protein food.

Handling Emergencies, **Activity D**, page 30
1. Apply pressure to stop any bleeding. Wash the cut with soap and water. Then apply an antiseptic solution and a bandage with a sterile dressing.
2. Immediately place the burned area under cold running water.
3. Do not move your mother. Make her as comfortable as possible and call a physician.
4. Call the poison control center and describe the product the child swallowed.
5. Immediately turn off the power and the water, then disconnect the mixer to avoid further danger of shock. Call for help. Since your sister is not connected to the power source, you can touch her and begin rescue breathing. Continue until help arrives.
6. Your friend is choking. Perform the abdominal thrust.
7. Cover the wound with a sterile cloth or clean handkerchief. Apply firm pressure and have someone take you to the hospital emergency room or your family doctor.
8. As an elderly person, your grandmother is at greater risk from the salmonellosis infection. You should take her to her doctor.

Teacher's Resources

Chapter 5 Test
1. B
2. C
3. D
4. F
5. E
6. G
7. T
8. T
9. T
10. F
11. T
12. F
13. T
14. F
15. T
16. T
17. A
18. C
19. B
20. C
21. B
22. (Student response. See page 94 in the text.)
23. (Student response. See pages 95-97 in the text.)
24. (Student response. See page 98 in the text.)
25. Use and care for equipment properly, follow good safety practices, and keep the kitchen clean.
26. (Student response. See pages 104-105 in the text.)

Safeguarding the Family's Health

Name _____

Date _____ Period _____ Score _____

Chapter 5 Test

Matching: Match the following first aid treatments with the injuries they are used to treat.

_____ 1. Place the injury under cold running water or in a cold bath.

_____ 2. Use the abdominal thrust.

_____ 3. Cover the injury with a sterile cloth and apply pressure to stop bleeding.

_____ 4. Avoid moving the victim if a broken bone is suspected.

_____ 5. Disconnect the power source and begin rescue breathing.

_____ 6. Call a poison control center and describe the poison taken.

A. broken bones
B. burns
C. choking
D. cuts
E. electric shock
F. falls
G. poisoning

True/False: Circle *T* if the statement is true or *F* if the statement is false.

T   F   7. Bacteria or toxins that bacteria produce cause most food-borne illnesses.

T   F   8. The bodies of healthy people can usually handle limited amounts of harmful bacteria.

T   F   9. Food service workers must follow strict standards for personal hygiene set by state and county health departments.

T   F   10. Meal managers who want to limit dirty dishes can safely use the same utensils for raw and cooked meats.

T   F   11. Chlorine bleach can be used to help kill bacteria found on kitchen counters and cutting boards.

T   F   12. Freezing temperatures kill all bacteria.

T   F   13. Large amounts of food take longer to heat or chill than small or average amounts of food.

T   F   14. The safety closures used on many medicines and household chemicals make the bottles impossible for children to open.

T   F   15. Always move a knife blade away from the body when cutting.

T   F   16. When lighting a gas range manually, light the match before turning on the gas.

Multiple Choice: Choose the best response. Write the letter in the space provided.

_____ 17. Double vision, inability to swallow, speech difficulty, and gradual respiratory paralysis are symptoms of _____.
A. botulism
B. perfringens poisoning
C. salmonellosis
D. staphylococcal poisoning

(Continued)

Name _____

_____ 18. For which of the following groups does food-borne illness pose the greatest health risk?
   A. School-age children.
   B. Teenagers.
   C. The elderly.
   D. All groups are at equal risk.

_____ 19. The temperature range known as the danger zone is _____.
   A. 40°-140°F (5°-60°C)
   B. 60°-126°F (16°-52°C)
   C. 140°-165°F (60°-74°C)
   D. None of the above.

_____ 20. Which of the following is not a safety precaution for preventing cuts?
   A. Wearing rubber gloves to pick up broken glass.
   B. Keeping knives sharp.
   C. Using knives to pry open cans.
   D. Disposing of can lids immediately.

_____ 21. Falls in the kitchen can be prevented by _____.
   A. standing on a chair to reach high places
   B. wiping up spills immediately
   C. covering the floor with throw rugs
   D. All of the above.

Essay Questions: Provide complete responses to the following questions or statements.

22. Give examples of two of the following causes of food-related illnesses: parasites, protozoa, viral diseases, natural poisons.
23. Give five tips for personal and kitchen cleanliness.
24. What are three characteristics you should look for in a restaurant and its employees to protect yourself from food-borne illness?
25. Give the three general guidelines for preventing all types of kitchen accidents.
26. Explain the safety procedure that should be followed when using two of the following: cabinets and drawers, aerosol cans, pressure cookers.

Career Opportunities

Objectives

After studying this chapter, students will be able to
■ describe three general career areas in the field of foods.
■ list the qualifications needed to work in each career area.
■ explain the steps involved in finding a job.

Bulletin Board

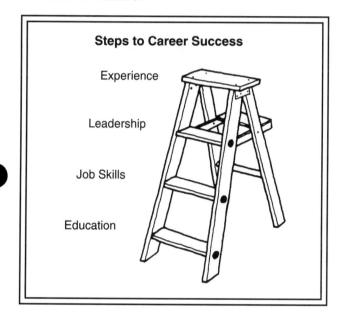

Steps to Career Success

Experience

Leadership

Job Skills

Education

Title: "Steps to Career Success"

Draw or cut out a large stepladder. Label the rungs of the ladder "education," "job skills," "leadership," and "experience" to indicate some of the important elements of success in the career world.

Teaching Materials

Text, pages 107-121
Student Activity Guide, pages 31-36
   A. *Career Self-Analysis*
   B. *Career Maze*
   C. *Careers in Foods*
   D. *Application Information*
   E. *You're the Boss*
Teacher's Resource Binder
   Food Industry Career Ladder, transparency master 6-1

Food-Related Careers, reproducible master 6-2
Preparing for an Interview, reproducible master 6-3
Catering Project Evaluation, reproducible master 6-4
Chapter 6 Study Sheet, reproducible master 6-5
Computers in the Food Industry, reproducible master 6-6
   Chapter 6 Test
Software, diskette for Part One
   Bingo, chapter review game

Introductory Activities

1. *Food Industry Career Ladder,* transparency master 6-1, TRB. Ask students what kinds of work situations might lead to career advancement. Ask them what characteristics of workers might facilitate career advancement. Then have students suggest food-related careers that might fall on different rungs on the career ladder. Write their suggestions on the transparency.
2. *Career Self-Analysis,* Activity A, SAG. Students are to complete a chart and answer questions to help them begin thinking about possible career interests.

Strategies to Reteach, Reinforce, Enrich, and Extend Text Concepts

Choosing a Career

3. **ER** Have each student use the *Dictionary of Occupational Titles* to find out about the three jobs that interest him or her most.
4. **ER** Have each student write to at least two schools (vocational schools, community colleges, or universities) for course catalogs and applications.
5. **RF** Have students practice filling out the application forms that they received through strategy 4.
6. **RF** Have students look through the catalogs they received through strategy 4. Have them take turns sharing examples of differ-

ent course offerings in family and consumer science and food industry programs. Discuss with students the variety of course work these various programs require.

7. **RF**   *Careers in Foods,* Activity C, SAG. Students are to answer questions about careers in the food industry.

8. **ER**   Have students interview someone working full-time in a food-related career. Students should find out how the interviewee's work schedule affects his or her family life.

9. **ER**   Panel discussion. Invite people working in a variety of food-related careers to speak to your class. Ask panelists to focus on any family and consumer science background they may have had and to highlight how it has helped them in their jobs. Job descriptions, educational requirements, and work experiences should also be part of their discussion.

10. **ER**   Guest speaker. Invite a school counselor to speak to your students about how to prepare for careers at various levels. Have the counselor describe any work-study programs that are available in your school. Also ask him or her to discuss aptitude tests and how to apply to postsecondary schools.

Skills for Success

11. **RF**   Have students list at least seven job skills and discuss the importance of each.

12. **EX**   Have students write case examples that illustrate how a lack of various job skills might result in problem situations.

13. **EX**   Have students role-play the case examples they wrote in strategy 12 to show how having various job skills can help prevent or correct the problems they had described.

14. **RF**   Have students discuss ways in which leadership skills would be used in work situations.

15. **EX**   Ask students to brainstorm a list of opportunities for leadership experiences of which they might be able to take advantage while they are still in high school.

The Food Service Industry

16. **ER**   Divide the class into four groups. Have each group prepare a presentation on one of the different areas of food service. Presentations should include a general description; examples of jobs; an outlook for numbers of new jobs; salary ranges; examples of entry-level, mid-level, and upper-

level positions; and educational background needed for each area.

17. **ER**   Field trip. Visit a hotel or hospital kitchen. Have your students ask questions they have prepared in advance about the food service opportunities available in this setting.

18. **ER**   Field trip. Visit a trade school or vocational school where students are training to be chefs. Have your students ask questions they have prepared in advanced about the requirements of the programs and the facilities of the institution.

The Food Handling Industry

19. **ER**   Have students visit a supermarket and make a list of all the food handling jobs they observe.

20. **ER**   Have each student draw a chart illustrating the path of a particular food from the farm to a grocery store shelf. Ask students to identify all the different people in the food handling industry who come in contact with the food along its path.

21. **ER**   Field trip. Visit a food processing plant. Have your students note what types of jobs are available. Ask your tour guide to describe to students the requirements for the different jobs.

Food-Related Careers in Education and Business

22. **RF**   Have students make a list of all the food-related careers in education and business. Then have them list the requirements for each career.

23. **RT**   *Food-Related Careers,* reproducible master 6-2, TRB. Review the handout with students and encourage them to consider listed options when planning their careers.

24. **ER**   Have students contact the American Dietetic Association to find out what registered dietitians have to do to obtain and maintain their credential.

25. **ER**   Arrange for your students to participate in a career shadowing experience. Have them each choose a food-related career in education and business and spend a typical working day with someone who has pursued that career.

Finding a Job

26. **EX**   Have students brainstorm a list of sources for learning about job openings.

27. **EX** *Preparing for an Interview,* reproducible master 6-3, TRB. Have students work in pairs to interview one another. The student conducting the interview in each pair should write the responses of the student he or she is interviewing. Give students an opportunity to review and evaluate their responses.
28. **EX** Have students role-play interview situations. If possible, videotape the mock interviews and replay them, giving students an opportunity to offer constructive criticism.
29. **RF** *Application Information,* Activity D, SAG. Encourage students to consider how they would fill out job applications by completing the personal fact sheet.

Entrepreneurship

30. **ER** Have students develop a list of questions about starting a business. Have each student use the list to interview an entrepreneur and share his or her findings in class.
31. **EX** Have each student head a piece of paper with the title "Entrepreneurship." Have students divide the paper into two columns. In the first column, have them list all the advantages they see to entrepreneurship. In the other column, have them list all the disadvantages they see. Then have students compare lists with classmates.
32. **EX** *You're the Boss,* Activity E, SAG. Students are to complete a worksheet to plan a food-related business.
33. **EX** *Catering Project Evaluation,* reproducible master 6-4, TRB. Have your class set up a catering business. Create a set of jobs that include positions in all four areas of food service. Appoint a few of your most responsible and creative students to be the managers of the business. (As an alternative, you might hold a class election to decide who will fill the managerial positions.) Have students interview with the managers for the other positions. Students will need to discuss the types of affairs they will be able to cater, making decisions about group sizes, types of foods, time schedules, appropriate dress, etc. Once this initial planning has taken place, a group of students will need to determine how to advertise the business and attract clients. (If you intend to make this a single learning experience rather than an ongoing project, you may wish to make advance arrangements for the class to cater a staff or par-

ent-teacher function.) Throughout the project, have students repeatedly evaluate their decisions and actions. Encourage them to modify their plans if their evaluations indicate a need to do so. At the completion of the project, have each student complete the handout.

Chapter Review

34. **RF** *Career Maze,* Activity B, SAG. Students are to complete statements about careers using terms from the chapter. Then they are to find and circle the words in a maze.
35. **RT** *Chapter 6 Study Sheet,* reproducible master 6-5, TRB. Have students complete the statements as they read text pages 108-119.
36. **RF** *Bingo,* Software, diskette for Part One. Have students play the chapter review game according to the instructions that appear on the screen.

Above and Beyond

37. **EX** Have your students plan a career day. You may wish to arrange to hold this event jointly with other departments or the entire school. Students should prepare booth displays, brochures, and posters describing various food-related careers in family and consumer sciences. Videotapes, slide presentations, and guest speakers could also be part of the event.
38. **RF** *Computers in the Food Industry,* reproducible master 6-6, TRB. Have students read the article and answer the questions about the use of computers in the food industry.
39. **ER** Have students investigate what software programs dietitians commonly use to analyze diets. If possible, obtain one of these programs for students to use in analyzing their diets.

Answer Key

Text

Review What You Have Read, page 121
1. (List five. Student response. See page 108 in the text.)
2. (List four:) school counselors, parents, teachers, people involved in a career you are interested in pursuing, college catalogs, career manuals
3. (List five:) ability to maintain a professional appearance, ability to communicate effectively, ability to get along with others, dedi-

cation to the job, knowledge of nutrition, artistic skills, leadership skills

4. leader
5. (Name the four types of jobs and give one example of each:) food preparation—assistant cook, cook, chef
customer service—busperson, waiter, host, head waiter, cashier
sanitation—dishwasher, pan scrubber, maintenance person
management—owner, manager, assistant manager, dietitian, executive chef
6. catering
7. (Give one example for each:) processing—positions involving such jobs as sorting, washing, peeling, slicing, drying, roasting, grinding, and packaging food products
transporting—truck, air freight, and train personnel, food brokers, distributors, food wholesalers, food retailers
retailing—stock personnel; dairy, produce, meat, and bakery managers; meat cutters and butchers; customer service personnel; advertising and marketing personnel; managerial personnel
8. true
9. food professional in business
10. (List two:) private industries, supermarkets, government agencies
11. (List three:) want ads; signs posted in windows of businesses; family members, friends, and neighbors; school guidance counselor or placement office
12. interview
13. entrepreneurs

Student Activity Guide

Career Maze, Activity B, pages 32-33

1. career ladder	12. dietitians
2. leader	13. care
3. food service	14. administration
4. preparation	15. nutritionist
5. customer	16. communications
6. sanitation	17. business
7. management	18. affairs
8. catering	19. research
9. handling	20. reference
10. teaching	21. interview
11. extension	22. entrepreneur

```
K U M E T S I N O I T I R T U N C N W A
M T L C A L B R S A N I T A T I O N N U
A D M I N I S T R A T I O N G I M H A E
A N K V C I O S Q O X F E U T K M B L L
F S T R E D D A L R E E R A C B U J J R
F J I E O N P L E E I V R H U J N U T T
A O D S R S R I A F F A F S S I I B O E
Y E R D L N D N D M P T I I T V C S M C
M H U O N A B A E E L N S G O C A H V M
A A E O B I Q E R E E I D G M A T N E B
H N N F Z T F P E S K Z N K E W I U C S
A D E A O I W J S Y M I B T R M O E N E
I L R P G T E D A X H N Y L E T N I E R
M I P P Q E R R H C R A E S E R S E R A
Z N E R C I M S A Y T Z O X R N V F E C
G G R B X D V E U C E U O V P E D I F L
A Y T G E X T E N S I O N X C S S G E H
V H N F G N I R E T A C O D I V Q E R W
A R E W D I D E P Z N W G Q N R E A R N
```

Teacher's Resources

Chapter 6 Test

1. G	13. F
2. B	14. F
3. C	15. T
4. I	16. F
5. A	17. T
6. H	18. T
7. F	19. D
8. D	20. C
9. T	21. D
10. T	22. B
11. F	23. C
12. T	

24. careers in the food service industry, careers in the food handling industry, food-related careers in business and education
25. (Name three:) coffee shops, snack bars, fast-food chains, restaurants, private clubs, school cafeterias, hotels, hospitals, other large institutions
26. (List five:) sorting, washing, peeling, slicing, packing, roasting, grinding
27. (List three:) nutritional care, administration, education, research, business and industry
28. What kind of business should I start? How much need is there for a business of this nature? Is it something I can manage? (Students may justify other responses.)

Career Opportunities

Name _____

Date _____ **Period** _____ **Score** _____

Chapter 6 Test

Matching: Match the following terms and identifying phrases.

_____ 1. A person who commands authority and takes a principal role in a group.

_____ 2. A business in which food and beverages are prepared for small and large parties, banquets, weddings, and other gatherings.

_____ 3. A member of the health care team who has knowledge and training in food and nutrition, the health sciences, and institution management.

_____ 4. A person that an employer can call to ask about a job applicant's capabilities as a worker.

_____ 5. A series of related jobs that form a career.

_____ 6. A registered dietitian who works directly in nutrition education.

_____ 7. A meeting between an employer and a job applicant help to discuss the applicant's qualifications for a job opening.

_____ 8. A person who sets up and runs his or her own business.

A. career ladder
B. catering
C. dietitian
D. entrepreneur
E. extension agent
F. interview
G. leader
H. nutritionist
I. reference

True/False: Circle *T* if the statement is true and *F* if the statement is false.

T F   9. Each job in a career ladder builds on the skills learned in the job below.

T F   10. A person's grooming habits influences the impressions he or she makes on the job.

T F   11. In large food service establishments, employees learn how to do many different food preparation tasks.

T F   12. Dietitians and executive chefs hold management positions in the food service industry.

T F   13. Caterers work in the food handling industry.

T F   14. Most food products are taken directly from the farmer to the consumer.

T F   15. Positions in the food handling industry include processing plant workers, truckers, and grocery store personnel.

T F   16. To teach family and consumer sciences at the high school level, a person must have a master's degree.

T F   17. Many supermarkets hire food professionals to answer consumer questions.

T F   18. A job application may require an applicant to specify expected wages and when he or she can start working.

(Continued)

Name _____

Multiple Choice: Choose the best response. Write the letter in the space provided.

_____ 19. Which of the following is the responsibility of a leader?
   A. Establishing priorities.
   B. Making decisions.
   C. Setting goals.
   D. All of the above.

_____ 20. Government figure show increasing needs for _____.
   A. dietitians
   B. extension agents
   C. food service workers
   D. supermarket managers

_____ 21. People employed in the customer service area of the food service industry might be _____.
   A. assistant managers
   B. cooks
   C. dishwashers
   D. waiters

_____ 22. Entry-level positions in the food handling industry might include _____.
   A. butchers
   B. food store checkers
   C. government inspectors
   D. plant managers

_____ 23. To make a good impression at a job interview, you should _____.
   A. wear casual clothes
   B. know your Social Security number
   C. have a positive attitude
   D. arrive a few minutes late

Essay Questions: Provide complete responses to the following questions or statements.

24. Name the three main groups of food careers.
25. Name three businesses in which food preparation jobs might be available.
26. Give examples of five processing steps that might take place at a food processing plant.
27. Name three areas in which dietitians work.
28. List three questions you should ask yourself if you are thinking about becoming an entrepreneur.

Kitchen and Dining Areas   Chapter 7

Objectives

After studying this chapter, students will be able to
- describe the three major work centers in a kitchen and the six basic kitchen floor plans.
- discuss considerations in kitchen and dining area design.
- identify different kinds of tableware and list selection factors applicable to each.
- set a table attractively.
- wait on a table correctly.

Bulletin Boards

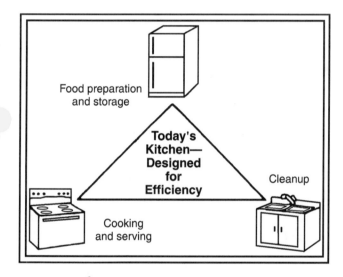

Food preparation and storage

Today's Kitchen— Designed for Efficiency

Cleanup

Cooking and serving

I. Title: "Today's Kitchen—Designed for Efficiency"

Draw a large triangle on the bulletin board and write the title inside it. Place drawings or photos of a refrigerator, a range, and a sink at the three corners of the triangle, as shown. Then label the points according to the area of the work triangle represented by the pictures—food preparation and storage, cooking and serving, and cleanup.

II. Title: "Get Set for Dining"

Place cutouts of table appointments on the bulletin board arranged as an overhead view of a table for two. Label the various types of table appointments—dinnerware, flatware, beverageware, holloware, table linens, and centerpiece.

Teaching Materials

Text, pages 125-143

Student Activity Guide
A. *Kitchen Floor Plans*
B. *Kitchen and Dining Area Design Crossword*
C. *Choosing Tableware*
D. *Setting the Table*
E. *Meal Service*

Teacher's Resource Binder
The Shape of Efficiency, transparency master 7-1
Low-Cost Decorating and Furnishing Ideas, reproducible master 7-2
Designing a Kitchen, reproducible master 7-3
Placing Tableware, transparency master with overlays 7-4A, 7-4B, 7-4C
Chapter 7 Study Sheet, reproducible master 7-5
Table Appointments, color transparency CT-7
Chapter 7 Test

Software, diskette for Part Two
The Matching Game, chapter review game

Introductory Activities

1. Ask students to brainstorm a list of activities that take place in the kitchen and dining area. Write their answers down one side of the chalkboard. Then go over the list one item at a time. Ask students to identify elements of kitchen and dining area design that are needed or desired for each of these activities.

2. Write the following types of meals on the chalkboard: a quick breakfast for one, a weekend brunch with the family, a quiet dinner shared by a couple, a pizza party for friends, and a holiday dinner shared by a large group of friends and relatives. Ask students to discuss how these various meals would differ in terms of the foods served and the space needed to store and prepare them. Also discuss where the foods would be eaten, the style of service, and the table appointments that would be set. Explain that in this chapter, students will learn how to

organize and design their kitchen space to make meal preparation and cleanup easier. Explain that they will also study how to design their dining area, select table appointments, set the table, and serve meals to create a variety of dining atmospheres.

Strategies to Reteach, Reinforce, Enrich, and Extend Text Concepts

Planning the Kitchen

3. **RF** Have students name the three basic kitchen work centers and describe the functions and requirements of each.

4. **RF** Have students describe the four optional work centers that may be found in a kitchen. Have them suggest where the activities of these centers might take place in homes that cannot accommodate these areas in the kitchen.

5. **EX** Have students divide a sheet of paper into three columns. Have them head the columns with the names of the three basic kitchen work centers. In the appropriate columns, have students list all the items located in each of the centers in their kitchens at home. Then have them circle any items on their lists that do not "belong" in the work centers in which they are placed. Have students use this sheet as the basis for a one-page summary report on how they might rearrange their kitchens at home to improve efficiency.

6. **ER** Have students measure the work triangle in their laboratory kitchens and evaluate the efficiency of the distance.

7. **ER** Have students measure the work triangles in their home kitchens and report their findings in class. Determine a class average and compare this figure with the ideal work triangle described in the text.

8. **RF** Prepare a cake from a packaged mix. Ask students to count the number of times you walk along each side of the work triangle. When you have finished, have students suggest ideas for simplifying your tasks and reducing the distance you walked.

9. **RT** *The Shape of Efficiency,* transparency master 7-1, TRB. Discuss the different kitchen floor plans with students, drawing in the work triangles for each on the transparency.

10. **RF** Have each student select a magazine picture of a kitchen and mount it on a sheet of paper. Have the student write a short paragraph describing, the arrangement of the cabinets and appliances in the picture. Collect the sheets and read the descriptions to the class. Ask students to identify the kitchen floor plans pictured based on the descriptions.

11. **RF** *Kitchen Floor Plans,* Activity A, SAG. Students are to complete exercises related to kitchen floor plans.

Planning the Dining Area

12. **RF** Have students find pictures of a variety of dining areas. Ask them to identify the type of each.

13. **RF** Have students list the advantages and disadvantages of kitchen eating areas, separate dining rooms, and attached dining areas.

14. **RF** Ask students to name areas in their homes that are used for eating aside from traditional dining areas and kitchen eating areas.

Kitchen and Dining Area Design

15. **RF** Have students visit a hardware store or home improvement center. Have them obtain brochures, catalogs, and samples of wall coverings, floor coverings, countertops, and cabinet materials that are suitable for kitchens and/or dining areas. Have them bring these items to class and use them in a discussion of the advantages and disadvantages of the various materials. (You may wish to obtain these items yourself and bring them to class for students to use.)

16. **ER** Have students make a kitchen and dining area design scrapbook that includes magazine photographs illustrating different uses of wall coverings, floor coverings, countertops, and cabinets.

17. **RF** Have students find pictures that illustrate the effects of good and poor lighting. Have them discuss their examples in class.

18. **ER** Have students locate the sources of ventilation in their kitchen laboratory. Ask them to evaluate the adequacy of these sources.

19. **ER** Have students check to see if the outlets in the classroom and in their home kitchens have neutral wires for grounding.

20. **ER** Have students check to see how many of the appliances in the foods lab have three-

pronged plugs. Ask them to explain the function of the third prong.

21. **EX** Have students develop a checklist of desirable characteristics for kitchen and dining area wall coverings, floor coverings, countertops, cabinets, lighting, ventilation, and electrical wiring. Have them use the checklist to determine how many of these positive design characteristics are found in the kitchens and dining areas at home.

22. **ER** Have students write a two-page paper describing what they would expect to find in kitchens or dining areas in the future. Submit two or three of the most creative papers to the school newspaper as part of an article about your study of kitchen and dining area design.

23. **ER** *Low-Cost Decorating and Furnishing Ideas,* reproducible master 7-2, TRB. Assign different students different tips from the handout. Have students investigate their assigned tips to find out what they might have to pay for various kitchen and dining area decorations and furnishings. Have students share their findings in class and give advantages and disadvantages of the options they investigated. Then discuss budgeting for the kitchen and dining area in a first apartment.

24. **EX** *Designing a Kitchen,* reproducible master 7-3, TRB. Have students use the graph paper and templates provided to design a kitchen for one of the households described. Then have them write a report describing decisions they made in planning their kitchens.

25. **RF** *Kitchen and Dining Area Design Crossword,* Activity B, SAG. Students are to complete statements about kitchen and dining area design and use the terms to fill in a crossword puzzle.

26. **ER** Guest speaker. Invite an interior designer to speak to your class about considerations in kitchen design.

Table Appointments

27. **RT** *Table Appointments,* color transparency CT-7, TRB. Use the transparency to introduce the different types of table appointments.

28. **RF** Have students list the different kinds of dinnerware materials and explain how each kind can be identified.

29. **RF** Have students list important points to consider when selecting dinnerware.

30. **RT** Display for students some of the less commonly used pieces of flatware, such as a soup/dessert spoon, salad fork, serrated fruit spoon, iced drink spoon, seafood fork, individual butter spreader, and demitasse spoon. (You may also wish to display serving pieces, such as a pierced serving spoon, cold meat fork, tablespoon, gravy ladle, dessert server, large serving spoon, sugar spoon, butter knife, and jelly spoon.) Explain to students when and how each item would be used.

31. **RF** Have students compare flatware made of sterling silver, silver plate, and stainless steel. Have them list the advantages and disadvantages of each material.

32. **EX** Have students compare the prices of several patterns of sterling silver, stainless steel, and silver-plated flatware. Have them use this comparison as the basis for a discussion of how the materials used and the intricacy of the designs influence the price.

33. **RT** Demonstrate for students the correct way to polish sterling silver and silver-plated flatware.

34. **RT** Display for students a variety of beverageware pieces, including on-the-rocks glasses, coolers, highballs, pilsners, juice glasses, shot glasses, champagne flutes, water goblets, brandy sifters, wine glasses, cordials, margaritas, and martini glasses. (You may wish to omit cocktail glasses from the display.) Explain the kinds of beverages and the kinds of meals for which each would be used.

35. **ER** Have students compare the cost and appearance of lead glass, lime glass, and plastic beverageware.

36. **RF** Have students list important points to consider when purchasing beverageware.

37. **RF** Show students place settings of the following types of tableware: china, stoneware, and plastic dinnerware; sterling silver, silver-plated, and stainless steel flatware; lead glass, lime glass, and plastic beverageware. Mix and match dinnerware, flatware, and beverageware pieces from the three different price levels. Give students the opportunity to identify how the styles of some pieces create a more unified table than others. Ask them to suggest occasions for which the different types of tableware might be most appropriate.

38. **RF** Have students use catalogs to make a list of as many holloware pieces as they can.

39. **ER** *Choosing Tableware,* Activity C, SAG. Students are to visit the tableware department of a department store. They are to select patterns of various types of tableware that they like. Then they are to record the pattern names, manufacturers, and pricing information on the worksheet and answer questions based on this information.

40. **RF** Divide the chalkboard into three columns headed "open stock," "place settings," and "by the set." Ask students to give advantages and disadvantages for each method of purchasing tableware. Write their responses on the chalkboard.

41. **RT** Show students examples of china sacks and protective separators. Demonstrate how to carefully pack china for storage.

42. **RT** Show students examples of flatware chests and tarnish-proof bags. Demonstrate how to carefully pack flatware for storage.

43. **EX** Have students find magazine pictures of different table linens. Have them note the table appointments used in each picture and comment on how they harmonize with the table linens.

44. **ER** Have students make two centerpieces using materials other than flowers.

45. **ER** Guest speaker. Invite a local florist to demonstrate how to arrange a floral centerpiece. If time allows, have fresh and dried flowers available for your students to practice what they have learned from the speaker. Ask the speaker to answer questions and assist students as they work.

46. **EX** Have students visit a party goods store and investigate the prices of disposable dinnerware, flatware, beverageware, table linens, and centerpieces. Have them use this information as they debate the topic, "Disposable tableware is the best option when having a party."

Meal Service

47. **ER** Have each student investigate when and where one of the styles of meal service developed. Have students share their findings in brief oral reports.

48. **EX** Give the class case examples of situations involving dinner guests. Be sure to specify the occasion, the menu, and the number of guests. Ask students what style of meal service they would use if they were hosting each event. Have them give reasons for their answers.

49. **ER** Working in small groups, have students use the table appointments available in lab to demonstrate Russian, English, and family service.

Setting the Table

50. **RT** *Placing Tableware,* transparency master with overlays 7-4A, 7-4B, 7-4C, TRB. Use master 7-4A to illustrate for students the placement of various pieces of tableware to fill a basic cover when setting the table. Explain that the menu items listed would all be served on the dinner plate and would be eaten with the basic set of utensils. Then use overlay 7-4B to illustrate the placement of additional pieces of dinnerware and beverageware that would be needed for the expanded menu shown. Explain to students what foods would be placed in or on the various pieces. Finally, add overlay 7-4C to illustrate the placement of additional pieces of flatware that would be used with the added pieces of dinnerware and beverageware.

51. **ER** Have each student write a menu for a meal of his or her choice. Collect the menus in a container. Have students take turns drawing a menu from the container, reading it to the class, and setting a lab table, using the appropriate table appointments for the menu he or she drew.

52. **RT** Demonstrate for students two ways a table could be set for a formal buffet.

53. **ER** *Setting the Table,* Activity D, SAG. Students are to draw an individual cover showing the correct placement of the dinnerware, flatware, beverageware, and linens needed by one person for each of the menus given.

Waiting on the Table

54. **EX** Have students role-play clearing and serving the table for a variety of courses according to menus you have written on the chalkboard.

55. **RF** *Meal Service,* Activity E, SAG. Students are to answer questions about styles of meal service and waiting on the table.

Chapter Review

56. **RT** *Chapter 7 Study Sheet,* reproducible master 7-5, TRB. Have students complete the statements as they read text pages 126-142.

57. **RF** *The Matching Game,* Software, diskette

for Part Two. Have students play the chapter review came according to the instructions that appear on the screen.

Above and Beyond

58. **EX** Have students plan a casual reception for faculty members. Have them plan a simple menu and choose dinnerware, flatware, beverageware, table linens, and a centerpiece that complement the food and the atmosphere being created. Have them choose what style of meal service they would like to use. Then have them set and wait on the tables accordingly.

Answer Key

Text

Review What You Have Read, page 143
1. food preparation and storage center, cooking and serving center, cleanup center
2. The U-shaped kitchen is the most desirable floor plan.
3. (Describe three. Student response. See pages 129-130 in the text.)
4. Floor coverings must be easy to clean. They must also provide walking comfort and be durable.
5. Lighting can be classified as natural or artificial. Natural light comes from the sun. Artificial light comes from electrical fixtures and candles.
6. Room size and the number and placement of windows and outside doors determine the amount of natural ventilation. The velocity and direction of the wind also affect ventilation.
7. china, stoneware, earthenware, pottery
8. tumblers and stemware
9. Tableware may be purchased open stock, in place settings, or by the set. Open stock pieces may be purchased individually. Place settings are sold in sets of all the pieces that would be used by one person. Items sold by the set include a number of the same piece or a number of place settings packages together.
10. tablecloths, place mats, table runners
11. American or family service is the style most often used in American homes.

12.

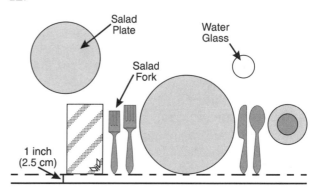

Student Activity Guide

Kitchen Floor Plans, Activity A, page 37
1. (The three points of the triangle should be labeled as:) food preparation and storage center, cooking and serving center, cleanup center
2. 21 feet (6.3 m)
3. mixing center, eating center, planning center, laundry center
4.

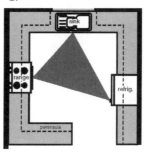

A. peninsula kitchen

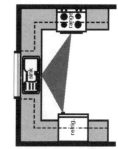

B. U-shaped kitchen

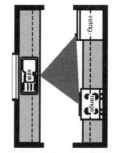

C. corridor kitchen

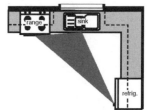

D. L-shaped kitchen

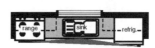

E. one-wall kitchen

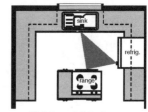

F. island kitchen

5. the U-shaped kitchen because of its compact work triangle

6. the peninsula kitchen
7. the corridor kitchen
8. the one wall kitchen (Give one disadvantage:) This floor plan generally does not give adequate storage or counter space; the work triangle is long and narrow.
9. the island kitchen
10. the L-shaped kitchen

Kitchen and Dining Area Design Crossword, Activity B, pages 38-39

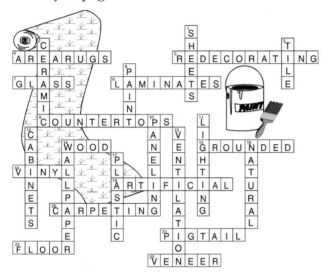

Setting the Table, Activity D, page 41

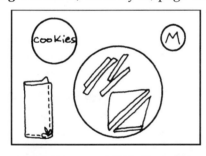

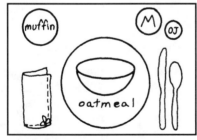

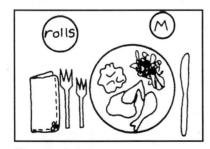

(Pie served when dinner is removed.)

Meal Service, Activity E, page 42

1. C	10. B
2. F	11. T
3. A	12. F
4. B	13. T
5. C	14. T
6. B	15. T
7. A	16. T
8. D	17. F
9. E	18. F

Teacher's Resources

Chapter 7 Test

1. D	14. F
2. G	15. F
3. C	16. T
4. E	17. C
5. A	18. D
6. B	19. D
7. T	20. D
8. F	21. D
9. T	22. C
10. F	23. B
11. T	24. B
12. F	25. A
13. T	26. D

27. The ideal work triangle is one that follows the normal flow of food preparation. Food is removed from the refrigerator or freezer and taken to the sink for cleaning. From the sink, it is taken to the range or oven for cooking. After cooking and eating, leftovers are returned to the refrigerator. The total distance from the range to the refrigerator to the sink should not exceed 21 feet (6.3 m).

28. Ventilation is needed in a kitchen to removed steam, heat, and cooking odors. Proper ventilation also helps maintain a comfortable dining atmosphere.

29. Circuit breakers may trip or fuses may blow frequently. Motor-driven appliances, such as mixers, may slow down during operation. Lights may dim when an appliance is being used. Appliances that heat, such as toasters, may take a long time to become hot.

30. durability, ease of laundering, colorfastness, and shrinkage

31. the occasion, the style of service, the size of the table, and the menu

Kitchen and Dining Areas

Name _____

Date _____ Period _____ Score _____

Chapter 7 Test

Matching: Match the following kitchen floor plans with their descriptions.

_____ 1. A kitchen floor plan in which all the appliances and cabinets are located along a single wall.

_____ 2. Floor plan in which all the appliances and cabinets are arranged in a continuous line along three adjoining walls.

_____ 3. Floor plan in which appliances and cabinets are arranged along two adjoining walls.

_____ 4. Floor plan in which a counter extending into the room can be used for storage or as an eating area.

_____ 5. Floor plan in which appliances and cabinets are arranged on two nonadjoining walls.

_____ 6. Floor plan in which a counter stands alone in the center of the room.

A. corridor kitchen
B. island kitchen
C. L-shaped kitchen
D. one-wall kitchen
E. peninsula kitchen
F. T-shaped kitchen
G. U-shaped kitchen

True/False: Circle *T* if the statement is true or *F* if the statement is false.

T   F   7. The likes, dislikes, and needs of all family members need to be considered when designing kitchen and dining areas.

T   F   8. The focal point of the food preparation and storage center is the range and oven.

T   F   9. The location of the dining area depends on the layout of the home, the size of the family, and the preferences of family members.

T   F   10. Ceramic tile is an inexpensive but durable kitchen wall covering and countertop material.

T   F   11. Kitchen and dining area lighting needs depend on the size of the room, the color of the walls, and the arrangement of furnishings and equipment.

T   F   12. Dinnerware includes plates, glasses, and silverware.

T   F   13. Stainless steel flatware does not tarnish, but foods like eggs, vinegar, and coffee can stain it.

T   F   14. The English style of meal service is the most formal style of service.

T   F   15. When setting the table, the dinner plate should be placed in the center of the cover flush with the table edge.

T   F   16. The order for serving a new course is the opposite of the order for removal of a course.

Multiple Choice: Choose the best response. Write the letter in the space provided.

_____ 17. In the cleanup center, a person would *not* find _____.
A. a dishwasher
B. a food waste disposer
C. a mixer
D. vegetables that do not need refrigeration

(Continued)

Name _____

_____ 18. Which of the following is an optional kitchen work center?
   A. Cleanup center.
   B. Cooking and serving center.
   C. Food preparation and storage center.
   D. Mixing center.

_____ 19. What type of dining area encourages the most gracious dining?
   A. Attached dining area.
   B. Kitchen eating area.
   C. Outdoor dining area on a patio or deck.
   D. Separate dining room.

_____ 20. Carpeting in kitchen and dining areas _____.
   A. provides good walking comfort and reduces noise
   B. is available in many patterns and colors
   C. is fairly expensive
   D. All of the above.

_____ 21. A moisture-resistant finish should be applied to cabinets made of _____.
   A. glass
   B. plastic laminates
   C. vinyl
   D. wood

_____ 22. Casual dinnerware that is lightweight, break-resistant, and colorful is made from _____.
   A. earthenware
   B. glass-ceramic
   C. plastic
   D. stoneware

_____ 23. Which of the following is *not* a stemware piece?
   A. Champagne glass.
   B. Cooler.
   C. Water goblet.
   D. Wine glass.

_____ 24. In which type of meal service do guests serve themselves from a table holding serving dishes and utensils, dinnerware, flatware, and napkins?
   A. Blue plate service.
   B. Buffet service.
   C. Compromise service.
   D. Family service.

_____ 25. If a salad will be eaten before the main course, the salad fork should be placed _____.
   A. to the left of the dinner fork
   B. to the right of the dinner fork
   C. on the salad plate
   D. to the right of the last spoon the on the right side of the plate

_____ 26. When serving a course, the last thing to be placed on the table is _____.
   A. flatware needed at each cover
   B. small items, such as cream and sugar, that will be needed
   C. dinnerware needed at each cover
   D. the food and/or beverage

(Continued)

Name _____

Essay Questions: Provide complete responses to the following questions or statements.

27. Describe the ideal work triangle.
28. Why is ventilation needed in kitchen and dining areas?
29. What are the warning signs of overloaded electrical circuits?
30. What four factors should be considered before purchasing table linens?
31. What four factors can help determine how a table should be set?

Choosing Appliances

Objectives

After studying this chapter, students will be able to
- list points to consider when choosing appliances.
- explain how to select, use, and care for major and portable kitchen appliances.

Bulletin Board

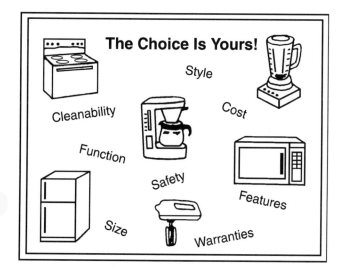

Title: "The Choice Is Yours!"

Draw or cut out pictures of a variety of major and portable appliances. Place the pictures randomly on the board interspersed with labels identifying some of the key factors used to make appliance purchase decisions, such as cost, size, style, features, etc.

Teaching Materials

Text, pages 145-169
Student Activity Guide
  A. *Major Appliance Shopper's Comparison*
  B. *Selecting Major Appliances*
  C. *Microwave Survey*
  D. *Portable Appliance Performance Comparison*
Teacher's Resource Binder
  Comparing Energy Efficiency, transparency master 8-1
  Microwave Generation, transparency master with overlay 8-2A, 8-2B
  How Microwaves Cook Food, transparency

master with overlay 8-3A, 8-3B
  Microwave Demonstration, reproducible master 8-4
  Portable Appliance Purchase Considerations Checklist, reproducible master 8-5
  Energy-Saving Tips for Kitchen Appliances, reproducible master 8-6
  Chapter 8 Study Sheet, reproducible master 8-7
  Induction Cooking, color transparency CT-8
  Chapter 8 Test
Software, diskette for Part Two
  Bingo, chapter review game

Introductory Activities

1. Have students define the term *appliance* in their words. Then have them compare their definitions with the definition given in the dictionary.
2. Ask students to complete the statement, "Appliance purchases should be considered carefully because . . ." Use their responses as the basis for a class discussion.

Strategies to Reteach, Reinforce, Enrich, and Extend Text Concepts

Safety and Service

3. **RF** Have students find the UL and AGA seals on various appliances in the lab. Have them explain what these seals indicate.
4. **EX** Obtain examples of full and limited warranties to distribute to students. Have them identify the differences between the two types of warranties.
5. **EX** Choose two teams of students to debate the topic, "Service Contracts are a Good Investment When Purchasing Major Appliances." Have students obtain copies of service contracts and warranties for various appliances to support their arguments.
6. **RT** *Comparing Energy Efficiency,* transparency master 8-1, TRB. Use the transparency to illustrate the various types of information

found on EnergyGuide labels. Ask students to suggest ways they could use this information.

7. **ER** Guest speaker. Invite an appliance repair technician to speak to your class about common appliance repair problems. Ask the speaker to emphasize ways students can avoid the need for repairs through proper use and care.

Major Kitchen Appliances

8. **RF** Have students list factors to consider when purchasing major appliances.

9. **ER** Have students contact a manufacturer of major kitchen appliances to find out what types of products are available to meet the needs of people with physical disabilities. Have students share their findings in class.

10. **ER** Obtain brochures and magazine ads on a variety of kitchen appliances. Have students use them to make a bulletin board display on current trends in appliances.

11. **ER** Have students visit appliance stores or appliance sales departments in department stores. Have them obtain brochures for a variety of major appliances. Have them compile their brochures into a major appliance product information file.

12. **EX** *Major Appliance Shopper's Comparison,* Activity A, SAG. Students are to visit an appliance dealer and compare two different, but comparable, models of a major appliance of their choice. Then they are to complete the worksheet and use it as the basis of an evaluation.

13 . **RF** *Selecting Major Appliances,* Activity B, SAG. Students are to illustrate the UL and AGA seals and then answer the questions about selecting major appliances.

Ranges

14. **RT** Demonstrate for students the use and care of a gas range and an electric range.

15. **RT** If your foods lab has a self-cleaning oven, discuss its operation with students.

16. **RF** Have students find pictures in magazines or catalogs that illustrate the various range styles.

Microwave Ovens

17. **RT** *Microwave Generation,* transparency master with overlay 8-2A, 8-2B, TRB. Use master 8-2A to illustrate how microwaves are

generated in a microwave oven by the magnetron tube. Then use overlay 8-2B to illustrate how microwaves are distributed throughout the oven cavity by the stirrer fan. Emphasize how the metal walls and floor of the oven reflect the microwaves so they can hit food from all angles.

18. **RT** *How Microwaves Cook Food,* transparency master with overlay 8-3A, 8-3B, TRB. Use master 8-3A to illustrate how microwaves penetrate food. Then use overlay 8-3B to illustrate how microwaves cause molecules within food to vibrate, thus creating heat through friction. Emphasize that it is this heat created within the food, rather than hot air surrounding the food, that cooks food in a microwave oven.

19. **RF** Have students find pictures in magazines or catalogs that illustrate the various styles of microwave ovens.

20. **ER** Divide the class into groups. Have each group investigate the functions of a different feature that can be purchased on some models of microwave ovens. Have the groups report their findings in class.

21. **ER** *Microwave Survey,* Activity C, SAG. Students are to use the questions provided to survey five people about their use of microwave ovens. Then students are to compile their results and write an article for your school paper.

22. **ER** *Microwave Demonstration,* reproducible master 8-4, TRB. Have students use the master to prepare a microwave cooking demonstration.

Convection Ovens and Induction Cooktops

23. **ER** Have students investigate the use of convection ovens in commercial bakeries and restaurants.

24. **RT** *Induction Cooking,* color transparency CT-8, TRB. Use the transparency to explain the principles of induction cooking.

25. **ER** Have students use a magnet to determine whether or not cookware pieces found in their lab kitchens could be used on an induction cooktop.

Refrigerators and Freezers

26. **ER** Have students determine the cubic footage of the refrigerator(s) in the foods lab. Have them divide this figure to determine the amount of cubic feet provided for each

student. Have them compare this figure with the amount of refrigerator storage space that should be provided for adult family members as given in the text.

27. **RF** Have students compare purchase and operation costs of manual defrost, automatic defrost, and frostless refrigerators.

28. **ER** Have a team of students demonstrate how to clean a refrigerator and refrigerator parts and accessories following guidelines given in the use and care manual.

29. **RF** Have students compare the advantages and disadvantages of chest and upright freezers.

Dishwashers

30. **ER** Have students investigate the differences in function and operation among various dishwasher cycles.

31. **RT** Demonstrate how to load a dishwasher properly. If your foods lab does not have a dishwasher, use dish drain racks to represent the racks in a dishwasher.

Food Waste Disposers and Trash Compactors

32. **RF** Have students list the advantages and disadvantages of continuous feed and batch feed food waste disposers.

33. **ER** Have students compare trash compactors with other means of trash disposal and summarize their findings in brief oral or written reports.

Portable Kitchen Appliances

34. **ER** Have each student make a portable appliance mobile. The mobile should include a picture or drawing of the appliance of each student's choice and tags labeled with purchase considerations for the appliance.

35. **ER** Have students prepare a simple food product to demonstrate the use and care of a appliance of his or her choice.

36. **EX** *Portable Appliance Performance Comparison*, Activity D, SAG. Students are to choose two portable appliances that perform the same basic tasks. They are to prepare the same simple food product with both appliances. Then they are to complete the chart and answer the questions to compare the two appliances.

37. **RF** Have students find portable appliance pictures and advertising copy in magazines or catalogs that illustrate current trends in portable appliances.

38. **EX** *Portable Appliance Purchase Considerations Checklist*, reproducible master 8-5, TRB. Have students complete the chart and answer the questions to evaluate how purchase considerations apply to portable appliances in the foods lab.

39. **EX** Have students prepare toast in the oven and using a toaster. Have them compare the appearance of the toast and the time and effort involved in preparation between the two methods.

40. **RF** Ask students to identify five mixing tasks for which a hand mixer would be suitable. Then have them identify five heavy-duty mixing tasks for which a standard mixer would be more appropriate.

41. **ER** Have students prepare milkshakes or fruit juice coolers in an electric blender.

42. **EX** Have students brew coffee using both an electric percolator and an automatic drip coffeemaker. Ask them to state which appliance they prefer and why.

43. **EX** Have students note the time and effort required to open a can using a manual can opener. Have them compare this with the time and effort required to open a can with an electric can opener.

44. **RT** Demonstrate for students the versatility of a food processor. Use the various cutting discs or blades to perform a variety of grinding, slicing, shredding, grating, kneading, and mixing tasks. Be sure to emphasize safety as you demonstrate.

45. **ER** Have each lab group prepare a dish that uses an electric skillet in a different way— frying, roasting, panbroiling, stewing, simmering, or baking.

46. **ER** Have one group of students make a loaf of yeast bread using traditional preparation methods. Have another group prepare a comparable recipe using an automatic bread machine. Ask students to compare the preparation experience as well as the taste and appearance of the bread.

47. **RT** *Energy-Saving Tips for Kitchen Appliances*, reproducible master 8-6, TRB. Discuss the economic and environmental advantages of conserving energy. Go over the tips listed on the handout with the students. Ask them which tips they are already employing in their homes. Encourage them to use the suggestions to make additional energy-saving adjustments.

Chapter Review

48. **RT** *Chapter 8 Study Sheet,* reproducible master 8-7, TRB. Have students complete the statements as they read text pages 146-168.
49. **RF** *Bingo,* Software, diskette for Part Two. Have students play the chapter review game according to the instructions that appear on the screen.

Above and Beyond

50. **ER** Arrange for your class to put on an appliance workshop for other students in the school. Divide the classroom into stations. Have students prepare displays, demonstrations, and presentations about current trends in appliances, styles and features, purchase considerations, safety and service, and use and care.

Answer Key

Text

Review What You Have Read, page 169

1. C
2. A full warranty states that a faulty product will be repaired or replaced free of charge. A limited warranty states conditions under which an appliance will be serviced, repaired, or replaced.
3. (List three:) more convenience features, space-saving models, energy conserving features, high-tech electronics, European styling
4. pilotless ignition
5. Self-cleaning ovens use very high temperatures to burn away oven spills. Continuous cleaning ovens have specially coated walls that allow food spills to oxidize over time during normal operation.
6. (List four:) temperature probe, child lock, automatic programming, automatic settings, turntables
7. A
8. single-door refrigerator, refrigerator-freezer, compact or portable refrigerator
9. false
10. continuous feed, batch feed
11. (List five. Student response. See page 162 in the text.)
12. true
13. false
14. false
15. true

Student Activity Guide

Selecting Major Appliances, Activity B, page 44

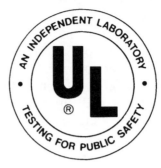 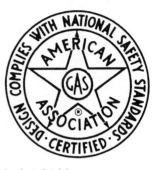

Seal: UL
Purpose: To indicate that an electrical appliance meets safety standards.

Seal: AGA blue star
Purpose: To indicate that a gas appliance meets safety, durability, and performance standards.

1.	T	5.	T	9.	F
2.	T	6.	T	10.	F
3.	F	7.	T	11.	T
4.	T	8.	F	12.	T

Teacher's Resources

Chapter 8 Test

1.	D	9.	F	17.	T
2.	B	10.	T	18.	F
3.	A	11.	F	19.	D
4.	F	12.	T	20.	C
5.	C	13.	T	21.	A
6.	I	14.	T	22.	D
7.	E	15.	F	23.	B
8.	G	16.	F		

24. EnergyGuide labels show an estimated yearly energy usage for major appliances. Consumers can use them to compare appliances of similar style and size. This will tell them which model is the most energy efficient and least costly to operate.
25. (Student response. See pages 151 and 153 of the text.)
26. (List three:) less energy is used; cooking times can be reduced by as much as 30 percent; many foods can be cooked at lower temperatures; foods cook more evenly; conventional utensils can be used
27. A thick layer of frost increases operating costs and can cause a refrigerator to break down because it must work so hard to remain cool.
28. (Student response. See page 161 of the text.)

Choosing Appliances

Name _____

Date _____ Period _____ Score _____

Chapter 8 Test

Matching: Match the following appliances with their descriptions.

_____ 1. May sharpen knives in addition to its primary function.

_____ 2. May be percolator or automatic drip type.

_____ 3. Can be used to prepare dough for pizza, rolls, and other yeast products.

_____ 4. Has a thermostat to control the temperature used for frying, roasting, panbroiling, stewing, and simmering.

_____ 5. Uses surgical steel blades to shred, chop, and puree foods.

_____ 6. Used to brown bread quickly on both sides.

_____ 7. Available in both standard and hand styles.

_____ 8. Can be used to knead dough, slice meats, grate cheese, and many other preparation jobs.

A. automatic bread machine
B. coffeemaker
C. electric blender
D. electric can opener
E. electric mixer
F. electric skillet
G. food processor
H. slow cooker
I. toaster

True/False: Circle *T* if the statement is true or *F* if the statement is false.

T F   9. Underwriters Laboratories is an organization that writes use and care booklets for appliances.

T F 10. An appliance owner might be charged for repairs on an appliance that is covered by a limited warranty.

T F 11. Purchasing major kitchen appliances is a long-term investment, so cost is not an important consideration.

T F 12. Modern appliances are designed to do more tasks in less space and with less energy than appliances of the past.

T F 13. In an electric range, the broiler is part of the oven; in a gas range, the broiler is often a separate unit.

T F 14. Microwave cooking can save up to 75 percent of the energy used by conventional ovens.

T F 15. Automatically defrosting refrigerators never have frost accumulation in the refrigerator or freezer.

T F 16. Food in a fully loaded freezer will remain frozen for up to a week during a power failure.

T F 17. Dishes washed in a dishwasher are more sanitary than dishes washed by hand.

T F 18. The water in the kitchen sink should not be running when a food waste disposer is in operation.

(Continued)

Name _____

Multiple Choice: Choose the best response. Write the letter in the space provided.

_____ 19. An insurance policy for major appliances that a consumer can buy from an appliance deal-
er is a(n) _____.
   A. EnergyGuide label
   B. full warranty
   C. limited warranty
   D. service contract

_____ 20. A range with unfinished sides that sits on a cabinet base is a _____.
   A. built-in range
   B. combination range
   C. drop-in range
   D. freestanding range

_____ 21. An induction cooktop cooks foods with _____.
   A. electromagnetic energy
   B. high pressure
   C. microwaves
   D. a stream of heated air

_____ 22. For efficient refrigerator operation _____.
   A. avoid unnecessarily opening the door
   B. defrost regularly
   C. clean the condenser
   D. All of the above.

_____ 23. When using a dishwasher _____.
   A. there is no need to scrape dishes before loading
   B. point knives, forks, and spoons down into the flatware basket
   C. a hand dishwashing detergent can be used if you run out of automatic dishwasher
      detergent
   D. remove dishes as soon as the dishwasher turns off

Essay Questions: Provide complete responses to the following questions or statements.

24. What are EnergyGuide labels and how can consumers use them?
25. Describe two special features that are available for microwave ovens.
26. List three advantages of convection cooking.
27. Why is it important to defrost a refrigerator regularly?
28. Describe three trends in portable appliances.

Kitchen Utensils

Objectives

After studying this chapter, students will be able to
■ identify various small kitchen utensils and discuss their functions.
■ explain how to select, use, and care for cooking and baking utensils.

Bulletin Board

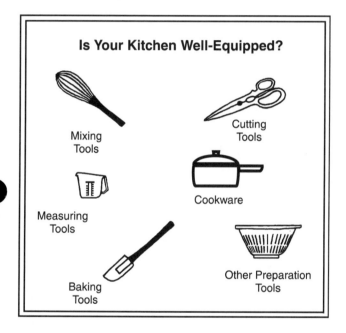

Title: "Is Your Kitchen Well-Equipped?"

   Draw or cut out pictures of a variety of pieces of small kitchen equipment, cookware, and bakeware. Arrange them on the bulletin board randomly with tags identifying some of the main concepts of the chapter.

Teaching Materials

Text, pages 171-184
Student Activity Guide
   A. *Small Equipment Identification*
   B. *Materials Comparison*
   C. *Microwave Cookware*
   D. *Equipment Review*
Teacher's Resource Binder
   Equipping Your Kitchen, reproducible master 9-1

   Utensils in Action, reproducible master 9-2
   Heat Conductivity of Cookware, reproducible master 9-3
   Chapter 9 Study Sheet, reproducible master 9-4
   Small Equipment Comparison, reproducible master 9-5
   Characteristics of Microwaves, color transparency CT-9
   Chapter 9 Test
Software, diskette for Part Two
   Tic Tac Toe, chapter review game

Introductory Activities

1. Demonstrate for students the functions of some less-common kitchen utensils, such as a lemon reamer, garlic press, cheese slicer, teaball mesh infuser, etc. As you demonstrate, mention to students that, although these items may be handy for special purposes, they are not essential to basic food preparation. Explain to them that this chapter will be focusing on basic kitchen utensils that are common in most kitchens.
2. Have students prepare a simple recipe, such as no-bake cookies, without using any hand-held utensils. Have them use their hands to "measure," mix, shape, and serve the food product they prepare. Discuss their experience in class. Ask them to explain how their preparation task might have been easier if they had been allowed to use utensils.
3. Guest speaker. Invite an antique specialist or museum curator to speak to your class about colonial kitchen utensils. If possible, have the speaker bring examples of some unique, special function utensils to show students.

Strategies to Reteach, Reinforce, Enrich, and Extend Text Concepts

Small Equipment

4. **EX** Have students visit the housewares section of a department store or a shop specializing in kitchen equipment. Have them make

a list of all the utensils available. Then have them evaluate each piece using the criteria given in the text.

5. **EX** Have students brainstorm lists of ingredients that they would measure with liquid measures, dry measures, and measuring spoons. Write their suggestions on the chalkboard. Discuss the differences among these three types of measuring tools.

6. **RF** Have students identify food products for which they would use wooden spoons, slotted spoons, and heavy metal spoons.

7. **RF** Ask students to describe the different uses of bent edge, straight edge, and rubber spatulas. Have them suggest food products that would require the use of each.

8. **RT** Discuss with students uses for the different sides of a grater.

9. **RF** Display for students the different types of knives that will be available in the lab. Ask them to identify the different types of cutting tasks for which they would use each of the knives.

10. **RF** Ask students to determine when they would use a strainer versus when they would use a colander.

11. **RF** *Small Equipment Identification*, Activity A, SAG. Students are to identify the name and type of each piece of small equipment pictured. They are also to describe the use of each piece and indicate whether it is located in their lab kitchens.

12. **RF** *Equipping Your Kitchen*, reproducible master 9-1, TRB. From the utensils pictured on the worksheet, have students select the ten they consider to be the most important and explain their choices.

13. **RF** *Utensils in Action*, reproducible master 9-2, TRB. Have students identify as many kitchen utensils as possible that would be needed to prepare this recipe. Have them describe how each of the utensils they listed would be used. Then have students share their answers in class. Write a list on the chalkboard of all the utensils students identified.

14. **ER** Guest speaker. Invite a cutlery or cookware sales representative to speak to your class and give a demonstration of the characteristics and functions of his or her products.

Cooking and Baking Utensils

15. **ER** Have students prepare a written report describing the materials used in the manufacture of cooking and baking utensils. Reports should include information on appearance, price range, durability, and the types of items made from each material.

16. **RT** *Characteristics of Microwaves*, color transparency CT-9, TRB. Use this transparency to illustrate the properties of microwaves in relation to various materials.

17. **RF** *Materials Comparison*, Activity B, SAG. Students are to complete a chart describing the advantages and disadvantages of the various cookware and bakeware materials listed. Then they are to answer the questions that follow.

18. **EX** *Heat Conductivity of Cookware*, reproducible master 9-3, TRB. Lightly grease and flour the bottoms of cookware pieces made from the various materials listed on the worksheet. Center each utensil over an electric element or a burner set for low heat. Heat the utensils just until the flour begins to brown. Do not move utensils around over the heat source while it is heating as this will reduce the clarity of any uneven conductivity. Have students look at the various utensils and sketch the heat pattern shown by the browned flour. Then have them evaluate what this indicates about the conductivity of each of the cookware materials.

19. **RF** *Microwave Cookware*, Activity C, SAG. Students are to explain why given statements about microwave cookware are false.

20. **EX** Have students prepare two recipes of a white sauce or pudding. Have them prepare one recipe in a saucepan and one recipe in a double boiler. Then have them compare the results of the two recipes and suggest food products for which it might be desirable to use a double boiler.

21. **RT** Prepare two recipes of a food product for students. Prepare one recipe in a regular saucepan and the other recipe in a pressure saucepan. Make students aware of the time savings involved in using the pressure saucepan. Demonstrate precautions they should take when using a pressure saucepan to ensure safe operation.

22. **ER** Have students prepare omelets using omelet pans.

23. **EX** Divide the glass into groups. Assign each group a recipe that requires the use of a different baking utensil. Allow students to sample each other's food products and eval-

uate the function and effectiveness of each piece of bakeware.

Chapter Review

24. **RF** Design a game similar to bingo called *Equip*. In the squares on each game card, write the names of various kitchen utensils. Be sure to choose a different set of items for each vertical row on the card and write them in random order in that row on each card. Then write five sets of questions identified by the letters *E, Q, U, I,* and *P* for which the items listed in the corresponding columns on the cards will be the answers. Randomly draw and read the questions, identifying the column to which each question relates. Have students state the answers and cover the appropriate squares if those answers appear on their cards. The first student covering five squares in a vertical, horizontal, or diagonal row wins.

25. **ER** Have each student in the class select a different piece of small equipment, cookware, or bakeware. Have each student give a one to two minute oral presentation to the class on the utensil he or she has selected. The presentation should include the name of the utensil, a description of its appearance, an explanation of how to use it, and a short list of food products it is used to prepare.

26. **RF** *Equipment Review,* Activity D, SAG. Students are to identify the various kitchen utensils being described using the clues given.

27. **RT** *Chapter 9 Study Sheet,* reproducible master 9-4, TRB. Have students complete the statements as they read text pages 172-183.

28. **RF** *Tic Tac Toe,* Software, diskette for Part Two. Have students play the chapter review game according to the instructions that appear on the screen.

Above and Beyond

29. **EX** *Small Equipment Comparison,* reproducible master 9-5, TRB. Have students complete the exercises described on the worksheet to help them evaluate the efficiency of various kitchen utensils. Have them present their findings in class and use this information as the basis for a class discussion.

30. **ER** Have students contact an appliance or utensil manufacturer to find out what recent produce innovations have been the result of input from family and consumer science professionals.

Answer Key

Text

Review What You Have Read, page 184
1. false
2. C
3. false
4. (List three:) snip herbs, trim vegetables, cut meat, cut dough, cut cookies, cut pizza, (poultry shears) cut through fowl and fish bones
5. B
6. colander
7. metal, ceramic, plastic
8. true
9. Saucepans generally have one handle. Pots have two handles.
10. B
11. true
12. (List three. Student response. See page 182 in the text.)

Student Activity Guide

Small Equipment Identification, Activity A, pages 47-49
1. measuring spoons; measuring tool
2. rubber spatula; baking tool
3. tongs; other preparation tool
4. vegetable peeler; cutting tool
5. straight edge spatula; baking tool
6. slotted spoon; mixing tool
7. liquid measures; measuring tool
8. whisk; mixing tool
9. French (chef's) knife; cutting tool
10. flour sifter; baking tool
11. rolling pin; baking tool
12. kitchen shears; cutting tool
13. grater; cutting tool
14. baster; other preparation tool
15. strainer; other preparation tool
16. pastry blender; baking tool
17. rotary beater; mixing tool
18. ladle; other preparation tool
19. dry measures; measuring tool
20. meat thermometer; thermometer (For descriptions of the use(s) of each piece of equipment, see pages 172-177 of the student text.)

Microwave Cookware, Activity C, page 51
1. Microwaves should be able to pass through microwave cookware to allow them to reach the food.

2. Microwaves can pass through materials such as ceramic, plastics, glass, wood, and paper. However, metal cookware reflects microwaves and prevents them from cooking food in a microwave oven.
3. Although metal cookware is generally not recommended for microwave use, some griddles and browning dishes with metal cooking surfaces are specially designed for microwave use.
4. Most people own conventional cookware pieces that can also be used for microwave cooking.
5. Disposable plastic containers from margarine and whipped toppings are not recommended for microwave cooking. They are made of soft plastics that may melt when they come in contact with hot food.
6. You should not use containers that absorb liquid, such as wooden bowls, when microwaving liquids. The moisture absorbed by such a container will attract microwave energy away from the food.
7. Although microwaves do not heat microwavable cookware, heat transferred from food can make cookware warm. Therefore, pot holders should be used when removing food containers from a microwave oven.
8. Round-shaped containers allow microwaves to hit food evenly.

Equipment Review, Activity D, page 52
1. whisk
2. stockinette
3. pastry brush
4. pastry blender
5. meat thermometer
6. grater
7. kitchen shears
8. rubber scraper
9. vegetable peeler
10. liquid measures
11. dry measures
12. measuring spoons
13. rotary beater
14. rolling pin
15. colander
16. French (chef's) knife
17. cutting board
18. strainer
19. sifter
20. double boiler
21. skillet
22. griddle
23. cookie sheet
24. muffin pan
25. baster

Teacher's Resources

Chapter 9 Test
1. F
2. B
3. C
4. E
5. G
6. K
7. A
8. I
9. J
10. D
11. T
12. F
13. T
14. F
15. T
16. T
17. F
18. F
19. F
20. F
21. A
22. C
23. D
24. D
25. C
26. liquid measures: 1 cup, 2 cups, 4 cups (250 mL, 500 mL, 1 L); dry measures: ¼ cup, ⅓ cup, ½ cup, 1 cup (50 mL, 125 mL, 250 mL); measuring spoons: ¼ teaspoon, ½ teaspoon, 1 teaspoon, 1 tablespoon (1 mL, 2 mL, 5 mL, 15 mL, 25 mL)
27. High-quality knives usually have hardwood handles. The handle should fit the hand comfortably. It also should be properly balanced and constructed for maximum safety. For safety, the tang should extend at least one-third of the way into the handle. The blade and handle should be joined with at least two rivets (three on larger knives).
28. (List two advantages for each:) stainless steel: resist stains, does not discolor, strong and durable; aluminum: lightweight, corrosion-resistant, conducts heat rapidly, reasonably priced
29. For maximum cooking efficiency, the bottoms of pots and pans should be about the same diameter as the surface unit.
30. A shiny or bright surface reflects part of the heat away from food. A dull or dark surface absorbs heat. Products baked in bright, shiny pans will have softer, lighter crusts. Products baked in dull, dark pans will have darker and crisper crusts.

Kitchen Utensils

Name _____

Date _____ Period _____ Score _____

Chapter 9 Test

Matching: Match the following utensils with their descriptions.

_____ 1. Used to beat, blend, and incorporate air into foods.

_____ 2. Used to drain fruits, vegetables, and pasta.

_____ 3. A small pan that fits into a larger pan.

_____ 4. Cooks food more quickly than conventional saucepans.

_____ 5. Used for making delicate desserts that are difficult to remove from the pan.

_____ 6. Preferred by chefs for preventing lumps from forming when preparing sauces.

_____ 7. Uses suction to collect juices from meat and poultry.

_____ 8. Used to separate liquid and solid foods.

_____ 9. Used for turning meats and handling corn on the cob.

_____ 10. Used to blend shortening with flour when making pie crust.

A. baster
B. colander
C. double boiler
D. pastry blender
E. pressure saucepan
F. rotary beater
G. springform pan
H. stockinette
I. strainer
J. tongs
K. whisk

True/False: Circle *T* if the statement is true or *F* if the statement is false.

T F 11. The construction of the handles should be considered when buying small equipment.

T F 12. Liquid measures may be made of glass or metal.

T F 13. A stockinette prevents dough from sticking to a rolling pin.

T F 14. A rubber spatula is a mixing tool.

T F 15. Using a vegetable peeler helps preserve nutrients.

T F 16. The tang of a knife should extend at least one-third of the way into the handle.

T F 17. Kitchen forks are used for eating salads and vegetables.

T F 18. Food and minerals may cause stainless steel to pit.

T F 19. Plastic utensils can be used in a microwave oven, in a conventional oven, or on the rangetop.

T F 20. An omelet pan is a skillet without sides.

(Continued)

Name _____

Multiple Choice: Choose the best response. Write the letter in the space provided.

_____ 21. Which of the following is used to stir thick mixtures?
A. Heavy metal spoon.
B. Slotted spoon.
C. Tablespoon.
D. Wooden spoon.

_____ 22. Which of the following is used to keep pastry from sticking to the counter while it is being rolled?
A. Pastry blender.
B. Pastry brush.
C. Pastry cloth.
D. Pastry peeler.

_____ 23. Which of the following knives is a good, all-around knife?
A. Chef or French knife.
B. Paring knife.
C. Slicing knife.
D. Utility knife.

_____ 24. A heat conducting core of copper or carbon steel sometimes is added to _____.
A. aluminum cookware
B. cast iron cookware
C. glass ceramic cookware
D. stainless steel cookware

_____ 25. Which of the following is a consideration when buying cooking utensils?
A. Pans should have rounded bottoms to keep foods from sticking.
B. Lids should fit loosely to allow steam to escape.
C. Utensils should be heavy enough to withstand warping.
D. All of the above.

Essay Questions: Provide complete responses to the following questions or statements.

26. List the available liquid and dry measures and measuring spoons in both conventional and metric sizes.
27. Describe a high-quality knife.
28. Stainless steel and aluminum are used in the manufacture of cookware.
29. What will maximize the cooking efficiency of pots and pans?
30. Why is it important to consider whether a baking utensil's surface is shiny or dull?

Planning Meals

Objectives

After studying this chapter, students will be able to
- plan nutritious menus using the Food Guide Pyramid and basic meal patterns.
- prepare a family food budget.
- plan menus with an appealing variety of flavors, colors, textures, shapes, sizes, and temperatures.
- discuss resources a meal manager can use as alternatives to time and energy.

Bulletin Board

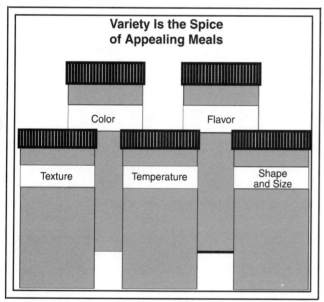

Title: "Variety Is the Spice of Appealing Meals"

Place cutouts of spice bottles in a spice rack on the bulletin board. Label each one of the spice bottles with one of the elements of satisfying meals—color, flavor, texture, temperature, and size and shape.

Teaching Materials

Text, pages 185-199
Student Activity Guide
    A. *Planning for Nutrition*
    B. *Planned Spending*
    C. *Planning Satisfying Menus*
    D. *Convenience Comparison*

Teacher's Resource Binder
    The Goals of Meal Management, transparency master 10-1
    Market Basket Comparison, reproducible master 10-2
    Planning a Food Budget, reproducible master 10-3
    Stretching Your Food Dollar, reproducible master 10-4
    Nongrocery Food Purchases, reproducible master 10-5
    Writing Menus, reproducible master 10-6
    Meal Management Tools, transparency master 10-7
    Microwaves Meet Meal Planning Goals, reproducible master, 10-8
    Chapter 10 Study Sheet, reproducible master 10-9
    Planning Meals for One, reproducible master 10-10
    Tasting Flavors, color transparency CT-10
    Chapter 10 Test
Software, diskette for Part Two
    The Matching Game, chapter review game

Introductory Activities

1. Ask students to complete the statement, "A meal manager's goal is to plan meals that ..."
2. *The Goals of Meal Management,* transparency master 10-1, TRB. Use the transparency to introduce students to the four goals of meal management. Briefly discuss with students how a meal manager will be able to determine when he or she has met these goals.

Strategies to Reteach, Reinforce, Enrich, and Extend Text Concepts

Provide Good Nutrition

3. **RF** Have students review the Food Guide Pyramid by making a chart that lists the amounts from each food group needed each day by each member in their family.
4. **EX** Have students use the basic meal patterns shown in chart 10-1 on page 186 of the

text to write three sample breakfast, lunch, and dinner menus. Have them plan the menus to meet the nutritional needs of a teenager. Then ask them to explain how they could modify the menus to meet the needs of an adult.

5. **EX** Have students analyze the nutritional value of one of the breakfast, one of the lunch, and one of the dinner menus written in strategy 4. Have them determine how close they have come to the guideline of breakfast supplying one-fourth of the day's total nutrient needs and lunch and dinner each supplying one-third. Then have them determine what nutrient needs remain to be supplied by snacks.

6. **RF** Have students write three nontraditional breakfast menus.

7. **EX** Take a poll to see how many students regularly eat breakfast. Ask those who do not eat breakfast why they skip this important meal. Then have students brainstorm solutions to the problems given by the noneaters.

8. **ER** Have students use cookbooks and their imaginations to come up with three lunch dishes that creatively use leftovers.

9. **EX** Divide the class into four groups. Assign each group the task of adding variety to a dinner menu in one of the following ways: find a new way of serving a typical set of menu items; plan a meal around an international theme; plan a cool, light, and nutritious menu for a hot summer evening; vary the preparation methods typically used for a set of dinner foods.

10. **EX** Have students plan and prepare a nutritious snack that would appeal to each of the following: a preschool child, a teenager, and an elderly person.

11. **RF** *Planning for Nutrition,* Activity A, SAG. Students are to use the terms listed to complete statements about planning nutritious meals.

Use Planned Spending

12. **RT** Discuss with students factors that would cause food budgets to differ from family to family.

13. **EX** Have students suggest foods that would meet the needs of each of the following people: an infant girl, a teenage boy on the swim team, a 110 pound (49 kg) woman, a 250 pound (112 kg) man, and an 80-year-old grandmother. Then have them analyze the costs of these various foods and explain how the weight, sex, age, and activity level of family members can affect a family's food needs.

14. **RT** Discuss with the class the six factors that affect the amount of money a meal manager spends for food.

15. **ER** *Market Basket Comparison,* reproducible master 10-2, TRB. Have students visit a grocery store and record the prices of all the items listed. Then have them answer the questions to compare the cost and nutritional value of the two similar sets of food products.

16. **EX** Have students use the USDA's family food plans and food budget figures for various economic levels to plan moderate cost menus for a family of four (a man, a woman, a 12-year-old boy, and a six-year-old girl) for three days.

17. **EX** Have students repeat strategy 16 using the low-cost plan. Have them identify the major differences between the moderate cost plan and the low-cost plan.

18. **EX** *Planning a Food Budget,* reproducible master 10-3, TRB. Have students use the information given to write a monthly budget and plan a weekly food budget.

19. **RF** Have students list five ways that a meal manager can save money at the grocery store without sacrificing good nutrition.

20. **RT** *Stretching Your Food Dollar,* reproducible master 10-4, TRB. In class, go over the tips listed on the handout. Ask students which of the listed suggestions they follow when they shop.

21. **RF** Have students compare the cost of a list of foods with built-in convenience with their less convenient counterparts. (Examples might include presliced or shredded cheese and bulk cheese, instant rice and long grain rice, and ready-made orange juice and frozen juice concentrate.)

22. **RF** *Nongrocery Food Purchases,* reproducible master 10-5, TRB. Students are to complete a chart listing all foods purchased for one week from restaurants, vending machines, concession stands, and other locations besides grocery stores. They are also to list the place of purchase and the cost of each item.

23. **EX** Have students brainstorm a list of nonfood items that may be included in the food budget. Ask them to estimate what percent-

age of a weekly grocery bill would be spent on these items.

24. **RF** *Planned Spending,* Activity B, SAG. Students are to indicate whether each statement about planned spending is true or false.

Prepare Satisfying Meals

25. **RF** Have each student make a list of his or her 10 favorite foods and a list of his or her 10 least favorite foods. Have students compare lists with their classmates. Write on the chalkboard a list of 10 foods that a majority of people like most and 10 foods that a majority of people like least.

26. **RT** *Tasting Flavors,* color transparency, CT-10, TRB. Use the transparency to describe to students how humans experience the sense of taste.

27. **RF** Have students name the four basic tastes and give examples of each.

28. **ER** Allow students to observe the role aroma plays in the flavors of foods. Blindfold students and have them hold their noses while sampling some familiar foods. See if they can identify the foods. Have them describe how the tastes of these foods differ from their usual flavors.

29. **RF** Have students name five flavor combinations that are compatible and five flavor combinations that are not compatible.

30. **ER** Have students use pictures cut from magazines to make posters illustrating good and poor uses of color, texture, shape, flavor, and temperature in meal planning.

31. **RT** Demonstrate for students how to make a variety of interesting and attractive garnishes.

32. **EX** *Planning Satisfying Menus,* Activity C, SAG. Students are to create an illustration of a satisfying meal. Then they are to evaluate it in terms of the variety of flavors, colors, textures, shapes, sizes, and temperatures it includes.

33. **RF** Have students plan a dinner menu following the steps given on page 195 of the text.

34. **ER** *Writing Menus,* reproducible master 10-6, TRB. Have students complete the menu writing exercises on the worksheet after studying the guidelines and examples given.

Control the Use of Time

35. **RT** *Meal Management Tools,* transparency master 10-7, TRB. Use this master to introduce students to the various resources meal managers have available. Discuss with students how the use of these resources must be planned and controlled. Also discuss how resources can be exchanged to help meal managers meet their goals of planning and preparing nutritious, appealing meals.

36. **RF** Have students list the factors that determine the amount of time needed for planning and preparing a meal.

37. **RF** As a class, discuss how the following resources can save time and/or energy: eating out, money, knowledge, skills, and time.

38. **RF** *Microwaves Meet Meal Planning Goals,* reproducible master 10-8, TRB. Prepare the recipe on the student handout. As you demonstrate, emphasize how microwave cooking aids nutrient retention through short cooking time and use of little or no cooking liquid. Allow students to sample how tasty and attractive microwaved foods can be. Allow them to observe the ease and speed of preparation. Emphasize the ease in cleanup due to the lack of pots and pans. Prepare a few extra vegetables and store them in a single-serving container to help illustrate the goal of staying within a budget by using leftovers. Have students answer the questions on the handout as they watch the demonstration.

39. **ER** Guest speaker. Invite someone who works as a cook or a professional shopper to speak to your class about how his or her services can save meal managers time and energy. Ask the speaker to give students a salary range for these types of services. Later, when evaluating the information presented by the speaker, ask students to compare this time-saving option with other options. Ask them when they feel the option of hiring additional help would be worthwhile.

40. **EX** Have students brainstorm a list of convenience food products. Write the list on the chalkboard. Then have students identify which of the products they named are finished foods and which are semiprepared foods.

41. **EX** Divide the class into two teams. Have them debate the topic, "Convenience Foods Are Time-Saving Products a Meal Manager Cannot Afford to Do Without."

42. **ER** Have students choose two different food products. Then have them visit a grocery store and find all the different forms of these products. Ask them to list the ingredients each contains, the amount of preparation required, and the cost. (Spaghetti with

meat sauce is an example of a food product with many forms. You could buy the pasta, ground beef, tomatoes, and seasonings needed for spaghetti with meat sauce made from scratch. You also could buy a boxed spaghetti dinner, canned spaghetti with meat sauce, or frozen spaghetti with meat sauce.)

43. **EX** *Convenience Comparison*, Activity D, SAG. Students are to choose a food product that is available in both semiprepared and finished forms. They are to prepare these convenience foods and their scratch counterpart. Then they are to complete a chart with information about product costs and preparation times and answer the evaluation questions that follow.

44. **RF** Have students list and discuss a variety of techniques for simplifying work in the kitchen.

Chapter Review

45. **RT** *Chapter 10 Study Sheet*, reproducible master 10-9, TRB. Have students complete the statements as they read text pages 186-198.

46. **RF** *The Matching Game*, Software, diskette for Part Two. Have students play the chapter review came according to the instructions that appear on the screen.

Above and Beyond

47. **EX** Have students develop three work simplification techniques. These techniques should demonstrate the simplification of time and energy by *(a)* developing a skill *(b)* changing a method *(c)* changing storage or placement of tools and equipment. Have students practice using these techniques in the preparation of food products in their homes. Then have them write a report describing how they used the techniques. The report should also include an evaluation of the effectiveness of the techniques. Students may choose to give an oral presentation instead of writing a report. They should prepare visual aids and give a demonstration of the techniques they developed if they choose this option.

48. **ER** *Planning Meals for One*, reproducible master 10-10, TRB. Have students read the information on the hand-out. Then have them visit a supermarket and identify 15 products in single-serving packages. Discuss their findings in terms of how manufacturers are responding to the greater number of single-person households.

Answer Key

Text

Review What You Have Read, page 199

1. Provide good nutrition to meet the needs of each family member.
   Use planned spending to make meals fit into the family food budget.
   Prepare satisfying meals that look and taste appealing.
   Control the use of time and energy involved in meal preparation.
2. Breakfast generally supplies one fourth of the day's total needs. Lunch and dinner each supply one third, and snacks supply the remaining needs.
3. false
4. (List four:) family income, meal manager's ability to choose foods that are within the food budget, meal manager's shopping skills and knowledge of the marketplace, amount of time the meal manager has to plan and prepare meals, food preferences of family members, family values
5. (Student response. See page 190 in the text.)
6. D
7. flavor, color, texture, shape, size, temperature (Examples are student response.)
8. (List four:) eating out, money, knowledge, skills, time
9. finished foods
10. Minimize hand and body motions. Organize work space and tools. Change the product or the method used to prepare the product.

Student Activity Guide

Planning for Nutrition, Activity A, page 53

1. meal patterns
2. Food Guide Pyramid
3. breakfast
4. vitamin C
5. lunch
6. dinner
7. protein
8. one-dish meals
9. snacks
10. calories (kilojoules)
11. appetizer
12. meal managers
13. nutrients
14. preparation methods
15. leftovers

Planned Spending, Activity B, page 54

1. F	11. T
2. T	12. F
3. F	13. F
4. F	14. T
5. T	15. T
6. T	16. T
7. F	17. F
8. F	18. T
9. T	19. T
10. T	20. T

Teacher's Resources

Chapter 10 Test

1. H	15. T
2. I	16. F
3. C	17. F
4. A	18. T
5. B	19. F
6. G	20. T
7. D	21. D
8. F	22. B
9. K	23. A
10. E	24. B
11. T	25. D
12. F	26. D
13. F	27. A
14. F	28. A

29. The Food Guide Pyramid helps a meal manager determine the number of servings each family member needs from each food group. It also provides information about how to select food within each group.
30. On a piece of paper, record your average monthly income. List your monthly fixed expenses and the cost of each. List your flexible expenses and their estimated monthly costs. Figure the total of your fixed and estimated flexible expenses. Compare this amount with your income and determine whether you need to make adjustments.
31. (Student response. See pages 190-192 in the text.)
32. (Student response should suggest texture and color improvements. Too many of the foods are crisp and brown or light in color.)
33. (Student response. See Chart 10-11 on page 197 in the text.)

Planning Meals

Name _____

Date _____ Period _____ Score _____

Chapter 10 Test

Matching: Match the following terms and identifying phrases.

_____ 1. Someone who uses resources to reach goals related to preparing and serving food.

_____ 2. A tool used for meal planning that is based on the kinds of foods usually served at a meal.

_____ 3. A food product that is ready for eating either immediately or after heating or thawing.

_____ 4. A plan for managing income and expenses.

_____ 5. A food product that has had some amount of service added to it.

_____ 6. Money received.

_____ 7. A regularly recurring cost in a set amount.

_____ 8. Attractive and complementary foodstuffs added to decorate a food or serving dish.

_____ 9. Act of performing tasks in the simplest way possible to conserve both time and energy.

_____ 10. A regularly recurring cost that varies in amount.

A. budget
B. convenience food
C. finished food
D. fixed expense
E. flexible expense
F. garnish
G. income
H. meal manager
I. meal pattern
J. semiprepared food
K. work simplification

True/False: Circle *T* if the statement is true or *F* if the statement is false.

T   F   11. All people need the same nutrients, but not necessarily in the same amounts.

T   F   12. Breakfast should supply one-third of the day's total nutrient needs.

T   F   13. High-income families usually spend a larger percentage of their income for food than low-income families.

T   F   14. Fixed expenses include food, clothing, and transportation.

T   F   15. Sight, smell, and touch as well as taste can affect food preferences.

T   F   16. The four basic tastes recognized by human beings are sweet, sour, salty, and spicy.

T   F   17. In most cases, menus are planned around the appetizer since it is served first.

T   F   18. Meal managers can use time to save time.

T   F   19. The majority of convenience foods cost less than their homemade counterparts.

T   F   20. Performing a task repeatedly can eventually result in reduced preparation time.

Multiple Choice: Choose the best response. Write the letter in the space provided.

_____ 21. Which of the following is *not* included in the basic meal pattern for breakfast?
   A. Bread.
   B. Main dish.
   C. Milk or other beverage.
   D. Occasional dessert.

(Continued)

Name _____

_____ 22. On the average, how much of their income do families in the United States spend for food?
  A. 15 percent.
  B. 20 percent.
  C. 35 percent.
  D. 50 percent.

_____ 23. Which of the following foods do *not* tend to have an increase in use when income increases?
  A. Beans and rice.
  B. Better cuts of meat.
  C. Convenience products.
  D. Milk and milk products.

_____ 24. Which of the following expenses is *not* considered a fixed expense?
  A. Car payment.
  B. Electric bill.
  C. Insurance premium.
  D. Mortgage payment.

_____ 25. The most costly group of foods is _____.
  A. breads and cereals
  B. dairy products
  C. fruits and vegetables
  D. protein foods

_____ 26. A meal consisting of chicken a la king over mashed potatoes, spinach soufflé, molded salad, and chocolate pudding is monotonous because _____.
  A. color is repeated
  B. flavor is repeated
  C. shape is repeated
  D. texture is repeated

_____ 27. Which of the following foods is a finished food?
  A. Brown-and-serve rolls.
  B. Chocolate cake mix.
  C. Instant pudding.
  D. Instant rice.

_____ 28. Serving boiled potatoes rather than mashed potatoes is an example of _____.
  A. changing the methods used to prepare the food product
  B. minimizing hand and body motions
  C. organizing work space and tools
  D. None of the above.

Essay Questions: Provide complete responses to the following questions or statements.

29. How can the Food Guide Pyramid help a meal manager plan nutritious meals?
30. Explain how to prepare a budget.
31. Give three suggestions for reducing food expenses.
32. Explain how you would improve the following meal: crispy fried chicken, French fries, raw vegetable relishes, bread sticks, vanilla ice cream, and sugar cookies.
33. What are two advantages and two disadvantages of using convenience foods?

The Smart Consumer

Objectives

After studying this chapter, students will be able to
- make wise decisions in the marketplace.
- organize a shopping list and comparison shop.
- explain how labeling, unit pricing, and generic products affect them as consumers.

Bulletin Boards

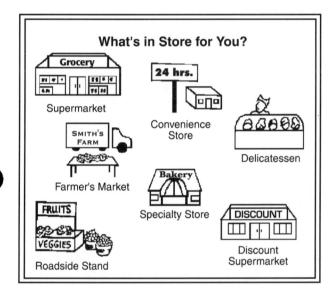

I. Title: "What's in Store for You?"

Make cutouts of the different types of stores discussed in the chapter—supermarkets, discount supermarkets, farmers' markets, twenty-four hour convenience stores, specialty stores, delicatessens, and roadside stands. Arrange the cutouts on the bulletin board. Beneath each cutout, place a list identifying the features offered by that particular type of store.

II. Title: "Smart Consumers Have More Than Food in Their Shopping Carts"

Draw a large outline of a shopping cart on the bulletin board. Fill the cart with cutouts of packages of various shapes and colors. Label the packages with consumer concepts from the chapter—food labeling, open dating, unit pricing, generic products, and UPC.

Teaching Materials

Text, pages 201-214
Student Activity Guide
    A. *Types of Stores*
    B. *Shopping for Food*
    C. *Using Food Advertisements*
    D. *Reading a Nutrition Label*
    E. *Help for Consumers*
Teacher's Resource Binder
    Chapter 11 Study Sheet, reproducible master 11-1
    Packaging and the Environment, reproducible master 11-2
    Nutrition News, color transparency CT-11
    Chapter 11 Test
Software, diskette for Part Two
    Reverse Thinking, chapter review game

Introductory Activities

1. Take a poll of your students to find out how many of them do at least occasional grocery shopping for their families. Ask them at which stores they prefer to shop. Find out when they are most likely to do their shopping. Ask them if they use coupons and shopping lists. Find out if they tend to be brand loyal or if they do comparison shopping. Tally their responses on the chalkboard. Explain to students that this chapter will focus on consumer tips that will help them get the most from their food dollars.

2. Go around the room giving each student a term or concept that they will study in this chapter, such as house brand, specialty store, and impulse buying. Ask each student to tell you the first thing that pops into his or her mind. Tape record this exercise for use with strategy 35.

Strategies to Reteach, Reinforce, Enrich, and Extend Text Concepts

Where and When to Shop

3. **RF** *Types of Stores*, Activity A, SAG. Students are to complete the chart by describing the

different types of food stores and listing the advantages and disadvantages of each.

4. **EX** Have students evaluate two food stores in your area by using the criteria given on page 202 of the text.

5. **ER** Have students investigate when local stores run their advertised specials and report their findings in class.

6. **ER** Guest speaker. Invite a local grocer to speak to your class about food product pricing, in-store marketing techniques, and advertised food specials.

What to Buy

7. **ER** Have students check the advertised food specials in a local newspaper. Ask them to go to the store at which the specials are valid and compare the nonsale prices with the special prices. Have them give brief oral reports in class evaluating the actual savings the use of sale items provides.

8. **ER** Have students set up a coupon exchange that students and faculty members throughout the school can use. Have them encourage people using the exchange to bring in coupons for products that they do not use and trade them for coupons for products they do use. Have students organize the coupons into categories and file them by expiration date. Have them periodically go through the file and throw away any coupons that are outdated.

9. **RF** Have students list guidelines for making a shopping list.

10. **EX** Have students compare the cost of national brand products purchased with coupons with the costs of similar house brand and generic products. Ask them to identify when the use of coupons is worthwhile.

11. **EX** Ask students to plan a dinner menu that includes a meat entree and a dinner menu that includes a meatless entree. Have them compare the costs of preparing the two menus.

12. **RF** Ask students to list marketing techniques grocery stores use to encourage impulse buying.

13. **ER** Have students prepare a brochure called "Shopping Tips That Can Save You Money" to distribute to parents, faculty members, and other students.

14. **ER** Have students choose 10 foods and list the forms in which each food is available.

Have them research the cost of each form and identify which form is usually the least expensive.

15. **EX** Have students plan menus for one day and determine the total cost of those menus. Then have them determine the cost for each person in a four-person family for each meal.

16. **RF** *Using Food Advertisements*, Activity C, SAG. Students are to use the food advertisements from a local store to make a shopping list organized according to areas of the store. Then they are to use these lists to plan menus for one day.

Organic Foods and Food Additives

17. **ER** Have students choose five foods that are available in both health food stores and supermarkets. Have them compare costs and report their findings to the class.

18. **RF** Have students list the four basic purposes of food additives. Then have them name an additive from each category and identify two foods in which each additive is found.

19. **RF** *Shopping For Food*, Activity B, SAG. Students are to complete the statements about shopping for food and then arrange circled letters to spell a term related to shopping for food.

Food Labeling

20. **RT** Nutrition News, color transparency CT-11, TRB. Use the transparency to illustrate for students the different types of information included on a nutrition label.

21. **EX** Have students compare nutrition information labels on regular food products with nutrition information labels on products labeled as dietetic, low cholesterol, or low sodium.

22. **RF** *Reading a Nutrition Label*, Activity D, SAG. Students are to answer questions about a given nutrition label.

23. **RF** Have students read three food product labels and look for the required information. Ask them to identify any additional information supplied by the manufacturer or food processor.

24. **ER** Have students read the ingredient list on a can of fruit cocktail. Then have them separate and weigh each type of fruit in the can to verify that the fruits are listed in the correct order on the label.

25. **ER** Have students make an educational poster illustrating the UPC lines, bars, and numbers found on a typical food package. Have them identify what the various parts of the code indicate.
26. **ER** Have students prepare a display using packaging from dated food products. The display should include at least one product representing each type of open dating discussed in the text.

Unit Pricing

27. **ER** Have students find examples of unit pricing in a grocery store. Have them use the unit prices to compare different brands and/or forms of the same product and report their findings to the class.
28. **RF** Have students choose 10 different ready-to-eat breakfast cereals. Have them use unit pricing to list the cereals in order from least expensive to most expensive.

Generic Products

29. **ER** Have students choose five food and two nonfood products. Have them compare the cost of the national brand, house brand, and generic brand of equivalent-sized packages of each product.
30. **EX** Have students compare the appearance, texture, and flavor of a generic, house, and national brand food product such as canned, sliced peaches.
31. **EX** Have students brainstorm a list of food items that are not available in generic packaging. Ask them to analyze why these items might not be available.

Sources of Consumer Information

32. **ER** Have each student identify a consumer issue about which he or she would like information. Have each student write to one of the sources of consumer information listed in the chapter (or some other appropriate source) to obtain the information in which he or she is interested.
33. **ER** Have students read two articles from recent issues of *Consumer Reports* and write a short report highlighting what they have read.
34. **RF** *Help for Consumers*, Activity E, SAG. Students are to complete exercises related to resources consumers can use to help them get the most value from their food dollars.

Chapter Review

35. **ER** Play the audiotape made in strategy 2. Stop the tape after the student response to each term or concept. Ask students to agree with, expand on, or correct the taped responses they gave before studying the chapter.
36. **ER** Field trip. Arrange with a local grocer to take your class to his or her store during an off-peak time. Talk to students about store layout. Show them examples of unit pricing. Have them observe UPC checkout. Allow students to examine generic products, house brand products, and national brand products. Show them examples of open dating and nutritional labeling. (This trip may facilitate the completion of several other learning experiences for this chapter.)
37. **RT** *Chapter 11 Study Sheet,* reproducible master 11-1, TRB. Have students complete the statements as they read text pages 202-213.
38. **RF** *Reverse Thinking,* Software, diskette for Part Two. Have students play the chapter review game according to the instructions that appear on the screen.

Above and Beyond

39. **EX** Have students ask a family member or friend to shop for groceries right after a meal and again right before a meal. Ask them to have the person save both shopping lists and lists of items actually purchased. Have students record the shopper's reactions to both shopping trips and compare the shopping lists with the lists of items actually purchased. Have them analyze the affect hunger has on purchase decisions and summarize their analysis in a written report. To reduce bias in the results, students should not inform shoppers of the reason for this study until after the study is completed.
40. **ER** *Packaging and the Environment*, reproducible master 11-2, TRB. Have students read the article on the handout. Then have them investigate some of the new uses being developed for recycled materials. Have them compile what they learn into a pamphlet that they can distribute throughout the school or community to encourage more people to recycle.

Answer Key

Text

Review What You Have Read, page 214

1. true
2. A shopping list helps a meal manager save time, avoid extra trips for forgotten items, and stick to the food budget.
3. Yes, two cans of green beans purchased at the regular price would cost $1.38. The sale price saves the consumer nine cents.
4. (List four. Student response. See pages 204 and 206 in the text.)
5. add nutrients, preserve quality, aid processing or preparation, enhance flavors or colors
6. Percent Daily Values listed on food labels are based on a 2,000 calorie diet. People who have higher or lower calorie needs will have higher or lower Daily Values, respectively.
7. true
8. (Student response. See pages 209-210 in the text.)
9. D
10. unit pricing
11. less money is spent on packaging and advertising, product may be of lower quality
12. (Name four:) Consumers Union, Consumers' Research Inc., Underwriters Laboratories, Better Business Bureaus, United States Department of Agriculture, Food and Drug Administration, Office of Consumer Affairs, Federal Trade Commission, magazines, newspapers, trade journals, family and consumer science professionals

Student Activity Guide

Shopping for Food, Activity B, page 58

1. additives
2. colors
3. convenience
4. coupons
5. delicatessen
6. discount
7. farmers'
8. house brand
9. impulse buying
10. national brand
11. nutrients
12. organic
13. organically processed
14. processing
15. roadside stand
16. shopping list
17. specialty
18. supermarkets

Circled letters: a, o, i, o, c, i, r, h, s, n, n, g, p, o, s, p, p, m

Comparison shopping involves evaluating different brands, sizes, and forms of a product before making a purchase decision.

Reading a Nutrition Label, Activity D, page 60

1. ½ cup (228 g)
2. 230 calories
3. 2 g
4. 10 percent
5. milligrams (mg)
6. 2,400 mg
7. 172 calories
8. 15 g
9. 10 g
10. 3 percent
11. calcium—it provides 35 percent of the Daily Value for calcium and only 1 percent of the Daily Value for iron
12. 7 servings
13. 30 g
14. 9 calories
15. (List two:) the common name and form of the food; the weight of the contents; the name and address of the manufacturer, packer, or distributor; a list of ingredients

Help for Consumers, Activity E, pages 61-62

1. B; canned foods
2. C; milk, ice cream, or cold cuts
3. A; yeast or baby food
4. D; bakery products
5. generic, frozen, 12 ounce
6. house brand, frozen
7. frozen
8. 16 ounce
9. 6 ounce
10. (List four:) canned products, pet food, staple items, cleaning agents, paper products
11. the name of the product; a list of ingredients; the net weight or contents; and the name and address of the manufacturer, packer, or distributor
12. Generic products generally cost consumers about 30 percent less than national brands and about 15 to 19 percent less than house brands.
13. Generic fruits and vegetables may have uneven sizes and shapes, and their colors and textures may vary. Generic paper products may be lighter in weight, and detergents may be less concentrated than brand name products.

14. when appearance or other quality factors are important
15. the product is a regular grocery item
16. the manufacturer
17. the products and its size, style, or form
18. (Student response. Students should base their answers on information in the section, "Sources of Consumer Information," found on pages 212-213 of the text.)

Teacher's Resources

Chapter 11 Test

1. G	15. F
2. C	16. F
3. A	17. F
4. B	18. T
5. E	19. C
6. F	20. C
7. T	21. B
8. T	22. C
9. F	23. B
10. T	24. D
11. F	25. C
12. F	26. C
13. F	27. A
14. T	28. D

29. (Student response. See page 202 in the text.)
30. (Student response. See pages 204 and 206 in the text.)
31. (Student response. See page 207 in the text.)
32. Unit pricing lists a cost per standard unit, weight, or measure. With this information, consumers can compare the cost of different forms, package sizes, and brands of products quickly and easily.
33. (Student response. See pages 212-213 in the text.)

The Smart Consumer

Name _____

Date _____ Period _____ Score _____

Chapter 11 Test

Matching: Match the following types of stores with their descriptions.

_____ 1. May charge higher prices to cover the cost of longer business hours.

_____ 2. Sells food grown by a group of farmers directly to consumers.

_____ 3. Specializes in ready-to-eat foods.

_____ 4. Sells food in large quantities at reduced prices.

_____ 5. Offers one specific type of product.

_____ 6. Carries both food and nonfood items; may offer special services.

A. delicatessen
B. discount supermarket
C. farmers' market
D. roadside stand
E. specialty store
F. supermarket
G. 24-hour convenience store

True/False: Circle *T* if the statement is true or *F* if the statement is false.

T F 7. Grocery stores are usually least crowded on weekday mornings and afternoons.

T F 8. A shopping list should include needed ingredients for recipes, staple items, and advertised specials.

T F 9. Saving money in the grocery store often requires sacrificing good nutrition.

T F 10. Most convenience foods cost more than homemade ones.

T F 11. Scientific evidence has shown that organic foods are more nutritious than foods produced by standard agricultural methods.

T F 12. Manufacturers started using food additives in the 1930s when scientists discovered that chemicals could be used to preserve foods.

T F 13. The first item listed under the "Nutrition Facts" heading on a food label is the servings per container.

T F 14. A consumer's Daily Values may be higher or lower than those listed on nutrition labels.

T F 15. Ingredients are listed alphabetically on food labels.

T F 16. The freshness date is the last day a food should be eaten or used.

T F 17. A generic food product usually is not as nutritious as a similar brand name product.

T F 18. The Food and Drug Administration prevents any hazardous foods from being sold across state lines.

Multiple Choice: Choose the best response. Write the letter in the space provided.

_____ 19. When do many food stores begin running their specials?
A. Monday.
B. Wednesday.
C. Thursday.
D. Saturday.

(Continued)

Name _____

_____ 20. A brand sold only by a store or chain of stores is a _____.
   A. bargain brand
   B. generic brand
   C. house brand
   D. national brand

_____ 21. Magazines and candy bars displayed by the checkout are examples of _____.
   A. advertised specials
   B. impulse items
   C. loss leader items
   D. None of the above.

_____ 22. Spices, MSG, and ultramarine blue are additives that _____.
   A. add nutrients
   B. aid processing or preparation
   C. enhance flavors or colors
   D. preserve quality

_____ 23. Which of the following is *not* required on a nutrition label?
   A. The number of calories per serving.
   B. The amount of potassium per serving.
   C. The amount of protein per serving.
   D. The amount of sodium per serving.

_____ 24. Which of the following is *not* required on all food product labels?
   A. The common name and form of the food.
   B. The weight of the contents.
   C. The name and address of the manufacturer, packer, or distributor.
   D. The price.

_____ 25. Which of the following consumer aids helps make comparison shopping easier?
   A. Generic products.
   B. Open dating.
   C. Unit pricing.
   D. Universal product code.

_____ 26. A jar of peanut butter costing $2.29 contains 16 servings. The cost per serving is about _____.
   A. $.07
   B. $.10
   C. $.14
   D. $.16

_____ 27. Which of the following statements about UPC is *not* true?
   A. The first five numbers of the code identify the product's price.
   B. Food manufacturers and store chains developed the UPC to save time and labor.
   C. As UPC codes are scanned, a computer prints a description of the items and their prices on the customer's receipt.
   D. The UPC computer system also functions as an automatic inventory system.

_____ 28. Which of the following sources of consumer information establishes grades for many products?
   A. Consumers Union.
   B. Federal Trade Commission.
   C. Office of Consumer Affairs.
   D. United States Department of Agriculture.

(Continued)

Name _____

Essay Questions: Provide complete responses to the following questions or statements.

29. List four factors that would help you decide where to shop if you had to choose among several grocery stores.
30. List five tips that can help consumers save money when shopping for food.
31. What are two factors a person should consider when choosing to eat organic foods?
32. How does unit pricing help consumers compare prices easily in the grocery store?
33. Name three government agencies, business organizations, or consumer groups and explain how each serves as a source of help for consumers.

Getting Started in the Kitchen

Objectives

After studying this chapter, students will be able to
- identify abbreviations and define cooking terms used in recipes.
- measure liquid and dry ingredients and fats for use in recipes.
- change the yield of a recipe.
- plan time-work schedules.
- follow a recipe to prepare a sandwich.

Bulletin Boards

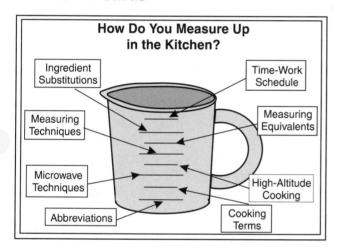

How Do You Measure Up in the Kitchen?

- Ingredient Substitutions
- Time-Work Schedule
- Measuring Techniques
- Measuring Equivalents
- Microwave Techniques
- High-Altitude Cooking
- Abbreviations
- Cooking Terms

I. Title: "How Do You Measure Up in the Kitchen?"

Place a cutout of a large liquid measuring cup in the center of the bulletin board. Place labels with various concepts from the chapter around the cup. Draw lines from each of the labels to a different measurement line on the cup, as shown.

II. Title: "Recipe for a Competent Cook"

Make the bulletin board look like a large recipe card. List various concepts from the chapter as the "ingredients" on the card. The "directions" for the recipe should read, "Combine all information. Allow knowledge to simmer gently, then blend in plenty of practice. Add equal measures of time and patience. Yield: One Competent Cook."

Teaching Materials

Text, pages 215-230

Student Activity Guide
- A. *Reading a Recipe*
- B. *Microwave Cooking*
- C. *Changing Recipe Yield*
- D. *Making a Time-Work Schedule*

Teacher's Resource Binder
Food Preparation Terms, reproducible master 12-1

Microwave Power Settings, reproducible master 12-2

The Multipurpose Microwave Oven, reproducible master 12-3

Measuring Basics, reproducible master 12-4

Sandwich Recipes, recipe master 12-5

Chapter 12 Study Sheet, reproducible master 12-6

Timing Foods in the Microwave, color transparency CT-12A

Promoting Even Microwave Cooking, color transparency CT-12B

Tips for Making Sandwiches, color transparency CT-12C

Chapter 12 Test

Software, diskette for Part Two
Chapter review game

Introductory Activities

1. Ask students to stand up if they have ever done each of the following activities in the kitchen:
   - made popcorn in the microwave oven
   - heated a frozen entree in the microwave oven
   - heated canned soup on top of the range
   - made macaroni and cheese from a packaged mix
   - made chocolate chip cookies from scratch
   - made an entree from scratch
   - made an entire meal from scratch
   - prepared all of the meals for your family for a week

   Student responses will help you evaluate the extent of their food preparation experience. Use this information to help you plan how you will cover chapter material.

2. Tell students that you want to make a batch of brownies. Have them coach you through the process. Ask them what you need to know or do each step of the way. Point out that studying this chapter will help students know how to go through a food preparation process.

Strategies to Reteach, Reinforce, Enrich, and Extend Text Concepts

Choosing a Recipe

3. **RT**   Have students find examples of seasonal food features in magazines and newspapers.

4. **RF**   Have students choose recipes for a dinner menu. Have them evaluate one of the recipes according to the criteria given in the text.

5. **RF**   Have students start a class recipe file. Ask them to clip recipes from magazines and newspapers that appeal to them to add to the file.

6. **RT**   *Food Preparation Terms*, reproducible master 12-1, TRB. Review the list of terms with students. Encourage students to keep the list posted inside a kitchen cabinet or tucked in a cookbook for easy reference when working in the kitchen.

7. **RF**   *Reading a Recipe*, Activity A, SAG. Students are to answer questions about a given recipe.

8. **RT**   *Microwave Power Settings*, reproducible master 12-2, TRB. Review the uses of typical microwave power settings listed on the handout. Encourage students to post the list near their microwave oven for easy reference.

9. **RT**   *Timing Foods in the Microwave*, color transparency CT-12A, TRB. Use this transparency to illustrate various factors that affect the speed at which foods cook in a microwave oven.

10. **RT**   *Promoting Even Microwave Cooking*, color transparency CT-12B, TRB. Use this transparency to illustrate various techniques for promoting even cooking in a microwave oven.

11. **EX**   Prepare two recipes of brownies. Place each recipe in a square microwavable pan. Shield the corners of one pan. Leave the other pan unshielded. Cook both recipes for the same amount of time in the microwave oven. Ask students to compare the two samples and note what effect the shields had.

12. **EX**   *Microwave Cooking*, Activity B, SAG.

Students are to read case studies and answer questions about microwave cooking problems.

13. **ER**   *The Multipurpose Microwave Oven*, reproducible master 12-3, TRB. Discuss with students how the microwave oven can save preparation time as well as cooking time. Divide the class into lab groups and have each group demonstrate one of the listed techniques.

Measuring Ingredients

14. **ER**   Set up a measuring lab. Have students practice measuring a variety of liquid and dry ingredients and fats in a variety of amounts using both measuring cups and measuring spoons. (Suggested ingredients include sifted flour, water, brown sugar, shortening, and margarine.)

15. **RT**   Demonstrate for students how to use the water displacement to measure solid fats.

Adjusting Recipes

16. **RT**   *Measuring Basics*, reproducible master 12-4, TRB. Review abbreviations, equivalents, and measuring techniques on the handout with students. Encourage students to save the handout for reference.

17. **RF**   Have students make a chart listing double and half amounts of all the measures listed in Chart 12-8 on page 224 in the text. Encourage students to tuck the chart into a cookbook for easy reference when adjusting recipes in the future.

18. **RF**   *Changing Recipe Yield*, Activity C, SAG. Students are to figure ingredient amounts for a half recipe and a double recipe and then answer questions about measuring and measurement equivalents.

19. **EX**   Have each student choose a conventional recipe. Ask students to identify specific ways they would modify their recipe for use with a microwave oven.

20. **EX**   Have students prepare some basic recipes, such as pudding and biscuits. Assign some lab group to prepare the recipes as written. Have other lab groups prepare the recipes using some of the ingredient substitutions listed in Chart 12-9 on page 225 of the text. Ask students to sample similar food products and compare them for taste, texture, and appearance. Have them note any differences created by the ingredient substitutions.

Using a Time-Work Schedule

21. **RT** Use food models to help you dramatize for students the need for a time-work schedule. Tell three or four students you are going to prepare lunch to reward them for their regular attendance or their performance on a recent project or test. Explain that you cannot join your guests for conversation because you are completing preparation tasks in the kitchen. Serve courses out of order. Serve some courses almost simultaneously. Allow large spans of time between other courses. Discuss your dramatization with the class. Explain how the use of a time-work schedule would have enabled you to spend more time with your guests and serve the meal in proper order.

22. **RT** Review on the chalkboard the steps for preparing a time-work schedule.

23. **EX** *Making a Time-Work Schedule,* Activity D, SAG. Students are to plan a menu and prepare a time-work schedule for preparing it using the forms provided.

24. **RT** Explain the concept of dovetailing to students. Give them several examples of how two or more food preparation tasks can be in progress at the same time, reducing the total amount of time needed to complete the tasks individually.

Preparing Simple Recipes

25. **RF** Have students name some of their favorite hot and cold sandwiches.

26. **RF** Ask students to list different types of bread that could be used to make sandwiches.

27. **RF** Have students look through cookbooks to make a list of sandwiches that could be made ahead and would be easy to serve at parties.

28. **RT** *Tips for Making Sandwiches,* color transparency CT-12C, TRB. Use this transparency as you discuss some basic suggestions for making sandwiches.

29. **ER** *Sandwich Recipes,* recipe master 12-5, TRB. Have students use the recipe master and additional recipes found in strategy 27 to plan a sandwich lab. Have each lab group complete a *Market Order Sheet* (TRB) and a *Time-Work Schedule* (TRB). Have groups share their sandwiches with the class. Then have each group complete a *Lab Evaluation Sheet* (TRB).

◗ Chapter Review

30. **RT** *Chapter 12 Study Sheet,* reproducible master 12-6, TRB. Have students complete the statements as they read text pages 216-229.

31. **RF** Software, diskette for Part Two. Have students play the chapter review game according to the instructions that appear on the screen.

Above and Beyond

32. **EX** Have students follow the time-work schedule they prepared in strategy 22 to prepare the menu they listed in that learning experience. Then have them evaluate the meal and discuss any scheduling problems they had in preparing it. Ask them to give suggestions for correcting these problems.

Answer Key

Text

Review What You Have Read, page 230

1. The recipe is written in a clear, concise manner. Ingredients are listed in the order in which they will be used. Amounts are easily measured. Directions are complete. Accurate baking or cooking time is given. Baking or cooking temperature is given. Pan size is given. Number of average servings is given.

2. A. cup
   B. ounce
   C. teaspoon
   D. tablespoon

3. A. blend
   B. dice
   C. grease
   D. preheat

4. Dehydration may occur when microwave cooking continues until foods are fully cooked due to the fact that many foods will continue to cook after the allotted time in the oven.

5. Pressure from steam can build up inside containers that are tightly covered with plastic.

6. The boiling point of water drops at high altitudes.

7. false

8. A. ¼ cup, 1 tablespoon
   B. ¾ teaspoon, 1 tablespoon
   C. $\frac{3}{8}$ cup (¼ cup plus 1 tablespoon), 1½ cups
   D. $\frac{5}{6}$ cup (½ cup plus $\frac{1}{3}$ cup), 3 $\frac{1}{3}$ cups

9. The time estimates for preparing menu items could be off target.

10. mayonnaise, hard-cooked egg white, jelly, lettuce or other raw vegetables

Student Activity Guide

Reading a Recipe, Activity A, page 63
1. (List five:) dry measures, French knife, cutting board, measuring spoons, can opener, liquid measures, kitchen shears, soup kettle
2. drain them
3. A. cup
   B. tablespoon
   C. teaspoon
   D. ounce
4. into small pieces
5. into very small cubes of even size
6. into very fine pieces
7. into small squares of equal size
8. in a small amount of hot fat
9. to cook in liquid that is barely at the boiling point
10. to cook in liquid over 212°F (100°C)
11. 1 hour
12. 10 servings

Microwave Cooking, Activity B, page 64
   (Student responses should be based on information under "Using Microwave Recipes" on pages 218 and 221 in the text.)

Changing Recipe Yield, Activity C, page 65
1. serves 3 to 4
2. ¾ pound
3. ¼ cup
4. ½ tablespoon
5. 1 teaspoon
6. ½ teaspoon
7. ¾ teaspoon
8. ¹/₆ cup
9. 1 tablespoon
10. ¾ cup
11. serves 12 to 16
12. 3 pounds
13. 1 cup
14. 2 tablespoons
15. 4 teaspoons
16. 2 teaspoons
17. 3 teaspoons
18. ²/₃ cup
19. 4 tablespoons
20. 3 cups
21. 1½ teaspoons
22. 2 tablespoons plus 2 teaspoons
23. 1 tablespoon plus 1 teaspoon
24. 1 tablespoon
25. ¼ cup
26. 50 mL
27. 2 mL
28. 15 mL
29. 175 mL
30. 5 mL
31. 75 mL
32. 250 mL
33. 150 mL
34. 50 mL

Teacher's Resources

Chapter 12 Test

1.	K	15.	T
2.	E	16.	F
3.	J	17.	F
4.	B	18.	T
5.	H	19.	T
6.	I	20.	T
7.	G	21.	A
8.	A	22.	D
9.	D	23.	C
10.	C	24.	C
11.	T	25.	B
12.	F	26.	D
13.	F	27.	D
14.	T	28.	C

29. (List three:) distributes heat more evenly, helps foods retain moisture, speeds cooking time, tenderizes foods, prevents spatters
30. (Student response. See pages 221-223 in the text. Students should mention that they will need a ¼ cup dry measure and a ½ cup dry measure to measure the flour.)
31. (Student response. See page 224 in the text.)
32. (Student response. See pages 225-226 in the text.)
33. bread, filling, extras (Examples are student response.)

Getting Started in the Kitchen

Name _____

Date _____ **Period** _____ **Score** _____

Chapter 12 Test

Matching: Match the following types of stores with their descriptions.

_____ 1. The average number of servings a recipe will make.

_____ 2. Instructions for preparing a particular food.

_____ 3. A unit used to measure the cooking power of microwave ovens.

_____ 4. Drying out.

_____ 5. The time during which foods finish cooking by internal heat after being removed from a microwave oven.

_____ 6. Leaving an opening through which steam can escape in the covering of food to be cooked in a microwave oven.

_____ 7. Using small pieces of foil to cover areas of a food to prevent them from overcooking in a microwave oven.

_____ 8. Sparking that occurs in a microwave oven when metal comes in contact with the oven walls.

_____ 9. Lifting a food off the floor of a microwave oven to allow microwaves to penetrate it from the bottom.

_____ 10. To overlap tasks to use time more efficiently.

A. arcing
B. dehydration
C. dovetail
D. elevating
E. recipe
F. rotating
G. shielding
H. standing time
I. venting
J. watt
K. yield

True/False: Circle *T* if the statement is true or *F* if the statement is false.

T F 11. A meal manager should read through a recipe before he or she begins to prepare it.

T F 12. Steep means to remove liquid from a food product.

T F 13. Microwave recipes are generally designed for ovens with a maximum wattage of 800 to 1000 watts.

T F 14. Uneven distribution of microwaves may cause some parts of a food product to be barely warm while other spots are very hot.

T F 15. Breads and cakes tend to rise more during baking at high altitudes.

T F 16. Brown sugar should be sifted before spooning it into a dry measuring cup.

T F 17. Two tablespoons of cornstarch can be substituted for one tablespoon of flour in a recipe.

T F 18. Time schedules differ depending on the menu.

T F 19. Rotating tasks on a time-work schedule from one time to the next gives everyone a range of kitchen experience.

T F 20. Garnishes can improve the appearance and food value of a sandwich.

(Continued)

Name _____

Multiple Choice: Choose the best response. Write the letter in the space provided.

_____ 21. Which of the following does *not* need to be included in a well-written recipe?
A. Abbreviations.
B. Directions.
C. Ingredients.
D. Yield.

_____ 22. Which of the following is the correct abbreviation for *ounce?*
A. O.
B. oc.
C. on.
D. oz.

_____ 23. Which of the following terms means to mix or blend two or more ingredients together?
A. Beat.
B. Blend.
C. Combine.
D. Cream.

_____ 24. What is the conventional equivalent of $1/3$ cup?
A. 3 teaspoons.
B. 4 tablespoons.
C. 5 $1/3$ tablespoons.
D. 10 $2/3$ tablespoons.

_____ 25. Which of the following steps should be taken when converting a conventional recipe for microwave use?
A. Increase the amount of liquid by one third.
B. Eliminate cooking oils and fats unless they provide flavor or consistency.
C. Double the amount of seasonings.
D. Use the defrost setting to cook most dishes.

_____ 26. Which of the following could be substituted for 1 cup buttermilk in a recipe?
A. ½ cup evaporated milk plus ½ cup water.
B. 1 cup reconstituted nonfat dry milk.
C. ¾ cup milk plus $1/3$ cup butter.
D. 1 tablespoon vinegar or lemon juice plus milk to make 1 cup.

_____ 27. What of the following is *not* a tool needed to make a time-work schedule?
A. A clock.
B. A pad of paper and a pencil.
C. A recipe or cookbook.
D. A set of measuring equipment.

_____ 28. Which of the following foods should *not* be used on sandwiches that are to be frozen?
A. Bologna.
B. Cheese.
C. Mayonnaise.
D. Peanut butter.

(Continued)

Name _____

Essay Questions: Provide complete responses to the following questions or statements.

29. What are three functions of covering food in a microwave oven?
30. Describe the correct way to measure each of the following ingredients:
    A. ¾ cup flour
    B. 1 cup milk
    C. ½ cup shortening
31. Explain how you would figure double and half amounts of recipe ingredients measured in fractions.
32. Explain the steps for making a time-work schedule.
33. Name the three types of ingredients used to make sandwiches and give two examples of each.

Meat

Objectives

After studying this chapter, students will be able to
- list factors affecting the selection of meats.
- describe how to properly store meats to maintain their quality.
- describe the principles and methods of cooking meat.
- prepare meats by moist and dry cooking methods.

Bulletin Boards

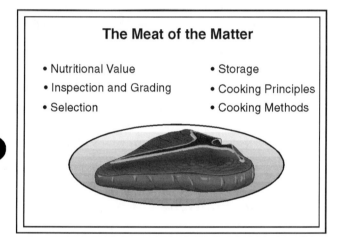

The Meat of the Matter

- Nutritional Value
- Inspection and Grading
- Selection
- Storage
- Cooking Principles
- Cooking Methods

I. Title: "The Meat of the Matter"

Place a large illustration of a meat entree on the bulletin board. List the main concepts of the chapter—nutritional value, inspection and grading, selection, storage, cooking principles, and cooking methods—under the title.

II. Title: "Cooking by Cut"

Draw an outline of an animal used for meat on the bulletin board. Divide the animal into wholesale cuts. Label each cut and identify if it should be cooked by moist or dry heat. (See page 69 of the *Student Activity Guide* for an example of the illustration.)

Teaching Materials

Text, pages 235-248
Student Activity Guide
   A. *Meat Inspection and Grading*

B. *Selection and Storage of Meats*
C. *Cooking by Cut*
D. *Meat Cookery Methods*

Teacher's Resource Binder
   Safe Food Handling Label, transparency master 13-1
   Evaluating Cooking Losses, food science master 13-2
   Meat Recipes, recipe master 13-3
   Chapter 13 Study Sheet, reproducible master 13-4
   Dry Heat Cooking Methods, color transparency CT-13A
   Moist Heat Cooking Methods, color transparency CT-13B
   Chapter 13 Test

Software, diskette for Part Three
   Hangman, chapter review game

Introductory Activities

1. Ask students to name their favorite meats or meat dishes.
2. Discuss with students why they think meat is so popular in the U.S. diet.

Strategies to Reteach, Reinforce, Enrich, and Extend Text Concepts

What Is Meat?

3. **RF** Ask students to give their definitions of *meat, beef, veal, pork,* and *lamb.* Compare their responses with the definitions given in the text.
4. **ER** Have students read a current health article on the relationship between the saturated fat and cholesterol found in red meats with heart disease. Then ask them to summarize what they have read in a brief oral report to the class.
5. **ER** Guest speaker. Invite a butcher to speak to your class about how animal carcasses are shipped. Have the speaker also discuss how the carcasses are divided into various wholesale and retail cuts.

6. **ER**   Field trip. Take your class to a meat packing plant to see how meat is processed and packaged for the retail market.

7. **EX**   Purchase three packages of ground beef having three degrees of leanness. Have students prepare one 4-ounce (113 g) patty from each package by panfrying it to the well done stage. Have the students weigh the cooked patties to measure the fat losses. Then have them compare the appearance, flavor, and juiciness of the samples on a *Food Product Evaluation Sheet* (TRB), and share their findings in class.

8. **ER**   Have students compare the retail cuts of beef and veal sold in a grocery store or butcher shop. Have them note the similarities and differences and report their findings in class.

9. **EX**   Set up a meat identification table. Select at least five cuts of beef, pork, veal, and lamb. Have students walk up to the table one at a time and try to identify the different meats. For each cut of meat, have students name the animal, the cut, and the location of the cut in the animal.

Inspection and Grading of Meat

10. **RT**   Have students discuss some of the factors used to determine meat grades.

11. **RF**   *Meat Inspection and Grading*, Activity A, SAG. Students are to answer questions related to meat inspection and grading.

12. **ER**   Field trip. Take your class to visit a stockyard to see how animals are kept and inspected before butchering.

13. **ER**   Guest speaker. Invite a meat inspector, USDA meat grader, or meat packer to speak to your class about the duties of his or her job.

Selecting Meat

14. **RT**   Have students describe the color of the lean and bone of high quality beef, pork, veal, and lamb.

15. **RF**   Have each student bring in a label from a retail meat package or record the label information from a retail meat label in the grocery store. Have them mount their labels or write their recorded information on a sheet of paper. Then have them identify the name of the meat, the wholesale cut, and the retail cut as shown on the labels.

16. **RF**   Have students determine how many pounds (kilograms) of the following cuts of meat they would need to buy to feed four

adults: rolled beef rump roast, lamb rib chops, pork spareribs, pork sausage links.

17. **ER**   Have students visit a grocery store or butcher shop to find examples of boneless cuts that cost less per serving than their "bone in" counterparts. Also have them find examples of boneless cuts that cost more per serving than their "bone in" counterparts.

18. **RF**   Have students determine the cost per serving of a cut of meat. Then have them determine the cost per serving of the same cut of meat when prepared with an extender, such as pasta, beans, or rice.

Storing Meat

19. **RT**   *Safe Food Handling Label*, transparency master 13-1, TRB. Use the transparency to point out to students the information found on perishable meat and poultry products.

20. **RF**   Have students make a chart showing how long various types of meat can be stored in the refrigerator and in the freezer.

21. **RT**   Demonstrate for students how to properly wrap meat in moistureproof and vaporproof paper for freezer storage.

22. **RF**   *Selection and Storage of Meats*, Activity B, SAG. Students are to complete statements with terms related to the selection and storage of meats.

Food Science Principles of Cooking Meat

23. **EX**   Purchase three identical cuts of beef. Have students roast each cut in a 325°F (160°C) oven. Using a meat thermometer for accuracy, have them cook their roasts to each of the following stages: medium rare, medium, and well done. Then have students compare the overall appearance, cooking losses, flavor, and texture on a *Food Product Evaluation Sheet* (TRB).

24. **RF**   Have students use a time chart to determine the cooking times of the following cuts of meat: 6 pound (3 kg) rolled beef roast (medium rare); 6 pound (3 kg) standing beef rib roast (medium rare); 4 pound (2 kg) rolled beef roast (medium), 4 pound (2 kg) sirloin steak (medium). Have students explain the differences in cooking times.

25. **EX**   *Evaluating Cooking Losses*, food science master 13-2, TRB. Have pairs of lab groups complete the experiment as directed on the master. This experiment is designed to be completed over a two-day period. On the

first day, students will record weights and prepare roasts for cooking. On the second day, you will place roasts in 325° and 450°F ovens and cook them to the medium stage (160°F) before class. Students will then calculate and compare cooking losses due to evaporation and drippings of roasts cooked at different temperatures.

Methods of Cooking Meat

26. **RT** *Dry Heat Cooking Methods,* color transparency CT-13A, TRB. Use the transparency to introduce students to the four basic dry heat cooking methods used to prepare protein foods.
27. **RT** *Moist Heat Cooking Methods,* color transparency CT-13B, TRB. Use the transparency to introduce students to the three basic moist heat cooking methods used to prepare protein foods.
28. **RF** Have students divide a sheet of paper into six columns, one column for each method for cooking meat. Then have them list the meat cuts found in the chart on page 237 of the text in the appropriate columns. (Be sure to inform students that some cuts will appear in more than one column.)
29. **ER** Have students broil, panfry, and braise three identical pork chops. Have them evaluate the overall appearance, flavor, tenderness, and juiciness on a *Food Product Evaluation Sheet* (TRB).
30. **RT** Demonstrate for students how to properly use a meat thermometer.
31. **ER** Have students prepare beef or lamb stew.
32. **ER** Assign each lab group a different variety meat and an appropriate cooking method for that meat. Ask students to sample and evaluate all the prepared variety meat dishes.
33. **EX** Purchase two of the same less tender cuts of beef. Have students prepare one with moist heat and the other with dry heat. Have them evaluate the appearance, texture, flavor, and shrinkage of each on a *Food Produce Evaluation Sheet* (TRB).
34. **RF** *Cooking by Cut,* Activity C, SAG. Students are to identify the illustrated beef wholesale cuts as tender or less tender. Then they are to identify the cooking methods to be used for various beef retail cuts.
35. **R** *Meat Cookery Methods,* Activity D, SAG. Students are to answer questions related to meat cookery methods.

36. **EX** *Meat Recipes,* recipe master 13-3, TRB. Have students use the recipe master to plan a meat cookery lab. Have each lab group complete a *Market Order Sheet* (TRB) and a *Time-Work Schedule* (TRB). After preparing their recipe and sampling their meat product, have each group complete a *Lab Evaluation Sheet* (TRB).

Chapter Review

37. **RT** *Chapter 13 Study Sheet,* reproducible master 13-4, TRB. Have students complete the statements as they read text pages 236-247.
38. **RF** *Hangman,* Software, diskette for Part Three. Have students play the chapter review game according to the instructions that appear on the screen.

Above and Beyond

39. **ER** Have each student select a culture and investigate the use of meat in that culture. Have each student prepare visual aids to use in giving a presentation to the class on the findings of his or her investigation. The presentation should include a listing of animals used for meat, a discussion of preparation techniques, and descriptions of popular meat dishes in that culture. The student should also mention any social customs or dietary restrictions related to the eating of meat in that culture. (Students may wish to begin their investigations using the information in Part Four of the text.)

Answer Key

Text

Review What You Have Read, page 248
1. (List five:) protein, iron, phosphorous, copper, thiamin, riboflavin, niacin, fat
2. (List three:) Choose lean cuts. Limit portion sizes. Trim visible fat before cooking. Use cooking methods that allow fat to drip away. Use nonstick pans. Skim fat after cooking.
3. Beef is usually bright cherry red with creamy white fat.
4. false
5. D
6. choice and select
7. Muscles located in areas of the animal that receive little exercise, such as rib and loin

muscles, are the most tender. Muscles located in areas of the animal that receive more exercise, such as leg and shoulder muscles, are less tender.

8. tenderness, amount of waste in the cut
9. three or four days
10. collagen
11. (List three for each:) overcooked—tough, dry, large amount of shrinkage, develops a hard crust, difficult to carve and eat
properly cooked—moist and juicy, tender, flavorful, easy to carve, smaller degree of shrinkage
12. Cooking losses are fat, water, and other volatile substances that evaporate from the surface of meat. Excessive cooking losses can cause tough, dry meat with a high degree of shrinkage, resulting in a reduced number of servings.
13. roasting—dry, broiling—dry, panbroiling—dry, frying—dry, braising—moist, cooking in liquid—moist
14. false
15. (List three:) Arrange meats with uniform shapes, such as patties or links, in a circle. Overlap sliced meats. Form ground meat into a doughnut-shaped loaf. Place meatier portions of cuts containing bone to the outside of the dish. Shield projections and edges on uneven cuts. Rotate, turn, and rearrange meats during cooking.

Student Activity Guide

Meat Inspection and Grading, Activity A, page 67
1. All meat shipped across state lines must be federally inspected.
2. An inspection stamp indicates that meat is wholesome and was processed under sanitary conditions.
3. Yield grades help wholesalers identify which carcasses will produce the most edible meat per pound. Quality grades assure consumers that meat has met set standards that predict taste appeal.
4. USDA
5. B
6. A
7. A
8. Prime, Choice, Select, Standard, Commercial, Utility, Cutter, Canner
9. Select
10. Prime

11. in manufactured meat products
12. Prime, Choice, Good, Standard, Utility, Cull
13. Acceptable, Utility
14. Prime, Choice, Good, Utility, Cull
15. carcasses that are expected to provide the tastiest meat

Selection and Storage of Meats, Activity B, page 68
1. meat
2. beef
3. wholesale cuts
4. retail cuts
5. hamburger
6. veal
7. pork
8. bacon
9. lamb
10. mutton
11. variety meats
12. tripe
13. wholesome
14. marbling
15. grade
16. bone
17. tender
18. exercise
19. URMIS
20. extenders

Cooking by Cut, Activity C, page 69
1. LT
2. T
3. T
4. T
5. LT
6. LT
7. LT
8. LT
9. roasting, broiling, panbroiling, frying
10. braising, cooking in liquid
11. M
12. D
13. D
14. M
15. M
16. E
17. D
18. D
19. E
20. E

Meat Cookery Methods, Activity D, page 70
1. G
2. B
3. F
4. D
5. A
6. C
7. 1 to 2 days for ground meats, 3 to 4 days for nonground products, 3 days for leftovers
8. discard it or bring it to a rolling boil for 1 minute before using it on cooked meat
9. brains, sweetbreads, and the liver and kidneys of young beef

10. in its original wrapper in the refrigerator
11. harmful microorganisms can grow that can result in food-borne illness
12. 50
13. this will prevent the outside from overcooking, before the inside is cooked
14. to keep them moist and tender and shorten the cooking time even further
15. tender, boneless cuts of uniform shape
16. large cuts and meat with a high fat content

26. Fresh beef will be bright, cherry red. Pork will be grayish-pink to rose. Veal will be light pink. Lamb will be pinkish-red.
27. blade bones, arm bone, and breast bones
28. the number of people you will serve, the amount of bone in the meat, whether or not you want leftovers
29. to destroy any harmful bacteria that may be present in raw meat, to improve flavor and digestibility, and sometimes for tenderization
30. roasting, broiling, panbroiling, and frying

Teacher's Resources

Chapter 13 Test

1. G
2. B
3. C
4. K
5. A
6. I
7. E
8. J
9. D
10. H
11. F
12. F
13. F
14. T
15. F
16. T
17. T
18. F
19. T
20. T
21. B
22. D
23. C
24. C
25. A

Meat

Name _____

Date _____ **Period** _____ **Score** _____

Chapter 13 Test

Matching: Match the following terms and identifying phrases.

_____ 1. The meat of swine.

_____ 2. A connective tissue in protein that can be softened by cooking.

_____ 3. Fat, water, and other volatile substances retained in pan drippings when meat is cooked.

_____ 4. Large cut of meat shipped to the retail grocery store.

_____ 5. Meat of cattle over 12 months of age.

_____ 6. Edible parts of animals other than muscle.

_____ 7. The meat of sheep less than one year old.

_____ 8. The meat of cattle less than three months of age.

_____ 9. A connective tissue in protein that cannot be softened by cooking.

_____ 10. Small cut of meat sold to consumers in retail stores.

A. beef

B. collagen

C. cooking losses

D. elastin

E. lamb

F. meat

G. pork

H. retail cut

I. variety meats

J. veal

K. wholesale cut

True/False: Circle *T* if the statement is true or *F* if the statement is false.

T F 11. Experts recommend that people stop eating red meat to eliminate saturated fat from their diet.

T F 12. Bacon comes from the pork leg.

T F 13. Veal is the smallest animal used for meat.

T F 14. All meat and meat products shipped across state lines must be federally inspected.

T F 15. Quality meats will have coarse, yellow fat.

T F 16. Muscles that are exercised the least are the most tender.

T F 17. Boneless meat will serve more people per pound than meat with bones.

T F 18. Ground meats and variety meats can be stored in a refrigerator two to three days longer than other meats.

T F 19. Heat coagulates protein.

T F 20. Large cuts and meat with a high fat content will brown naturally in a microwave oven.

(Continued)

Name _____

Multiple Choice: Choose the best response. Write the letter in the space provided.

_____ 21. The top quality grade of beef found in supermarkets is usually _____.
A. Prime
B. Choice
C. Select
D. Standard

_____ 22. Which of the following are clues to meat tenderness?
A. Amount of marbling.
B. Bone shape.
C. Location of the meat in the animal.
D. All of the above.

_____ 23. Which of the following does not affect the cooking time of meat?
A. Desired degree of doneness.
B. Oven temperature.
C. Salting the meat before cooking.
D. Size and shape of the cut.

_____ 24. Beef liver would most likely be prepared by _____.
A. braising
B. cooking in liquid
C. frying
D. roasting

_____ 25. Which of the following is true about frozen meats?
A. They should be thawed in the refrigerator.
B. They cook faster than thawed meats.
C. They should be placed closer to the heat source for broiling.
D. None of the above.

Essay Questions: Provide complete responses to the following questions or statements.

26. What is the characteristic color of fresh beef, veal, pork, and lamb?
27. What bone shapes indicate that a cut of meat should be cooked by moist heat?
28. What factors affect the amount of meat you need to buy?
29. Why is meat cooked?
30. Name the dry heat cooking methods used to prepare tender cuts of meat.

Poultry

Objectives

After studying this chapter, students will be able to
- list tips for buying poultry.
- describe how to properly store poultry to maintain its quality.
- describe the principles and methods for cooking poultry.
- prepare poultry by moist and dry cooking methods.

Bulletin Board

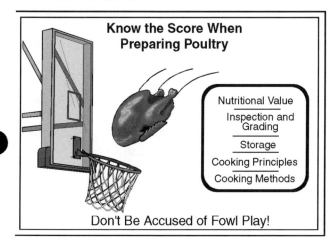

Know the Score When Preparing Poultry

Nutritional Value

Inspection and Grading

Storage

Cooking Principles

Cooking Methods

Don't Be Accused of Fowl Play!

Title: "Know the Score When Preparing Poultry"

At one side of the bulletin board, place a drawing or cutout of a large basketball hoop. Draw or cut out a picture of a roasted chicken or turkey and place it so it appears to be going into the hoop. List concepts from the chapter down the other side of the board. Across the bottom of the board place the subtitle, "Don't Be Accused of Fowl Play!"

Teaching Materials

Text, pages 249-258
Student Activity Guide
 A. *Poultry Pointers*
 B. *Poultry Selection and Storage*
 C. *Poultry Cookery*
Teacher's Resource Binder
 Fat Distribution in Poultry, food science master 14-1

 Boning a Chicken Breast, transparency master 14-2
 Boning a Chicken Thigh, transparency master 14-3
 Poultry Recipes, recipe master 14-4
 Chapter 14 Study Sheet, reproducible master 14-5
 Buying Poultry, color transparency CT-14
 Chapter 14 Test
Software, diskette for Part Three
 Tic Tac Toe, chapter review game

Introductory Activities

1. Have students investigate how poultry was served in colonial America.
2. Use a blind taste test to see if students can identify the flavor of turkey, chicken, duck, and goose.

Strategies to Reteach, Reinforce, Enrich, and Extend Text Concepts

Nutritional Value of Poultry

3. **ER** Have students make a chart comparing the saturated fat and cholesterol in chicken and turkey with that in red meat.
4. **EX** Have students sample poultry-based luncheon meats and compare them with their red meat counterparts for appearance, texture, and flavor on a *Food Product Evaluation Sheet* (TRB).
5. **EX** *Fat Distribution in Poultry*, food science master 14-1, TRB. This experiment is designed to be completed over a two-day period. On the first day, students will stew two chicken breast halves, one with skin and one without. On the second day, students will compare the chilled broth from the two breast halves in terms of fat content.

Buying Poultry

6. **RF** Have students read a current news article about quality control in the poultry industry.

7. **ER** Have students go to a grocery store to investigate the variety of ways frozen and fresh-chilled poultry is packaged. Have them share their findings in class.
8. **RF** Have students explain why it is more economical to purchase poultry whole than cut into pieces.
9. **RT** *Buying Poultry,* color transparency CT-14, TRB. Use the transparency to review basic guidelines to follow when shopping for poultry.
10. **ER** Divide the class into groups. Assign each group a category such as frozen entrees, ethnic dishes, canned soups, etc. Have the groups visit a grocery store and list all the available products in their category that contain poultry. Have the groups share their findings with the class.
11. **RF** Have students read the labels on a variety of processed food products that contain poultry. Ask them to identify the types of poultry products used. See if they can determine whether poultry skin was included in each product.
12. **EX** Have students investigate the price per pound (kilogram) of the various purchase forms of chicken and turkey. Ask them to analyze which forms would be the best buys in terms of servings.

Storing Poultry

13. **RT** Review with students the food sources, symptoms, and prevention of salmonellae.
14. **RT** Demonstrate for students how to properly wrap poultry for refrigerator and freezer storage. Discuss the cause of freezer burn and how it can be prevented.
15. **RF** *Poultry Pointers,* Activity A, SAG. Students are to fill in a word puzzle by completing sentences about poultry selection and storage.
16. **RF** *Poultry Selection and Storage,* Activity B, SAG. Students are to choose answers that best complete statements about poultry selection and storage.

Food Science Principles of Cooking Poultry

17. **RF** Have students describe the methods that can be used to determine the degree of doneness of cooked poultry.
18. **RF** Have students explain why it is important to cook poultry to the well-done stage.

Ask them also to describe color changes that may occur in the flesh and bones of poultry during cooking.

Methods of Cooking Poultry

19. **RF** Have students name the methods that can be used to cook poultry and define each.
20. **RT** Demonstrate for students trussing and stuffing a whole turkey.
21. **EX** Purchase four roasting chickens of equal size. Have students stuff one and roast it in a 325°F (160°C) oven until it tests done. Have them roast another at the same temperature unstuffed. Have them roast the third chicken by wrapping it completely in foil and roasting it in a 450°F (230°C) oven. Have them roast the fourth chicken in an oven cooking bag. Have them compare the cooking times required for the four birds.
22. **ER** Have students prepare recipes using giblets.
23. **ER** Have students sample breaded fried chicken and battered fried chicken to see which coating they prefer.
24. **ER** Have students sample fried chicken and oven-fried chicken. Have them describe the differences between the two methods and decide which they would prefer to make and which they would prefer to eat.
25. **RT** Demonstrate for students the proper way to shield poultry for microwave cooking.
26. **RF** Have students describe acceptable methods for thawing frozen poultry.
27. **RT** *Boning a Chicken Breast,* transparency master 14-2, TRB. Use the transparency to explain to students the steps for boning a chicken breast. If possible, allow students to practice the technique for some of the recipes to be prepared in strategy 29.
28. **RT** *Boning a Chicken Thigh,* transparency master 14-3, TRB. Use the transparency to explain to students the steps for boning a chicken thigh. If possible, allow students to practice the technique for some of the recipes to be prepared in strategy 29.
29. **EX** *Poultry Recipes,* recipe master 14-4, TRB. Have students use the recipe master to plan a poultry lab. Have each lab group complete a *Market Order Sheet* (TRB) and a *Time-Work Schedule* (TRB). After preparing their recipe and sampling their poultry product, have each group complete a *Lab Evaluation Sheet* (TRB).

30. **RF** *Poultry Cookery,* Activity C, SAG. Students are to answer questions about poultry cookery.

Chapter Review

31. **RT** *Chapter 14 Study Sheet,* reproducible master 14-5, TRB. Have students complete the statements as they read text pages 250-256.
32. **RF** *Tic Tac Toe,* Software, diskette for Part Three. Have students play the chapter review game according to the instructions that appear on the screen.

Above and Beyond

33. **ER** Several animals, including rabbit, frog, squirrel, snake, and alligator, are reported to have meat that tastes like chicken. Have students obtain one or more of these meats and investigate how to prepare it. Have them prepare the meat and distribute samples to the class. Ask students to compare the flavor, texture, and appearance with chicken.
34. **ER** Have students prepare one or more of the less common types of poultry, such as guinea hen, Rock Cornish hen, pigeon, quail, or pheasant. Have them distribute samples and ask the class to evaluate the flavor, texture, and appearance of the meat.
35. **ER** Have students contact the USDA for information about the education and training requirements for poultry inspectors.

Answer Key

Text

Review What You Have Read, page 258
1. chicken, turkey, goose, duck
2. true
3. Poultry contains more bone in proportion to muscle than red meat.
4. two to three days
5. false
6. true
7. washing the bird under cold running water and patting it dry with paper towels
8. trussing
9. Place bony portions to the center, arrange drumsticks like the spokes of a wheel, and shield wing and leg tips of whole birds.
10. Poultry may contain harmful bacteria that can get on the cutting board and utensils. Thoroughly washing the cutting board and utensils can help avoid the possibility of transferring these harmful bacteria to other foods.

Student Activity Guide

Poultry Pointers, Activity A, page 71
1. phosphorus
2. frozen
3. young
4. salmonellae
5. poultry
6. freezer burn
7. quality

Poultry Selection and Storage, Activity B, page 72
1. B
2. B
3. A
4. A
5. A
6. A
7. B
8. B
9. A
10. A
11. A
12. A
13. A
14. B

Poultry Cookery, Activity C, pages 73-74
1. Poultry should be cooked at low temperatures using careful timing. Poultry that is cooked at too high a temperature or cooked too long is tough, dry, and flavorless.
2. Grasp the drumstick gently. If the bird is cooked, the drumstick will twist easily at the thigh joint. The breast will pierce easily with a fork, and juices will be clear.
3. (dry heat methods:) roasting, broiling, frying, oven-frying (moist heat methods:) braising, stewing
4. It will be easier to carve.
5. Trussing prevents the wing and leg tips from overbrowning. It also makes the bird easier to handle and more attractive to serve.
6. The bird should be stuffed immediately before it is put into the oven. The bird should not be stuffed until this time to prevent the growth of harmful bacteria that can cause food-borne illness.
7. at least 165°F (75°C)
8. Make a tent out of aluminum foil. Cover the breast with the foil when the bird is about half cooked.
9. Cooking bags use steam to help cook the bird.
10. 4 to 5 inches
11. about 40 minutes
12. Pieces are rolled in flour, egg, and bread crumbs or dipped in a batter.
13. about ½ inch

14. baking
15. Uncover the pan for the last 10 minutes of cooking.
16. carrots, celery, seasonings
17. Stewed poultry can easily be removed from the bone and used in soups and casseroles.
18. (List three:) Poultry comes out tender and juicy. Poultry cooked in a microwave oven generally cooks in much less time than poultry cooked in a conventional oven. Poultry can be defrosted quickly in a microwave oven. Poultry can be partially cooked before being prepared by another method, such as grilling.
19. like the spokes of a wheel with the bony portions toward the center and the meaty ends toward the outside
20. before cooking
21. Frozen poultry can be wrapped in a tightly closed plastic bag and placed in a sink full of cold water. The water should be changed about every 30 minutes until the bird is defrosted.
22. Boning chicken yourself can save you money.

Teacher's Resources

Chapter 14 Test

1. E		11. F	
2. B		12. T	
3. C		13. T	
4. A		14. F	
5. F		15. T	
6. T		16. A	
7. T		17. C	
8. F		18. B	
9. T		19. D	
10. F		20. B	

21. (List two:) Choose chicken or turkey over duck and goose. Choose young birds over older birds. Choose light meat over dark meat. Remove the skin before cooking or eating.
22. (Student response. See page 251 in the text.)
23. Remove store wrapping and rewrap bird loosely in waxed paper. Wrap and store giblets separately. Place poultry in the coldest part of the refrigerator and use within two to three days.
24. Low temperatures and careful timing are important. Cooking poultry for too long or at too high a temperature can make it tough, dry, and flavorless.
25. Stuffing should be packed loosely into the body cavity of the bird just before roasting. Extra stuffing should be baked in a casserole dish.

Poultry

Name _____

Date _____ **Period** _____ **Score** _____

Chapter 14 Test

Matching: Match each of the following methods of cooking poultry with its description.

_____ 1. Place the bird breast side up in a shallow pan, season the cavity, and place the pan in a 325°F (160°C) oven.

_____ 2. Place poultry pieces on a pan, brush them lightly with melted margarine, and place the pan 4 to 5 inches (10 to 12 cm) from the heat source.

_____ 3. Cut the bird into pieces, coat the pieces with breading or batter, and brown them in ½ inch (1.5 cm) of hot fat.

_____ 4. Add a small amount of water to a skillet containing browned poultry pieces. Then cover the skillet tightly and cook over low heat until poultry is tender.

_____ 5. Put the bird in a big kettle and cover it completely with water. Then cover the kettle and simmer until poultry is tender.

A. braising
B. broiling
C. frying
D. oven-frying
E. roasting
F. stewing

True/False: Circle *T* if the statement is true or *F* if the statement is false.

T   F   6. Dark meat is slightly higher in fat than light meat.

T   F   7. Chicken and turkey can be flavored and processed to resemble hot dogs, ham, and other luncheon meats.

T   F   8. All poultry sold in interstate commerce must be graded.

T   F   9. Poultry contains more bone in proportion to muscle than does red meat.

T   F   10. Poultry can be stored in the freezer for up to one year.

T   F   11. Cooked poultry with dark-colored bones should not be eaten.

T   F   12. Cooking bags use steam to shorten cooking time when roasting poultry.

T   F   13. To ensure even cooking in a microwave oven, poultry pieces should be arranged with the bony portions to the center.

T   F   14. Commercially stuffed frozen turkeys should be thawed before cooking.

T   F   15. Boning chicken at home can save money over buying boned chicken pieces.

(Continued)

Name _____

Multiple Choice: Choose the best response. Write the letter in the space provided.

_____ 16. Poultry is a good source of all the following nutrients *except* _____.
   A. carbohydrates
   B. phosphorus
   C. proteins
   D. thiamin

_____ 17. Which type of bird usually has the most fat?
   A. Chicken.
   B. Duck.
   C. Goose.
   D. Turkey.

_____ 18. A pink color in cooked poultry indicates _____.
   A. the bird is overcooked
   B. a harmless chemical reaction has taken place
   C. the bird is spoiled and unsafe to eat
   D. the bird was stuffed several hours before cooking

_____ 19. Large birds should be trussed before roasting to _____.
   A. prevent the wing and leg tips from overbrowning
   B. make the bird easier to handle
   C. make the bird more attractive to serve
   D. All of the above.

_____ 20. For quick thawing, poultry can be _____.
   A. left at room temperature until defrosted
   B. wrapped in a tightly closed plastic bag and placed in a sink full of cold water
   C. placed directly into a hot oven for cooking
   D. None of the above.

Essay Questions: Provide complete responses to the following questions or statements.

21. Give two suggestions for choosing and preparing poultry to be included in a reduced-fat diet.
22. Give three guidelines to follow when buying poultry.
23. How should poultry be wrapped for refrigerator storage?
24. What are the basic cooking principles for preparing poultry?
25. How should poultry be stuffed?

Fish and Shellfish

Objectives

After studying this chapter, students will be able to
- list factors affecting the selection of fish and shellfish.
- describe how to properly store fish to maintain its quality.
- describe the principles and methods for cooking fish and shellfish.
- prepare fish by moist and dry cooking methods.

Bulletin Board

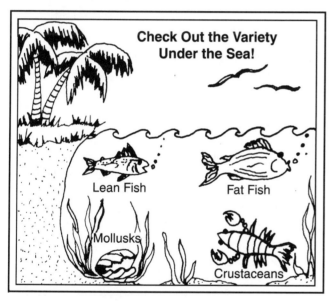

Title: "Check Out the Variety Under the Sea!"

Use cutouts to show an underwater scene. Place drawings or cutouts of lean fish, fat fish, mollusks, and crustaceans under the water with appropriate labels, as shown.

Teaching Materials

Text, pages 259-269
Student Activity Guide
    A. *Selecting Fish and Shellfish*
    B. *Finfish Cookery*
    C. *Fish Maze*
    D. *Investigating Shellfish*
Teacher's Resource Binder
    Criteria for Selecting Fish, transparency master 15-1

Comparing Cooking Methods for Fish, food science master 15-2
    Filleting Fish, transparency master 15-3
    Finfish Recipes, recipe master 15-4
    Shellfish Recipes, recipe master 15-5
    Chapter 15 Study Sheet, reproducible master 15-6
    Chapter 15 Test
Software, diskette for Part Three
    Reverse Thinking, chapter review game

Introductory Activities

1. Have students find out which varieties of fish are most commercially important in the United States.
2. Describe to students how fish are caught and processed for the retail market.

Strategies to Reteach, Reinforce, Enrich, and Extend Text Concepts

Classification of Fish and Shellfish

3. **ER** Have students do research to identify varieties of fish and shellfish, other than those identified in the text, that fit into the classes of lean fish, fat fish, crustaceans, and mollusks.
4. **ER** Field trip. Visit a fish market or fish section of the supermarket. Have students make a list of the different kinds of finfish and shellfish available in your area. Have them check the availability of canned and frozen varieties, too.
5. **ER** Have students compare the cholesterol and fat content of several varieties of fish and shellfish with those of several cuts of meat.

Selecting and Purchasing Fish and Shellfish

6. **RT** Ask students to list characteristics on which quality grades of fish are based.
7. **RT** *Criteria for Selecting Fish,* transparency master 15-1, TRB. Use the master to illustrate for students signs of quality they should use when selecting fresh fish.

8. **RF** Have students compare the costs of fresh and frozen finfish. Ask them to explain what factors help determine the differences in price.

9. **ER** Have students compare the cost per pound of various forms of fresh finfish. Then have them compute cost per serving to identify which forms are most economical.

10. **ER** Have students contact a fish market to find out the number of jumbo, large, large-medium, medium, and small shrimp needed to weigh 1 pound.

11. **ER** Have students examine samples of fresh shellfish for the signs of quality outlined on pages 262-263 of the text.

12. **RF** *Selecting Fish and Shellfish,* Activity A, SAG. Students are to complete exercises about selecting fish and shellfish.

13. **RT** Demonstrate for students how to properly wrap fish for refrigerator and freezer storage.

14. **RF** *Fish Maze,* Activity C, SAG. Students are to complete statements about the selection and storage of fish. Then they are to find and circle the terms in a word maze.

Cooking Finfish

15. **ER** Select two halibut steaks. Broil one steak to the proper degree of doneness. Overcook the other. Have students compare the appearance, flavor, and texture of the two steaks on a *Food Product Evaluation Sheet* (TRB).

16. **RT** Demonstrate for students how to poach whole fish and how to broil fish fillets or steaks.

17. **RF** Have students find five recipes for lean fish prepared by broiling. In each recipe, have them identify how the fish is prevented from becoming dry.

18. **ER** Have students prepare identical portions of fish by panfrying, oven-frying, and deep-frying. Have them sample the three fish products. Ask them to identify the one they prefer to prepare and the one they prefer to eat. Have them give reasons for their choices.

19. **EX** *Comparing Cooking Methods for Fish,* food science master 15-2, TRB. Have lab groups complete the experiment as directed on the master. Students will be comparing dry and moist heat cooking methods for preparing lean and fat fish. For each lab group, you will need to purchase two lean fish fillets and two fat fish fillets from the options on the supply list. All four fillets for each group should be of similar thickness. Tell students what varieties of fish they are preparing. However, allow them to use their reading and observations to determine which is fat and which is lean.

20. **RT** *Filleting Fish,* transparency master 15-3, TRB. Use the transparency to explain to students the steps for filleting fish. If possible, allow students to practice the technique for some of the recipes to be prepared in strategy 21.

21. **EX** *Finfish Recipes,* recipe master 15-4, TRB. Have students use the recipe master to plan a finfish lab using several varieties of fish. Have each lab group complete a *Market Order Sheet* (TRB) and a *Time-Work Schedule* (TRB). After preparing their recipes and sampling their finfish product, have each group complete a *Lab Evaluation Sheet* (TRB).

22. **RF** *Finfish Cookery,* Activity B, SAG. Students are to answer questions about cooking finfish.

Principles and Methods of Cooking Shellfish

23. **RT** Demonstrate for students how to cook various types of live shellfish.

24. **ER** *Investigating Shellfish,* Activity D, SAG. Students are to use library resources and supermarket research to write a brief report about one type of shellfish on the form provided.

25. **ER** Have students devein and parboil shrimp. Then have them use three different cooking methods to prepare a shrimp appetizer, salad, and main dish. Remind them to select the best size shrimp for each use.

26. **ER** Have students cook a live lobster. When cool, have them detach the claws and remove the meat from the lobster for use in an entree.

27. **EX** *Shellfish Recipes,* recipe master 15-5, TRB. Have students use the recipe master to plan a shellfish lab. Have each lab group complete a *Market Order Sheet* (TRB) and a *Time-Work Schedule* (TRB). After preparing their recipes and sampling their shellfish product, have each group complete a *Lab Evaluation Sheet* (TRB).

Chapter Review

28. **RT** *Chapter 15 Study Sheet,* reproducible master 15-6, TRB. Have students complete the statements as they read text pages 260-267.

29. **RF** *Reverse Thinking,* Software, diskette for

Part Three. Have students play the chapter review game according to the instructions that appear on the screen.

Above and Beyond

30. **ER** Field trip. Take students on a fishing trip to a local waterway. Have students inspect the quality characteristics of the fresh fish they catch. If fish are large enough to keep, have students clean and dress their fish and prepare them by one of the methods described in the text.
31. **ER** Have students prepare an oral presentation on one of the following topics:
    A. how fish flour is made and how and where it used.
    B. how one of the by-products of the fishing industry, such as fish liver oil or whale bone, is obtained and used.
    Students should prepare visual aids for use in their presentations.

Answer Key

Text

Review What You Have Read, page 269
1. true
2. crustaceans (shellfish)
3. (List three:) phosphorous, iron, calcium, iodine
4. (List three:) scales firmly affixed; firm flesh; bright, clear eyes; shiny skin; internal body walls bright in color; no bones protruding; no strong odor
5. A
6. shrimp sold without the intestinal tract
7. true
8. Wrap fresh fish tightly in waxed paper or foil and place it in a tightly covered container.
9. The flesh will be firm, and it will flake easily with a fork.
10. fat fish
11. Brush the pieces of fish with melted butter or a sauce.
12. Wrap the fish in cheesecloth or parchment paper or place it on a rack before poaching.
13. false
14. true

Student Activity Guide

Selecting Fish and Shellfish, Activity A, pages 75-76

Lean fish have very little fat in their flesh. Their flesh is white.

(Examples:) cod, flounder, haddock, halibut, red snapper, swordfish

Fat fish have flesh that is fattier than that of lean fish. They usually are pink, yellow, or gray in color.

(Examples:) catfish, mackerel, salmon, trout

Mollusks have soft bodies that are partially or fully covered by hard shells.

(Examples:) clams, oysters, scallops

Crustaceans are covered by crustlike shells and have segmented bodies.

(Examples:) crabs, lobster, shrimp

1. steaks
2. drawn fish
3. whole (round) fish
4. single fillet
5. dressed fish
6. B or E
7. B or E
8. F
9. C
10. A
11. D

Finfish Cookery, Activity B, page 77
1. poaching
2. broiling
3. baking
4. steaming
5. frying
6. microwaving
7. Broiling and baking are recommended methods for cooking fat fish.
8. Frying, poaching, and steaming are recommended methods for cooking lean fish.
9. Fish, including stuffed and rolled fish, is measured at its thickest point. It should be cooked about 10 minutes for every inch (2.5 cm) of thickness. This guide does not apply when deep-frying or microwaving fish.
10. (Student response.)

Fish Maze, Activity C, pages 78-79

1. finfish
2. shellfish
3. lean
4. fat
5. mollusk
6. crustacean
7. flour
8. iodine
9. inspection
10. odor
11. whole
12. drawn
13. dressed
14. steak
15. fillet
16. shrimp
17. deveined
18. shucked
19. lobster
20. scallop
21. broil
22. bake
23. fry
24. poach
25. steam
26. parboil

```
D D N T P O A C H Z R F A L A I B C D D
A R A S E R C S S B I O D O R G P B E E
C A E B E S D N Y L I O R B Q C P P K V
L W L S X D H A L A R F E S T E A M C E
T N R E S C T E E Q U A G T R L R F U I
Q I K W X E T C L O O I T E S O B E H N
F A G A J Z D A Z L L A Y R F H O D S E
B V M I E U I T Y L F A H T H W I M Y D
P V U O U T K S N E E I A S C A L L O P
U O S D H K S U L L O M S L U O I P J U
S H R I M P L R X N I L K H S I F N I F
O T I N S P E C T I O N W J V K S M P O
W N E E K M R X Y L N J T L I M R N H N
```

Teacher's Resources

Chapter 15 Test

1. G
2. A
3. E
4. B
5. F
6. C
7. F
8. T
9. F
10. F
11. F
12. T
13. T
14. F
15. T
16. T
17. B
18. B
19. B
20. C
21. B

22. appearance, odor, flavor, and lack of defects
23. (List four:) The shell covering shrimp should be firmly attached. Shrimp should be odorless. The tail of a live lobster should snap back quickly after it is flattened. A fresh deep sea scallop should be white. A fresh bay scallop should be creamy white or pink. Live oyster and clam shells should be tightly closed or they should close when you touch them. Shucked oysters and clams should be plump, creamy in color, and odorless.
24. Wrap fresh fish tightly in waxed paper or foil. Place it in a tightly covered container in the coldest part of the refrigerator and use it within a day or two.
25. Gently insert the tines of a fork into the flesh of the fish and lift slightly. If the flesh separates into distinct layers, the fish is cooked to the proper degree of doneness.
26. because fresh, uncooked shellfish deteriorates very rapidly

Fish and Shellfish

Name _____

Date _____ **Period** _____ **Score** _____

Chapter 15 Test

Matching: Match the following terms and identifying phrases.

_____ 1. Fish with shells instead of backbones.

_____ 2. A shellfish with a segmented body that is covered by a crustlike shell.

_____ 3. Fish that have very little fat in their flesh.

_____ 4. Fish that have a higher level of fat in their flesh.

_____ 5. A shellfish that has a soft body that is fully or partially covered by a hard shell.

_____ 6. Fish that have fins and backbones.

A. crustacean
B. fat fish
C. finfish
D. fish fillet
E. lean fish
F. mollusk
G. shellfish

True/False: Circle *T* if the statement is true or *F* if the statement is false.

T F 7. All finfish are considered lean.

T F 8. Most fish have fewer calories (kilojoules) and less saturated fat and cholesterol than moderately fat red meat.

T F 9. Fish that are sold across state lines must be federally inspected.

T F 10. A fresh fish should have a limp body, pink gills, and glazed eyes.

T F 11. Crabs and lobsters are the most important shellfish in the United States in terms of the amount eaten.

T F 12. Shrimp are marketed according to the number needed to weight 1 pound (450 g).

T F 13. Fish steaks yield more servings per pound than whole or dressed fish.

T F 14. Tenderization is a major goal of finfish cookery.

T F 15. Poached fish are cooked in simmering liquid.

T F 16. Shellfish cooked in a microwave oven require the same timing whether cooked in or out of the shell.

Multiple Choice: Choose the best response. Write the letter in the space provided.

_____ 17. Saltwater fish are one of the most important sources of _____.
   A. calcium
   B. iodine
   C. niacin
   D. vitamin D

_____ 18. A fish that has the entrails, head, fins, and scales removed is a _____.
   A. drawn fish
   B. dressed fish
   C. fish fillet
   D. fish steak

(Continued)

Name _____

_____ 19. Which of the following cooking methods is least suitable for lean finfish?
A. Baking in a sauce.
B. Broiling.
C. Panfrying in butter.
D. Poaching.

_____ 20. Coating fish with crumbs or a batter and frying it in a small amount of fat until browned describes _____.
A. deep-frying
B. oven-frying
C. panfrying
D. stir-frying

_____ 21. Shellfish should be cooked for a _____.
A. short time at high temperatures
B. short time at moderate temperatures
C. long time at low temperatures
D. long time at moderate temperatures

Essay Questions: Provide complete responses to the following questions or statements.

22. On what factors are quality grades of fish based?
23. Give four signs of freshness to look for when buying shellfish.
24. How should fresh fish be stored in the refrigerator?
25. Describe how to test if a fish is cooked to the proper degree of doneness.
26. Why should shellfish purchased in the shell be cooked live?

Eggs

Objectives

After studying this chapter, students will be able to
■ list factors affecting the selection of eggs.
■ describe the principles and methods for cooking eggs.
■ cook eggs properly for breakfast menus and use eggs as ingredients in other foods.

Bulletin Board

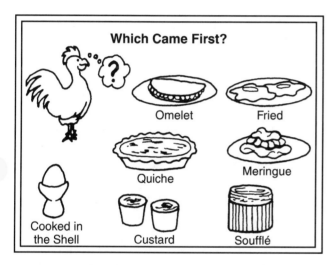

Which Came First?

Omelet   Fried
Quiche   Meringue
Cooked in the Shell   Custard   Soufflé

Title: "Which Came First?"

In the upper left corner of the bulletin board, place a drawing or cutout of a chicken with a thought cloud indicating that the bird is puzzled. Then randomly arrange pictures of various egg dishes on the board with appropriate labels.

Teaching Materials

Text, pages 271-284
Student Activity Guide
   A. *Selection and Storage of Eggs*
   B. *Functions of Eggs*
   C. *Egg Dishes*
   D. *Scrambled Eggs*

Teacher's Resource Binder
   Cooking Soft Custard, food science master 16-1
   Egg Recipes, recipe master 16-2
   Chapter 16 Study Sheet, reproducible master 16-3
   Anatomy of an Egg, color transparency CT-16

Chapter 16 Test
Software, diskette for Part Three
   Hangman, chapter review game

Introductory Activities

1. Have students list as many foods as they can that contain eggs.
2. Discuss with students why eggs are used in so many food products.
3. *Anatomy of an Egg,* color transparency CT-16, TRB. Use the transparency to identify for students the various parts of an egg.

Strategies to Reteach, Reinforce, Enrich, and Extend Text Concepts

Selecting and Storing Eggs

4. **ER** Have students investigate ways that food products containing eggs can be prepared to lower their cholesterol content.
5. **RT** Have students describe how eggs are graded and sized.
6. **RF** Have students find the medium weight per dozen for eggs of each of the six sizes.
7. **ER** Have students find out which breeds of chickens lay white-shelled eggs and which lay brown-shelled eggs.
8. **ER** Have students investigate the reason for storing eggs large end up.
9. **ER** Break into a dish an egg that has just been purchased, one that has been stored for one week, and one that has been stored for three weeks. Have students compare the appearance and quality of the three eggs.
10. **RF** Have students find recipes calling only for egg whites and recipes calling only for egg yolks.
11. **RF** *Selection and Storage of Eggs,* Activity A, SAG. Students are to complete exercises related to the selection and storage of eggs.

Eggs as Ingredients

12. **ER** Have students prepare a permanent and a temporary emulsion.

139

13. **ER**   Have students practice separating eggs.

14. **ER**   Have students compare the ease of separating cold eggs and eggs at room temperature.

15. **ER**   Have students compare the volume of an egg white foam produced from a cold egg with the volume of an egg white foam from a room temperature egg.

16. **ER**   Beat egg whites to the foamy stage, the soft peak stage, the stiff peak stage, and the overbeaten stage. Have students compare the volume and appearance.

17. **RF**   Have students describe the effects of adding fat, acid, and sugar to an egg white foam.

18. **ER**   Have students prepare a fruit-flavored gelatin and chill it to the syrupy stage. Then have them use a rubber spatula to practice folding two stiffly beaten egg whites into the gelatin.

19. **EX**   Have students prepare three batches of a sauce or pudding recipe that is thickened by both eggs and starch. For one batch, have them add the eggs with the other ingredients and cook the product over low to moderate heat until thickened. Have them prepare a second batch by stirring a small amount of the hot food product into the beaten eggs and then adding the warmed eggs to the remainder of the hot mixture. Have them prepare the third batch by adding the beaten eggs all at once to the hot mixture. Have them compare the appearance, texture, and flavor of the three products on a *Food Product Evaluation Sheet* (TRB).

20. **RF**   *Functions of Eggs,* Activity B, SAG. Students are to complete a chart describing the various functions performed by eggs and give examples of food products in which eggs perform each function.

21. **ER**   Have students prepare scrambled eggs from fresh eggs and from an egg substitute. Ask them to compare flavor, texture, and appearance on a *Food Product Evaluation Sheet* (TRB).

Food Science Principles of Cooking Eggs

22. **EX**   Have students scramble one egg over low to moderate heat for a short cooking time. Have them scramble another egg over high heat for a long cooking time. Have them compare the size and texture of the two products.

23. **EX**   Have students compare the coagulation temperatures of eggs without added ingredients and eggs individually prepared with salt, milk, sugar, and acid.

Methods of Cooking Eggs

24. **EX**   On a *Food Product Evaluation Sheet* (TRB), have students compare the flavor, texture, and appearance of scrambled eggs prepared on a rangetop with scrambled eggs prepared in a microwave oven.

25. **ER**   Have students prepare hard-cooked eggs by both the cold water method and the hot water method. Have the students explain which method they prefer to use.

26. **ER**   Have students use the hard-cooked eggs prepared in strategy 24 in a variety of recipes, such as egg salad and deviled eggs.

27. **ER**   Have students prepare both plain and puffy omelets with a variety of fillings.

28. **EX**   Have students plan a breakfast buffet. Each lab group should prepare eggs using a different method.

29. **ER**   Have students prepare a variety of dessert and main dish soufflés.

30. **EX**   *Cooking Soft Custard,* food science master 16-1, TRB. Have lab groups complete the experiment as directed on the master. Students will be applying principles of cooking eggs to the preparation of soft custard.

31. **ER**   Have students prepare a pie shell and fill it with a custard made with egg yolks. Have them use the egg whites to make a meringue. Have them seal the meringue to the pastry, and brown the meringue in the oven. Ask them to note any signs of weeping or beading.

32. **ER**   Have students prepare a soft custard and a baked custard. Ask them to explain how overcoagulation of the egg proteins can be prevented in each product.

33. **EX**   *Egg Recipes,* recipe master 16-2, TRB. Have students use the recipe master to plan an egg lab. Have each lab group complete a *Market Order Sheet* (TRB) and a *Time-Work Schedule* (TRB). After preparing their recipe and sampling their egg product, have each lab group complete a *Lab Evaluation Sheet* (TRB).

34. **RF**   *Egg Dishes,* Activity C, SAG. Students are to indicate whether various statements about cooking eggs are true or false.

Chapter Review

35. **RF** *Scrambled Eggs,* Activity D, SAG. Students are to unscramble letters and use the words to complete statements about eggs.
36. **RT** *Chapter 16 Study Sheet,* reproducible master 16-3, TRB. Have students complete the statements as they read text pages 272-280.
37. **RF** *Hangman,* Software, diskette for Part Three. Have students play the chapter review game according to the instructions that appear on the screen.

Above and Beyond

38. **EX** Have students design an experiment or demonstration that illustrates one of the functions of eggs as ingredients. Have them present their projects to the class using visual aids that they have made.

Answer Key

Text

Review What You Have Read, page 284
1. to quality-grade eggs
2. extra large, large, medium
3. in their original carton, large end up
4. (List five:) emulsifiers; a means of incorporating air (as foams); thickeners; binding agents; interfering agents; as nutrient, flavor, and color additives
5. (List four:) temperature, beating time, fat, acid, sugar
6. (List three:) soft and hard meringues, angel food and sponge cakes, soufflés, puffy omelets
7. false
8. (Describe two. Student response. See pages 277-278 in the text.)
9. cooking in simmering liquid
10. Remove eggs from the shell and gently puncture yolks with a fork or toothpick.
11. beading
12. Hard meringues contain a higher proportion of sugar and are baked at a lower temperature for a longer time than soft meringues.
13. Soft custards contain a smaller proportion of eggs to milk and are stirred more than baked custards.
14. C

Student Activity Guide

Selection and Storage of Eggs, Activity A, page 81
1. large
2. protein
3. cholesterol
4. candling
5. AA
6. A, B, C, E
7. grade and size
8. because they are usually used in the preparation of other food products
9. Eggs are sized on the basis of a medium weight per dozen.
10. medium or large
11. Shell color is determined by the breed of chicken.
12. Eggs should be stored in their original carton, large end up.
13. four to five weeks
14. Cover yolks with cold water and refrigerate in tightly covered container. Refrigerate whites in a tightly covered container.

Functions of Eggs, Activity B, page 82
(Descriptions:) Emulsifier—an ingredient that keeps oil droplets suspended in a water-based liquid to form a permanent emulsion.
Foam—the result of beating air into egg whites.
Thickener—an ingredient added to some cooked foods that causes them to thicken.
Binding agent—an ingredient used to hold other foods together.
Interfering agent—an ingredient that inhibits a reaction that would otherwise take place in a food product.
Structure agent—an ingredient that gives stability to baked products.
Nutrient additive—an ingredient that increases the nutritional value of a food product.
Flavoring additive—an ingredient that is used to flavor a food product.
Coloring agent—an ingredient that adds appealing color to a food product.
(Food products are student response.)

Egg Dishes, Activity C, page 83
1. E (true)
2. M (false)
3. U (false)
4. L (true)
5. S (true)
6. I (true)
7. F (false)
8. Y (false)

9. I (true)
10. N (true)
11. G (false)
12. A (false)
13. G (false)
14. E (true)
15. N (false)
16. T (true)

Correct answers spell *emulsifying agent.*

Scrambled Eggs, Activity D, page 84

1. stiff peak
2. interfering agent
3. omelet
4. beading
5. folding
6. poaching
7. emulsion
8. shirred
9. syneresis
10. soufflé
11. weeping
12. meringue
13. coagulum
14. candling
15. custard

Teacher's Resources

Chapter 16 Test

1. E		13. T	
2. B		14. T	
3. G		15. T	
4. D		16. T	
5. A		17. F	
6. F		18. F	
7. F		19. C	
8. T		20. C	
9. T		21. B	
10. T		22. D	
11. F		23. A	
12. F			

24. condition of the shell, size of the air cell, clearness and thickness of the egg white, and condition of the yolk
25. A Grade AA egg has a clean, unbroken shell and a small air cell. When broken into a dish, it has a thick, clear white that covers a small area. The yolk is thick and stands high above the white.
26. because extra ingredients dilute the proteins found in eggs
27. A greenish-colored ring around the yolk of a hard-cooked egg is caused by a chemical reaction between the iron in the egg yolk and hydrogen sulfide in the egg white. This discoloration takes place when eggs are overcooked.
28. Baked custard is tested by inserting the tip of a knife into the center of the custard. If the knife comes out clean, the custard is baked. Soft custards are tested with a metal spoon. A properly thickened soft custard will coat the back of the spoon.

Eggs

Name _____

Date _____ **Period** _____ **Score** _____

Chapter 16 Test

Matching: Match the following terms and identifying phrases.

_____ 1. Fluffy mixture of beaten egg whites and sugar that may be soft or hard.

_____ 2. Mixture of milk, eggs, sugar, and flavoring that is baked until firm or stirred and cooked until thickened.

_____ 3. Fluffy baked dish made with a starch-thickened sauce into which egg whites are folded.

_____ 4. Mixture that forms when oil and a water-based liquid are combined.

_____ 5. A smooth, thickened mass that forms when eggs are cooked.

_____ 6. A beaten egg mixture that is cooked without stirring and served folded in half.

A. coagulum
B. custard
C. egg foam
D. emulsion
E. meringue
F. omelet
G. soufflé

True/False: Circle *T* if the statement is true or *F* if the statement is false.

T   F   7. Most shoppers buy medium-sized eggs.

T   F   8. Many experts urge people to limit the number of egg yolks they eat because egg yolks are high in cholesterol.

T   F   9. Grade B eggs are rarely sold in food stores.

T   F   10. Eggs of any size can be Grade AA.

T   F   11. The color of an eggshell is a sign of quality.

T   F   12. Eggs should be stored small end up.

T   F   13. Eggs may be safely stored in a refrigerator for four to five weeks.

T   F   14. Mayonnaise is an example of a permanent emulsion.

T   F   15. When scrambling eggs, adding too much liquid will cause the coagulum to be small and firm.

T   F   16. When cooking eggs in the shell, the water should never be allowed to boil.

T   F   17. Eggs can be scrambled, poached, and cooked in the shell in a microwave oven.

T   F   18. After being cooked over medium heat, plain omelets are baked in an oven.

Multiple Choice: Choose the best response. Write the letter in the space provided.

_____ 19. An oil and vinegar dressing is an example of a _____.
   A. permanent emulsion
   B. semipermanent emulsion
   C. temporary emulsion
   D. None of the above.

(Continued)

Name _____

_____ 20. Which of the following inhibits the formation of an egg white foam?
   A. Acid.
   B. Cream of tartar.
   C. Fat.
   D. Sugar.

_____ 21. Egg whites that have reached full volume and have peaks that bend at the tips have been beaten to the _____.
   A. foamy stage
   B. soft peak stage
   C. stiff peak stage
   D. overbeaten stage

_____ 22. The layer of moisture that sometimes forms between a meringue and a pie filling is called _____.
   A. beading
   B. candling
   C. syneresis
   D. weeping

_____ 23. In which of the following products is syneresis likely to occur?
   A. Baked custard.
   B. Cheese soufflé.
   C. Poached egg.
   D. Soft meringue.

Essay Questions: Provide complete responses to the following questions or statements.

24. What four quality factors are used to determine egg grades?
25. Describe the appearance of a Grade AA egg.
26. Why does the addition of other ingredients change the coagulation temperature of eggs?
27. What causes a greenish ring around the yolks of hard-cooked eggs?
28. How are baked and soft custards tested for doneness?

Dairy Products

Objectives

After studying this chapter, students will be able to
- list factors affecting the selection of dairy products.
- describe guidelines for preventing adverse reactions when cooking with milk.
- prepare many different dishes using milk, cream, cheese, and other dairy products.

Bulletin Board

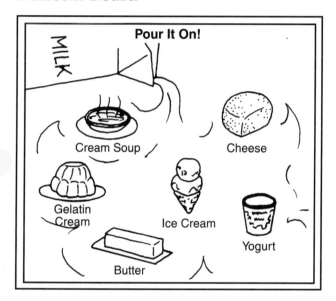

Title: "Pour It On!"

Draw a large milk carton in the upper left corner of the bulletin board with a stream of milk pouring from it down the length of the board. Show a variety of milk products, such as yogurt, cheese, ice cream, and butter, coming from the stream of milk.

Teaching Materials

Text, pages 285-303
Student Activity Guide
- A. *Dairy Product Variety*
- B. *Cheese Tasting*
- C. *Milk Cookery*
- D. *Dairy Products Crossword*
- E. *Dairy Desserts*

Teacher's Resource Binder
    Scum Formation on Milk, food science master 17-1
    Cream of Variety Soup, reproducible master 17-2
    Dairy Dessert Recipes, recipe master 17-3
    Cheese Recipes, recipe master 17-4
    Chapter 17 Study Sheet, reproducible master 17-5
    Factors Affecting Cost of Dairy Products, color transparency, CT-17
    Chapter 17 Test
Software, diskette for Part Three
    Bingo, chapter review game

Introductory Activities

1. Go around the room asking each student to name his or her favorite food. Make a list on the chalkboard. Then go through the list and have students identify all the foods that contain dairy products.
2. *Dairy Product Variety*, Activity A, SAG. Use this exercise to help students increase their awareness of the variety of dairy products available and the frequency with which people include them in the diet. Students are to identify the dairy products and foods containing dairy products in the menus on the worksheet. Then they are to write a shopping list of all the dairy products they would need to buy to prepare the menus and suggest snacks that can be made from some of these dairy products.

Strategies to Reteach, Reinforce, Enrich, and Extend Text Concepts

Selecting and Storing Dairy Products

3. **ER** Field trip. Take your class to visit a dairy farm or a creamery to see milk or milk product production.
4. **ER** Have students compare the flavor and body of goat's milk and goat's milk cheeses with the flavor and body of cow's milk and cow's milk cheeses.

5. **ER**   Allow students to sample UHT processed milk. Ask them to evaluate the flavor compared to milk from the dairy case. Then have them analyze the packaging of the UHT product.

6. **ER**   Have students make yogurt. Allow them to taste and evaluate samples of homemade and commercial yogurt.

7. **RF**   Have students read the ingredient labels on nondairy coffee whitener, nondairy whipped topping, and imitation sour cream. Have them compare these products with their dairy counterparts.

8. **ER**   Have students evaluate the appearance of evaporated milk and nonfat dry milk. Then reconstitute these products and have students compare the flavor and body of each product with the flavor and body of fluid, fresh milk.

9. **ER**   Have students visit the frozen food aisle of a grocery store and make a list of all the types of frozen dairy desserts that are available. Have students record the percentage of milkfat found in each type of product. Have them report their findings in class.

10. **ER**   Using baking powder biscuits or unsalted crackers as a base, have students sample salted butter, sweet butter, whipped butter, margarine made with corn oil, margarine containing animal fat, and whipped margarine. Have them evaluate the appearance, flavor, and texture of the products on a *Food Product Evaluation Sheet* (TRB).

11. **ER**   Have students prepare two basic shortened cakes. Have them use butter in the first cake and margarine in the second cake. Have them compare the flavor and color of the two cakes to see if they can detect a difference.

12. **EX**   Have students compare the nutrition and ingredient labels of several brands of margarine. From this comparison, have students write a brief conclusion about the link between margarine ingredients and saturated fat, polyunsaturated fat, and cholesterol content of margarine products.

13. **RF**   Have students find the cost of 8 ounces (250 mL) of fluid whole milk, lowfat milk, skim milk, buttermilk, diluted evaporated milk, and reconstituted nonfat dry milk to determine which product is the most economical.

14. **RF**   Have students make a bar graph illustrating the length of time various dairy products can be stored in the refrigerator.

15. **RT**   *Factors Affecting Cost of Dairy Products,* color transparency CT 17-1, TRB. Use the transparency as you discuss the various factors that affect the cost of dairy products.

16. **RF**   *Cheese Tasting,* Activity B, SAG. Students are to sample a variety of cheeses and complete a chart by describing the appearance, texture, and flavor of each cheese. Then they are to identify how the various cheeses would be used for cooking and eating.

17. **RF**   Have students compare the costs of American cheese sold in bulk, sliced, individually wrapped, and shredded. Ask them to explain why the different forms of American cheese vary in cost.

18. **RF**   *Dairy Products Crossword,* Activity D, SAG. Students are to review all the information on selection and storage of dairy products by completing the crossword puzzle.

Making the Lowfat Choice

19. **ER**   Have students visit a grocery store and make a list of the lowfat and nonfat dairy products available. Have students share their findings in class. Then take a poll to see which of the available products students have tried.

20. **ER**   Have each student use nutrition labels to prepare a chart comparing nutrients in a lowfat or nonfat dairy product with its whole milk or cream counterpart.

21. **ER**   Have students sample a variety of lowfat and nonfat diary products and compare their flavor and texture with whole milk and cream products.

Cooking with Milk and Cream

22. **RF**   Have students explain what causes the following undesirable reactions when heating milk: scum formation, boiling over, scorching, and curdling.

23. **EX**   *Scum Formation on Milk,* food science master 17-1, TRB. Have lab groups complete the experiment as directed on the master. Students will be comparing the effectiveness of various methods for preventing scum formation on the surface of milk during heating.

24. **EX**   *Cream of Variety Soup,* reproducible master 17-2, TRB. Divide the class into lab groups. Have each group prepare one of the soup recipes described on the master and then answer the evaluation questions at the

bottom of the page. If desired, have each lab group complete a *Time-Work Schedule* (TRB) before beginning to work in the lab.

25. **EX**   Have students prepare hot cocoa beverages using fresh fluid milk, reconstituted nonfat dry milk, and evaporated milk. Ask students to evaluate the products in terms of appearance, texture, and flavor. Ask them if they noticed any differences in the way the three products handled during cooking. Have them identify the beverage they prefer and explain why they prefer it.

26. **RF**   Have students describe the changes that take place when heavy cream is whipped. Then ask them to explain why milk and light cream will not behave in the same way.

27. **EX**   Have students whip samples of heavy whipping cream, light whipping cream, nonfat dry milk, and evaporated milk. Divide the samples in half. Refrigerate half of the samples. Evaluate the other half. Thirty minutes later, evaluate the refrigerated samples. Compare the stability and flavor with the first set of samples.

Preparing Common Milk-Based Foods

28. **RF**   Have students describe the cooking principles that are important in the preparation of a white sauce.

29. **ER**   Have lab groups prepare dishes made from each of the four different thicknesses of white sauce—thin, medium, thick, and very thick.

30. **RF**   *Milk Cookery,* Activity C, SAG. Students are to identify problems that occur when cooking with milk and suggest a method that could be used to prevent each problem. Then they are to identify the correct order of steps for preparing a white sauce.

31. **EX**   Have students use cookbooks to find a variety of recipes for thickened cream soups, bisques, and chowders. Have them use these recipes to plan a cream soup lab. Have each lab group complete a *Market Order Sheet* (TRB) and a *Time-Work Schedule* (TRB). After preparing their recipe and sampling their soup, have each group complete a *Lab Evaluation Sheet* (TRB).

32. **ER**   Divide the class into laboratory groups. Assign one of the following puddings to each group: cornstarch pudding, tapioca pudding, rice pudding, bread pudding, and Indian pudding. Have students identify what important cooking principles apply to each of these products.

33. **ER**   Have students prepare homemade chocolate cornstarch pudding, packaged chocolate pudding and pie filling, and packaged instant chocolate pudding. Place chilled samples of the puddings on an evaluation table along with samples of canned chocolate pudding and commercial refrigerated pudding. Have students compare the appearance, consistency, and flavor of the products on a *Food Product Evaluation Sheet* (TRB). Then have them give each product a final score on overall quality.

34. **ER**   Discuss with students the importance of hydration when cooking with gelatin. Then have them prepare a Spanish cream, a Bavarian cream, and a charlotte.

35. **RT**   Demonstrate for students how to unmold a gelatin cream.

36. **RT**   Have students define the terms *ice cream, sherbet, parfait,* and *mousse.*

37. **RF**   Have each student find a recipe for a frozen dessert that can be frozen in a typical kitchen freezer. Have students identify the interfering substances used in their recipe to keep ice crystals small.

38. **RF**   *Dairy Desserts,* Activity E, SAG. Students are to complete statements about dairy desserts.

39. **EX**   *Dairy Dessert Recipes,* recipe master 17-3, TRB. Have students use the recipe master to plan a dairy dessert lab. Have each lab group complete a *Market Order Sheet* (TRB) and a *Time-Work Schedule* (TRB). After preparing their recipe and sampling their dessert product, have each group complete a *Lab Evaluation Sheet* (TRB).

Cooking with Cheese

40. **ER**   Divide the class into laboratory groups. Assign one of the following cheese sauce products to each group: medium white sauce and sharp Cheddar cheese, medium white sauce and mild Cheddar cheese, medium white sauce and pasteurized process cheese, medium white sauce and pasteurized process cheese food, and condensed cheese soup used as a cheese sauce. Have students compare the appearance, texture, and flavor of the products on a *Food Product Evaluation Sheet* (TRB).

41. **ER**   As a demonstration of melting qualities, place two pieces of bread on a cookie sheet. Place one slice of Cheddar cheese on one piece of bread and one slice of pasteurized process cheese on the other. Cut each piece of bread into quarters. Place the cookie sheet in an oven set at 325°F (160°C). Remove one quarter from each piece of bread after 5 minutes, another after 10 minutes, another after 15 minutes, and the last after 20 minutes. Allow students to evaluate the appearance, flavor, and texture of the various samples.

42. **EX**   *Cheese Recipes,* recipe master 17-4, TRB. Have students use the recipe master to plan a cheese lab. Have each lab group complete a *Market Order Sheet* (TRB) and a *Time-Work Schedule* (TRB). After preparing their recipe and sampling their cheese product, have each group complete a *Lab Evaluation Sheet* (TRB).

Chapter Review

43. **RT**   *Chapter 17 Study Sheet,* reproducible master 17-5, TRB. Have students complete the statements as they read text pages 286-302.

44. **RF**   *Bingo,* Software, diskette for Part Three. Have students play the chapter review game according to the instructions that appear on the screen.

Above and Beyond

45. **ER**   Have students write a report or give a class presentation on one of the following topics:
   A. milk production
   B. product development in the dairy industry
   C. milk products and osteoporosis
   D. lactose intolerance
   E. use of dairy products in other cultures and animals used for milk production in those cultures

Answer Key

Text

Review What You Have Read, page 303
1. (List two for each. Student response.)
2. (Name and describe three. Student response. See pages 287-288 in the text.)
3. pasteurization
4. C
5. false
6. false
7. (Student response. See page 291 in the text.)
8. Ripened cheeses contain controlled amounts of bacteria, mold, yeast, or enzymes and are stored at specific temperature to develop texture and flavor. Unripened cheeses are prepared for marketing as soon as the whey has been removed.
9. true
10. by using low temperatures and fresh milk and by thickening either the milk or the acid before combining milk with an acid food
11. Sugar should be added to whipped cream a little bit at a time after thickening has begun. If sugar is added at the beginning of beating, it will increase beating time considerably.
12. (List four:) other sauces, gravies, cream soups, creamed vegetables, creamed meats, soufflés, croquettes
13. false
14. to keep the ice crystals that form during freezing small so the frozen dessert will have a smooth and creamy texture
15. (List three:) whipped cream, whipped evaporated milk, whipped gelatin, beaten egg whites
16. to prevent overcoagulation of the proteins that will make the cheese tough and rubbery

Student Activity Guide

Dairy Product Variety, Activity A, page 85
Students should underline the following menu items:

Day 1	Day 2
Breakfast	
milk	cream cheese
	chocolate milk
Lunch	
grilled American cheese sandwiches	grilled ham and Swiss sandwiches
cream of tomato soup	yogurt dressing
Dinner	
Cheddar cheese sauce	cottage cheese
whipped cream	butter pecan ice
milk	cream

   (Students may justify underlining additional menu items in which dairy products might be used. For instance, whole wheat toast could be underlined because it might be spread with butter. Inclusion of such items should also be reflected in the shopping list.)

Shopping List

milk	chocolate milk
American cheese	Swiss cheese
Cheddar cheese	yogurt
whipping cream	cottage cheese
cream cheese	butter pecan ice cream

(Snacks are student response.)

Milk Cookery, Activity C, page 87

Problem 1: Curdling. This problem can be prevented by using low temperatures and fresh milk.
Problem 2: Scum formation. This problem can be prevented by stirring the milk during heating, beating the milk with a rotary beater, or covering the pan.
Problem 3: Scorching. This problem can be prevented by using low heat or by heating the pudding in the top of a double boiler.

1. C
2. R
3. E
4. A
5. M
6. S
7. O
8. U
9. P
10. (List five:) a base for other sauces, cream soups, gravies, casseroles, soufflés, creamed vegetables, croquettes

Dairy Products Crossword, Activity D, pages 88-89

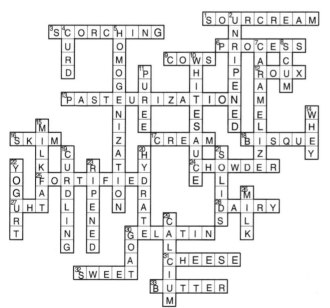

Dairy Desserts, Activity E, page 90

1. sherbet
2. Bavarian creams
3. bread pudding
4. charlottes
5. Indian pudding
6. ice cream
7. frozen yogurt
8. parfaits
9. cornstarch pudding
10. mousses
11. tapioca pudding
12. Spanish creams

Teacher's Resources

Chapter 17 Test

1.	A	13.	F	25.	F
2.	B	14.	F	26.	D
3.	F	15.	T	27.	A
4.	G	16.	T	28.	D
5.	C	17.	T	29.	B
6.	K	18.	T	30.	C
7.	H	19.	F	31.	A
8.	I	20.	T	32.	B
9.	D	21.	T	33.	A
10.	E	22.	F	34.	A
11.	F	23.	T	35.	B
12.	T	24.	T		

36. to destroy any harmful bacterial that may be present
37. Ripened cheeses are made by adding controlled amounts of bacteria, mold, yeast, or enzymes to the milk mixture and storing the finished cheeses at a specific temperature for a certain period of time.
38. Boiling over usually is caused by scum formation. A scum layer forms, pressure builds up under the layer as the milk heats, and the scum layer prevents the pressure from being released as steam. When the pressure becomes great enough, the milk will boil over.
39. Sugar decreases both the volume and stiffness of whipped cream. It also increases beating time if added before the cream has begun to thicken.
40. Mixing the cornstarch, sugar, and salt together thoroughly then adding a small amount of cold milk to form a paste will prevent lumping by separating the starch granules. Adding a small amount of hot pudding to beaten eggs before adding the diluted egg mixture to the rest of the hot pudding will prevent lumps due to coagulated egg proteins.

Dairy Products

Name _____

Date _____ Period _____ Score _____

Chapter 17 Test

Matching: Match the following terms with their definitions.

_____   1. To heat sugar until it changes into a brown, bitter substance.

_____   2. Solid portion of coagulated milk.

_____   3. To cause a substance to absorb water.

_____   4. Portion of milk containing most of the vitamins, minerals, proteins, and sugar.

_____   5. Milk to which nutrients have been added in amounts greater than would naturally occur.

_____   6. Liquid part of coagulated milk.

_____   7. Process by which dairy products are heated to destroy harmful bacteria.

_____   8. A product made from various cheeses.

_____   9. A gummy substance made from animal bones and connective tissues.

_____   10. A mechanical process that prevents cream from rising to the surface of milk.

A. caramelize
B. curd
C. fortified milk
D. gelatin
E. homogenization
F. hydrate
G. milk solids
H. pasteurization
I. process cheese
J. scorching
K. whey

True/False: Circle *T* if the statement is true or *F* if the statement is false.

T   F   11. All milk and milk products sold in the United States must be homogenized.

T   F   12. Yogurt and buttermilk are cultured milk products.

T   F   13. Salted butter is more perishable than sweet butter.

T   F   14. Ripened cheeses are ready for marketing as soon as the whey has been removed.

T   F   15. Stirring or beating milk during heating will help prevent scum formation.

T   F   16. Milk and milk products are generally microwaved on lower settings to prevent curdling.

T   F   17. Cream containing 30 percent milkfat will produce a stable whipped product.

T   F   18. A roux is a cooked fat and flour mixture used as the thickening agent in white sauce.

T   F   19. Indian pudding is thickened with tapioca.

T   F   20. Both protein and starch cooking principles are used in the preparation of puddings.

T   F   21. A Spanish cream is a molded custard.

T   F   22. When preparing a gelatin cream, the unflavored gelatin must first be soaked in a hot liquid.

T   F   23. Parfaits are not stirred during freezing.

T   F   24. Frozen desserts made in an ice cream freezer have better flavor if allowed to ripen for a short time.

T   F   25. Cheese is high in carbohydrates, so it must be cooked at a very low temperature.

(Continued)

Name _____

Multiple Choice: Choose the best response. Write the letter in the space provided.

_____ 26. Milk that is heated to a higher temperature than regular pasteurized milk to increase its shelf life is _____.
   A. fortified milk
   B. homogenized milk
   C. lactose reduced milk
   D. UHT processed milk

_____ 27. Whole milk that has had some of the water removed and a sweetener added is called _____.
   A. condensed milk
   B. dried whole milk
   C. evaporated milk
   D. nonfat dry milk

_____ 28. Choosing lowfat or nonfat dairy products in place of whole milk and cream products can help you _____.
   A. reduce your fat intake
   B. reduce your calorie intake
   C. follow dietary guidelines
   D. All of the above.

_____ 29. When heating milk, which of the following is caused by acids, tannins, enzymes, and salts?
   A. Boiling over.
   B. Curdling.
   C. Scorching.
   D. Scum formation.

_____ 30. When whipping cream, sugar should be added _____.
   A. at the start of beating
   B. after cream has reached maximum stiffness
   C. after cream has begun to thicken
   D. after soft peaks has formed

_____ 31. Which of the following ingredients is *not* part of a white sauce?
   A. Eggs.
   B. Fat.
   C. Flour.
   D. Milk.

_____ 32. Which of the following would be used to prepare a soufflé?
   A. Medium white sauce.
   B. Thick white sauce.
   C. Very thick white sauce.
   D. Cornstarch-thickened sauce.

_____ 33. A rich, milk-based soup in which light cream often replaces all or part of the milk is a _____.
   A. bisque
   B. chowder
   C. puree
   D. thickened cream soup

(Continued)

Name _____

_____ 34. A milk-based dessert made by folding beat egg whites, whipped cream, and flavorings or fruit purees into a whipped, thickened gelatin is called a _____.
   A. Bavarian cream
   B. charlotte
   C. gelatin cream
   D. Spanish cream

_____ 35. If you were making chocolate ice cream, which of the following ingredients would *not* be an acceptable interfering agent?
   A. Beaten egg whites.
   B. Melted chocolate.
   C. Whipped cream.
   D. Whipped evaporated milk.

Essay Questions: Provide complete responses to the following questions or statements.

36. Why is milk pasteurized?
37. How are ripened cheeses made?
38. How are the problems of boiling over and scum formation related?
39. How does sugar affect the whipping properties of cream?
40. How can you prevent a cornstarch pudding from lumping?

Fruits

Objectives

After studying this chapter, students will be able to
- describe how to properly select and store fruits.
- discuss the principles and methods of fruit cookery.
- prepare fruits, preserving their color, texture, flavor, and nutrients.

Bulletin Board

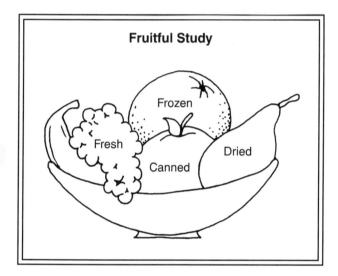

Fruitful Study

Title: "Fruitful Study"
    Use cutouts of large pieces of fruit filling a fruit bowl. Place labels on some of the pieces of fruit to indicate the various forms in which fruit can be purchased.

Teaching Materials

Text, pages 305-314
Student Activity Guide
    A. *Fruit Scramble*
    B. *Mixed Fruit*

Teacher's Resource Binder
    Evaluating Fruit Ripeness, food science master 18-1
    Fruit Recipes, recipe master 18-2
    Chapter 18 Study Sheet, reproducible master 18-3

    Are Pesticides Bugging the Environment? reproducible master 18-4
    Selecting Fresh Fruits and Vegetables, color transparency CT-18A
    Peak Seasons for Fresh Fruits, color transparency CT-18B
    Chapter 18 Test
Software, diskette for Part Three
    Tic Tac Toe, chapter review game

Introductory Activities

1. Review with students the number of daily servings needed from the fruit group of the Food Guide Pyramid. Ask students what important nutrients fruits supply.
2. Have students suggest ways that fruits can be included in meals throughout the day.

Strategies to Reteach, Reinforce, Enrich, and Extend Text Concepts

Choosing Fresh Fruit

3. **ER** Field trip. Take your class to a pick-your-own orchard or berry patch.
4. **ER** Guest speaker. Invite a produce manager from a grocery store to speak to your class about the seasonal availability of fruit. Ask the manager to describe how fruits are shipped and handled to maintain their quality.
5. **ER** Have students visit the produce section of a supermarket and make a list of the fruits that are available. Have them make another list of fruits that will be available in six months.
6. **ER** Display for students a banana that is at its peak of quality, an overripe banana, and an underripe banana. Allow the students to sample the three bananas and compare them for appearance, flavor, and texture.
7. **EX** *Evaluating Fruit Ripeness,* food science master 18-1, TRB. Have lab groups complete the two-part experiment as directed on the master. In the first part of the experiment, students will be comparing fruit in various stages of ripeness. For this part, you will

need to provide one underripe peach, one top quality peach, and one overripe peach for each lab group. Use masking tape labels to randomly label the peaches for each group as A, B, and C. Allow students to use their reading and observations to determine the correct level of ripeness of each peach. In the second part of the experiment, students will be evaluating the effects of refrigeration on the ripening of fruit following a three-day storage period. For this part, you will need to provide two underripe peaches and two top quality peaches for each lab group. Both parts of this experiment require students to test the pH of fruit with litmus paper. You may wish to review the concept of pH and proper testing procedure with students before beginning the experiment.

8. **RT** *Selecting Fresh Fruits and Vegetables,* color transparency CT-18A, TRB. Use the transparency to review basic guidelines to follow when buying fresh produce.

9. **RT** *Peak Seasons for Fresh Fruits,* color transparency CT-18B, TRB. Use the transparency to illustrate the peak seasons for buying popular fruits.

10. **RF** *Fruit Scramble,* Activity A, SAG. Students are to unscramble the names of various fruits and identify the classification to which each fruit belongs.

Choosing Canned, Frozen, and Dried Fruit

11. **RF** Have students make a list of those fruits that are available in all four forms—fresh, canned, frozen, and dried.

12. **EX** Have students compare the cost and appearance of generic, house brand, and national brand canned peaches. Ask them to suggest appropriate uses for each of the three products.

13. **ER** Have students compare the cost of a canned fruit with its fresh and frozen counterparts to determine which form is the most economical. Have them do this with a fruit that is in season as well as with a fruit that is not in season.

14. **ER** Have students sample canned pineapple packed in juice and canned pineapple packed in syrup. Ask students to identify which product they prefer and explain why.

15. **EX** Have students compare the texture of a thawed frozen fruit with its fresh counterpart. Have them suggest uses for the frozen

fruit in which its inferior texture qualities would not matter.

16. **ER** Have students use Appendix B (Nutritive Values of Foods) on pages 617-634 of the text to calculate the difference between the percentage of water in fresh and dried apples, apricots, peaches, prunes (plums), and raisins (grapes).

17. **EX** Have students use Appendix B (Nutritive Values of Foods) on pages 617-634 of the text to calculate the number of calories per gram provided by fresh and dried apples, apricots, peaches, prunes (plums), and raisins (grapes). Ask students to evaluate what this indicates about including dried fruits in the diet.

Preparing Fruits

18. **EX** Slice an apple into rings. Divide the rings evenly between two saucers. Dip the slices on one saucer into lemon juice. Allow both groups of apple slices to stand uncovered for one hour. Have students record their observations and give explanations.

19. **RF** Have students find appetizer, salad, and dessert recipes made with raw fruits.

20. **ER** Have students practice sectioning raw citrus fruits for use in a fruit salad.

21. **RT** Demonstrate for students different ways they can cut raw fruits to create interesting and appealing shapes in fruit dishes.

22. **ER** Have students prepare a fresh fruit tray including a variety of tropical fruits that they have not tried before.

23. **ER** Have students reconstitute a dried fruit. Have them use a *Food Product Evaluation Sheet* (TRB) to compare it with its fresh, canned, and frozen counterparts in terms of flavor, texture, appearance, and cost.

24. **ER** Divide the class into lab groups. Have each group prepare peach crisp using a different form of the fruit—fresh, canned, frozen, or dried. Have students sample each version and compare the appearance, flavor, and cost of the finished products.

25. **EX** Divide the class into three groups. Assign one of the following fruit preparations to each group: fruit cooked without sugar for 12 minutes; fruit cooked with ¼ cup (50 mL) sugar added before cooking and then cooked for 12 minutes; fruit cooked with ¼ cup (50 mL) sugar added after the first eight minutes of cooking, followed by

four additional minutes of cooking. In each instance, use 1 cup (250 mL) fresh rhubarb cut into ½ inch pieces. Have students display rhubarb with its cooking liquid for observation. Have them compare the appearance, texture, and sweetness of the samples and explain their observations.

26. **EX** *Fruit Recipes*, recipe master, TRB. Have students use the recipe master and additional recipes, as desired, to prepare a variety of cooked fruits using each of the methods described in the text. Have each lab group complete a *Market Order Sheet* (TRB) and a *Time-Work Schedule* (TRB). Serve the fruits buffet style. Have each lab group complete a *Lab Evaluation Sheet* (TRB) based on the product they prepared.

27. **ER** Have students use cookbooks found in the library and in the classroom to find at least six recipes for products made with dried fruits. Have students prepare at least three of the products. Evaluate the products as a class.

Chapter Review

28. **RF** *Mixed Fruit*, Activity B, SAG. Students are to describe how to select, store, and prepare the various fruits listed on the activity sheet.

29. **RT** *Chapter 18 Study Sheet*, reproducible master 18-3, TRB. Have students complete the statements as they read text pages 306-313.

30. **RF** *Tic Tac Toe*, Software, diskette for Part Three. Have students play the chapter review game according to the instructions that appear on the screen.

Above and Beyond

31. **EX** Have each student plan and prepare a marketing campaign for the fruit of his or her choice. Each campaign should involve the development of two of the following promotional materials:
   A. magazine ad
   B. poster or billboard
   C. informational leaflet for consumers
   D. radio or television ad
   E. newspaper food page
   Promotional materials may include harvesting information, selection and storage tips, serving suggestions, recipe ideas, etc. Encourage students to choose an angle, such as vitamin or fiber content, seasonal availability, or cooking versatility, to use as the focus of their campaign. Have students identify to whom their campaign is geared—teens, homemakers, children, etc. Have students give a marketing presentation to the class or write a report summarizing why they chose the strategies they did. Have them explain why they think those strategies would be successful in getting consumers to buy the fruit. You may wish to ask a panel of teachers or community members to judge the campaigns and award prizes for those that are most creative.

32. **EX** *Are Pesticides Bugging the Environment?* reproducible master 18-4, TRB. Have students read the article. Then have them form two teams to debate the use of pesticides. Both teams should conduct research to support the arguments they will be raising.

Answer Key

Text

Review What You Have Read, page 314
1. berries, drupes, pomes, citrus fruits, melons, tropical fruits (For examples, see page 306 in the text.)
2. C
3. Underripe fruits are fruits that are full size but have not yet reached peak eating quality. They will ripen at room temperature. Immature fruits have not reached full size and will not improve in quality when left at room temperature.
4. (List three. Student response. See page 307 in the text.)
5. true
6. during their peak growing season
7. fruit juice, light syrup, heavy syrup, extra heavy syrup
8. enzymatic browning
9. (Describe three:) Cellulose softens and makes fruit easier to digest. Colors change. Heat-sensitive and water-soluble nutrients may be lost. Flavors become less acidic and more mellow.
10. true
11. two to one
12. fritters
13. (List three:) type of fruit, size, ripeness, moisture content

14. Dried fruits are usually soaked in hot water for about an hour before cooking.

Student Activity Guide

Fruit Scramble, Activity A, page 91
1. oranges, citrus fruits
2. apples, pomes
3. bananas, tropical fruits
4. pineapples, tropical fruits
5. cantaloupe, melons
6. blueberries, berries
7. strawberries, berries
8. grapefruit, citrus fruits
9. grapes, berries
10. papaya, tropical fruits
11. kiwifruit, tropical fruits
12. cherries, drupes
13. honeydew, melons
14. pears, pomes
15. tangerines, citrus fruits
16. apricots, drupes
17. lemons, citrus fruits
18. watermelon, melons
19. plums, drupes
20. peaches, drupes
21. figs, tropical fruits
22. avocado, tropical fruits
23. cranberries, berries
24. limes, citrus fruits
25. casaba, melons

Mixed Fruit, Activity B, page 92
1. Use: (Student response.)
   Selection: Packages should be clean, undamaged, and frozen solid.
   Storage: Store in the coldest part of the freezer. Store thawed, unused berries in a tightly covered container in the refrigerator.
   Preparation: (Student response.)
2. Selection: Fruit should be firm, have a bright color, and be free from defects.
   Storage: Ripen at room temperature. Refrigerate ripened fruit.
   Preparation: Dip cut bananas in lemon, orange, grapefruit, or pineapple juice to prevent enzymatic browning and make them look more appealing.

3. Use: (Student response.)
   Selection: Cans should be free from dents, bulges, and leaks.
   Storage: Store cans in a cool, dry place. Cover and refrigerate fruit after opening.
   Preparation: (Student response.)
4. Selection: Fruit should be soft and pliable.
   Storage: Store unopened package in cool, dark, dry place. After opening, store in tightly covered container.
   Preparation: Soak in hot water for about an hour before cooking to soften and rehydrate.

Teacher's Resources

Chapter 18 Test

1. B	12. F
2. F	13. T
3. C	14. F
4. A	15. T
5. G	16. T
6. E	17. C
7. F	18. A
8. F	19. D
9. T	20. C
10. T	21. D
11. T	

22. ripeness and maturity
23. Berries should be covered loosely and refrigerated. They should not be washed until ready to be used.
24. to make fruit more palatable and easier to digest, to add variety to a meal, and to make use of overripe fruits
25. Fruits that undergo enzymatic browning will retain their colors if cooked with a small amount of lemon or orange juice. Water-soluble nutrients will be retained if the fruit is cooked in a small amount of water just until tender. Natural flavors will be retained if the fruit is not overcooked. Shape will be retained if the fruit is cooked in a sugar syrup instead of plain water.
26. because frozen fruits that are completely thawed are often soft and mushy

Fruits

Name _____

Date _____ **Period** _____ **Score** _____

Chapter 18 Test

Matching: Match the following classifications of fruits with their descriptions.

_____ 1. Have thick rinds and thin membranes separating the flesh into segments.

_____ 2. Have a central, seed-containing core surrounded by a thick layer of flesh.

_____ 3. Have a skin covering a soft flesh that surrounds a single, hard pit.

_____ 4. Are small and juicy and have a thin skin.

_____ 5. Are grown in warm climates and are considered to be somewhat exotic.

_____ 6. Are in the gourd family and are large and juicy with a thick skin and many seeds.

A. berries
B. citrus fruits
C. drupes
D. immature fruits
E. melons
F. pomes
G. tropical fruits

True/False: Circle *T* if the statement is true or *F* if the statement is false.

T   F   7. Fruits are only available fresh during the short time of year when they are in season.

T   F   8. Cherries, apricots, and plums belong to the group of fruits known as pomes.

T   F   9. Fruits are good sources of vitamins and fiber.

T   F   10. When pressed gently, ripe fruits should give slightly.

T   F   11. Some fruits can be purchased underripe.

T   F   12. Berries, melons, and grapes can be stored longer than apples and citrus fruits.

T   F   13. Fruits may lose some texture qualities during freezing.

T   F   14. Fresh fruits should be soaked before serving.

T   F   15. When making a fruit sauce, adding sugar at the end of the cooking will thin the product.

T   F   16. Fruits covered with a tight skin should be pierced if they are to be microwaved whole.

Multiple Choice: Choose the best response. Write the letter in the space provided.

_____ 17. Which of the following is a good source of vitamin A?
  A. Apples.
  B. Cherries.
  C. Peaches.
  D. Pears.

_____ 18. Which of the following should *not* be purchased?
  A. Immature pears.
  B. Plump, firm cherries.
  C. Slightly soft plums.
  D. Underripe bananas.

(Continued)

Name _____

_____ 19. Which of the following would *not* be used as a packing liquid for canned fruit?
   A. Fruit juice.
   B. Heavy syrup.
   C. Light syrup.
   D. Water.

_____ 20. Which of the following fruits is *not* subject to enzymatic browning?
   A. Apples.
   B. Bananas.
   C. Oranges.
   D. Peaches.

_____ 21. Fruits coated with a batter and deep-fried are called _____.
   A. beignets
   B. croquettes
   C. crullers
   D. fritters

Essay Questions: Provide complete responses to the following questions or statements.

22. What two factors determine the quality of fresh fruit?
23. How should berries be handled after they are purchased?
24. Why are fruits cooked?
25. Give guidelines for helping cooked fruits retain their colors, nutrients, flavors, and shapes.
26. Why should frozen fruits be served with a few ice crystals remaining in them?

Vegetables

Objectives

After studying this chapter, students will be able to
- explain how to properly select and store vegetables.
- discuss food science principles of cooking vegetables.
- describe methods for cooking vegetables.
- prepare vegetables, preserving their color, texture, flavor, and nutrients.

Bulletin Board

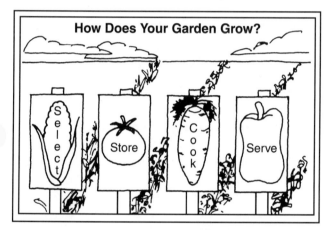

Title: "How Does Your Garden Grow?"

Sketch the background of the bulletin board to look like a vegetable garden. In the foreground, use cutouts of vegetables to make row markers. Label each of the markers with a key concept from the chapter, such as selection, storage, cooking, and serving.

Teaching Materials

Text, pages 315-326
Student Activity Guide
    A. *Vegetable Selection and Storage*
    B. *Vegetable Maze*
    C. *Cooking Vegetables by Class*

Teacher's Resource Binder
    Testing Acidity of Vegetables, food science master 19-1
    Vegetable Recipes, recipe master 19-2
    Chapter 19 Study Sheet, reproducible master 19-3

    Peak Seasons for Fresh Vegetables, color transparency CT-19
    Chapter 19 Test
Software, diskette for Part Three
    Tic Tac Toe, chapter review game

Introductory Activities

1. Ask students if they like vegetables. If you receive a favorable response, find out what their favorite vegetables are and ask the students how they like to have these vegetables prepared. If you receive a negative response, ask students why they do not like vegetables. Try to see if you can change some of these negative opinions through the study of this chapter.
2. Bring in samples or pictures of some of the more "exotic" vegetables, such as bok choy, radicchio, cilantro, etc. See how many of these vegetables students are able to identify. Allow them to try samples of these vegetables.

Strategies to Reteach, Reinforce, Enrich, and Extend Text Concepts

Choosing Fresh Vegetables

3. **ER** Field trip. Take your class to a farmers' market to see the variety of seasonal vegetables that are available. If possible, have students ask the people selling the vegetables about the growth and productivity of various vegetable crops.
4. **RF** Have each student divide a piece of paper vertically into eight columns and head each column with the name of one vegetable group—bulbs, flowers, fruits, stems, leaves, seeds, tubers, and roots. Then have students fill in each column with the names of vegetables that belong to that particular group. You may also wish to have them include pictures of as many vegetables as possible.
5. **ER** Have students visit the produce section of a grocery store. Have them make a list of the vegetables that are available now. Then

have them make another list of vegetables that will be available in six months.

6. **RF**   Have students describe how the following fresh vegetables should be stored: potatoes, tomatoes, sweet corn, onions, green beans, and acorn squash.

Choosing Canned, Frozen, and Dried Vegetables

7. **ER**   Divide the class into six lab groups. Assign each group one of the following vegetables: corn, carrots, potatoes, green beans, spinach, and beets. Have each group cook the fresh, canned, and frozen forms of their assigned vegetable. Display the vegetables buffet style. Have students evaluate samples of all the vegetables in terms of appearance, flavor, color, and texture on a *Food Product Evaluation Sheet* (TRB). For each vegetable, have students identify which form they prefer and explain why.

8. **ER**   Have students visit the frozen food section of a grocery store. Have them compare the cost per serving of plain and specialty frozen vegetables (for example, plain chopped spinach and creamed spinach).

9. **ER**   Have students make a showcase display of dried legumes available in your area. Have them identify each legume in the display and list a few of its uses.

10. **RF**   *Vegetable Selection and Storage*, Activity A, SAG. Students are to rewrite false statements about vegetables to make them true.

Preparing Vegetables

11. **RT**   Demonstrate for students how to prepare fresh vegetables. Select a number of vegetables that are often served raw. Wash them thoroughly and cut them into attractive shapes for serving. Arrange them on a tray and serve them with a dip.

12. **EX**   Prepare three samples of fresh broccoli. Cook each sample in a small amount of water. Begin timing when the water has returned to a boil. Cook the first sample for 3 minutes, the second sample for 10 minutes, and the third sample for 15 minutes. Drain each sample, reserving the cooking liquid in a glass container. Have students evaluate the samples, comparing the appearance, flavor, and texture of the vegetable and the color of the cooking liquid. Have students explain their observations.

13. **EX**   Divide the class into four lab groups. Have each group prepare one of the following vegetables: carrots, broccoli, red cabbage, and cauliflower. Have each group prepare four samples as follows: lid on, lid off, 1 teaspoon (5 mL) vinegar added to cooking water, ½ teaspoon (2 mL) baking soda added to cooking water. Students should use a small amount of water for all samples. Have students compare the colors and textures of all vegetables and explain their observations.

14. **EX**   *Testing Acidity of Vegetables*, food science master 19-1, TRB. Have lab groups complete the experiment as directed on the master. Students will be preparing an indicator solution and using it to compare the acidity of the cooking liquid from various vegetables.

15. **EX**   Divide the class into three lab groups. Have each group prepare one of the following vegetables: peas, green cabbage, and onions. Have each group prepare four samples as follows: lid on, small amount of water, cook until crisp-tender; lid on, small amount of water, cook 20 minutes; lid off, large amount of water, cook until crisp-tender; cook by steaming until crisp-tender. Have students compare the color, flavor, and texture of each sample on a *Food Product Evaluation Sheet* (TRB) and explain their observations.

16. **EX**   *Vegetable Recipes*, recipe master 19-2, TRB. Have students use the recipe master to plan a vegetable lab. Have each lab group complete a *Market Order Sheet* (TRB) and a *Time-Work Schedule* (TRB). After preparing their recipe and sampling their vegetable product, have each group complete a *Lab Evaluation Sheet* (TRB).

17. **RF**   *Cooking Vegetables by Class*, Activity C, SAG. Students are to identify cooking methods recommended for vegetables of different pigments and flavor strengths.

18. **EX**   Divide the class into four lab groups. Assign one of the following potato preparations to each group: baked, mashed, boiled, and fried. Have each group prepare three samples, using different varieties of potatoes: waxy, all-purpose, and mealy. Set up an evaluation table. Have students compare the appearance, texture, and flavor of the samples on a *Food Product Evaluation Sheet* (TRB). Then have them categorize each variety of potato according to its best use.

19. **ER** Have each lab group find a recipe and prepare a meatless main dish using dried legumes as a meat substitute.
20. **ER** Have lab groups use a variety of vegetables and cooking methods to prepare a vegetable buffet. Serve the vegetables with an assortment of toppings and sauces.

Chapter Review

21. **RF** *Vegetable Maze,* Activity B, SAG. Students are to use terms related to vegetables to complete statements. Then they are to find and circle the terms in a maze.
22. **RT** *Chapter 19 Study Sheet,* reproducible master 19-3, TRB. Have students complete the statements as they read text pages 316-324.
23. **RF** *Tic Tac Toe,* Software, diskette for Part Three. Have students play the chapter review game according to the instructions that appear on the screen.

Above and Beyond

24. **ER** Have each student select a vegetable. Have students investigate the planting, tending, and harvesting requirements for the vegetables they have chosen. (During the winter, students should limit their selections to vegetables that can be grown indoors.) Then have students obtain seeds or starter plants and plant their vegetables. Students should record their observations and sketch their plants periodically during the growing period. Have students harvest their vegetables and bring them in to show the class. Students whose plants did not successfully produce vegetables should give a brief report explaining why based on their observations. (You may want to arrange for an agriculture teacher or a horticulture or biology teacher to serve as a resource person on this project.)

Answer Key

Text

Review What You Have Read, page 326
1. bulbs, flowers, fruits, stems, leaves, seeds, tubers, roots (For examples, see page 316 in the text.)
2. succulents
3. (List three. Student response. See page 316 in the text.)
4. It is important to wash fresh vegetables to remove dirt, bacteria, and pesticide residues. Use cool running water or several changes of cool water and a brush to get into crevices and cracks. Handle vegetables carefully and never soak them.
5. (List three:) Cellulose softens. Starch absorbs water and swells. Flavors change. Colors change. Some nutrients may be lost.
6. false
7. D
8. mild—cook in a small amount of water, with the pan covered for a short time
   strong—cover with water and cook in an uncovered pan for a short time
   very strong—cover with water and cook in an uncovered pan for a longer time
9. (List four:) cooking in water, steaming, pressure cooking, baking, frying, broiling, microwaving (For descriptions, see pages 321-323 in the text.)
10. served with the vegetables or added to gravies, soups, or sauces
11. a mealy or all-purpose variety
12. true

Student Activity Guide

Vegetable Selection and Storage, Activity A, page 93
1. Vegetables are often grouped according to the part of the plant from which they come.
2. Broccoli, green peppers, and raw cabbage are excellent sources of vitamin C.
3. When selecting vegetables select those that are medium in size.
4. Fresh vegetables lose quality quickly, so buy only what you will use within a short time.
5. Vegetables that are in season usually are high in quality and low in price.
6. Wash vegetables quickly and shake to remove excess water. Soaking vegetables will result in a loss of water-soluble nutrients.
7. Choose cans that are free from dents, bulges, and leaks. Choose house brands and lower qualities of products to save money.
8. Frozen vegetables retain the appearance and flavor of fresh vegetables better than canned and dried vegetables.
9. Choose packages that are clean and solidly frozen. A heavy layer of ice on the package may indicate that the vegetables were thawed and refrozen.
10. Dried vegetables of greatest commercial importance are peas, beans, and lentils.

Vegetable Maze, Activity B, pages 94-95

1. stem
2. brush
3. succulents
4. water-soluble
5. root
6. bulb
7. cellulose
8. crisp
9. tuber
10. anthocyanin
11. seed
12. canned
13. chlorophyll
14. baking soda
15. carotene
16. new
17. alkali
18. flavones
19. blanching
20. soaked
21. acid
22. color
23. flowers
24. skins
25. peak

Cooking Vegetables by Class, Activity C, page 96

1. chlorophyll
   Cook green vegetables in a small amount of water. Use a short cooking time and keep the pan lid off for the first few minutes of cooking. Then cover the pan for the remainder of the cooking period.
2. carotene
   Cook most yellow vegetables in a small amount of water with the pan covered.
3. flavones
   Avoid overcooking to prevent undesirable color changes.
4. anthocyanin
   Cook most red vegetables in a small amount of water, with the pan lid on, just until tender.
5. peas, green beans, spinach, corn, beets, parsnips
   Cook most mildly flavored vegetables in a small amount of water, with the pan covered, for a short time.
6. cabbage, broccoli, Brussels sprouts, yellow turnips
   Cover strongly flavored vegetables with water. Cook them in an uncovered pan for a short time.
7. leeks, onions
   Cover very strongly flavored vegetables with water. Cook them in an uncovered pan for a longer time.

Teacher's Resources

Chapter 19 Test

1. C
2. H
3. F
4. I
5. E
6. G
7. B
8. D
9. T
10. T
11. F
12. T
13. F
14. T
15. F
16. T
17. F
18. T
19. C
20. D
21. A
22. C
23. B
24. Vegetables that are very small can be immature and lack flavor. Very large vegetables can be overmature and tough.
25. (List five:) navy beans, lima beans, split peas, lentils, pinto beans, red beans, black-eyed peas, garbanzo beans, kidney beans, soybeans
26. Wash them carefully, trim any bruised areas, wilted leaves, and thick stems; and peel with a vegetable scraper or floating edge peeler, if desired.
27. The cellulose (fiber) softens to make chewing easier; the starch absorbs water, swells, and becomes easier to digest; colors and flavors change; and nutrients may be lost.
28. in a small amount of water, for a short time, with the pan lid off for the first few minutes of cooking

Vegetables

Name _____

Date _____ **Period** _____ **Score** _____

Chapter 19 Test

Matching: Match the following vegetables with the part of the plants they represent.

_____ 1. Artichokes and cauliflower.

_____ 2. Asparagus and celery.

_____ 3. Carrots and radishes.

_____ 4. Potatoes.

_____ 5. Lettuce and spinach.

_____ 6. Corn and peas.

_____ 7. Garlic and onion.

_____ 8. Tomatoes and peppers.

A. berries
B. bulbs
C. flowers
D. fruits
E. leaves
F. roots
G. seeds
H. stems
I. tubers

True/False: Circle *T* if the statement is true or *F* if the statement is false.

T F 9. A greater variety of fresh vegetables are now available in grocery stores for longer periods of time than were available years ago.

T F 10. Most vegetables are low in calories (kilojoules).

T F 11. Most vegetables do not need to be stored in the refrigerator.

T F 12. Most vegetables are canned in water.

T F 13. Because heat kills germs, vegetables do not need to be washed before cooking.

T F 14. Most yellow vegetables should be cooked in a small amount of water, in a covered pan, just until crisp-tender.

T F 15. Mildly flavored vegetables are covered with water for cooking.

T F 16. Baking vegetables takes longer than other cooking methods.

T F 17. Vegetables cooked in a microwave oven are less nutritious than vegetables prepared by other methods.

T F 18. Potatoes are classified on the basis of appearance and use.

Multiple Choice: Choose the best answer and write the corresponding letter in the blank.

_____ 19. Which of the following vegetables does *not* need to be stored in the refrigerator?
A. Brussels sprouts.
B. Green beans.
C. Onions.
D. Sweet corn.

_____ 20. Which of the following vegetables contains pigments called *flavones?*
A. Beets.
B. Broccoli.
C. Carrots.
D. Cauliflower.

(Continued)

Name _____

_____ 21. Which of the following vegetables should be cooked in a large amount of water, in an uncovered pan, for a short time?
   A. Brussels sprouts.
   B. Leeks.
   C. Onions.
   D. Parsnips.

_____ 22. Which of the following vegetables should be cooked in a small amount of water, in a covered pan, for a short time?
   A. Broccoli.
   B. Green cabbage.
   C. Peas.
   D. Turnips.

_____ 23. Which of the following potato varieties is best suited for potato salad?
   A. Baking potato.
   B. Round red potato.
   C. Russet potato.
   D. None of the above.

Essay Questions: Provide complete responses to the following questions or statements.

24. Why should you choose fresh vegetables that are medium in size?
25. Name five kinds of legumes.
26. How should fresh vegetables be prepared for eating raw or cooking?
27. What changes take place in vegetables during cooking?
28. How should green vegetables be cooked in order to preserve their bright color?

Salads, Casseroles, and Soups

Objectives

After studying this chapter, students will be able to
- prepare attractive and nutritious salads and three basic dressings.
- prepare casseroles and stock-based soups.

Bulletin Board

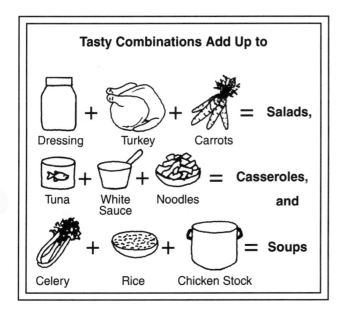

Tasty Combinations Add Up to

Dressing + Turkey + Carrots = **Salads,**

Tuna + White Sauce + Noodles = **Casseroles,**

and

Celery + Rice + Chicken Stock = **Soups**

Title: "Tasty Combinations Add Up to Salads, Casseroles, and Soups"

Make drawings or cutouts of three rows of three ingredients that could be combined both horizontally and vertically to make a salad, a casserole, or a soup.

Teaching Materials

Text, pages 327-337
Student Activity Guide
- A. *Salads*
- B. *Casserole Preparation Guide*
- C. *Stock Soups*
- D. *Herbs, Spices, and Blends*

Teacher's Resource Binder
Salad Recipes, recipe master 20-1
Salad Dressing Recipes, recipe master 20-2
Casserole Recipes, recipe master 20-3
Stock Soup Recipes, recipe master 20-4

Seasoning Cooked Food, food science master 20-5
Chapter 20 Study Sheet, reproducible master 20-6
Casserole Ingredients, color transparency CT-20
Chapter 20 Test
Software, diskette for Part Three
Tic Tac Toe, chapter review game

Introductory Activities

1. Write the word *combination* vertically on the chalkboard. Have students try to think of a salad, casserole, or soup that begins with each letter.
2. Studies have shown that salads, soups, and combination dishes are among the least liked foods. Ask students if they agree with those study findings and have them explain why or why not.

Strategies to Reteach, Reinforce, Enrich, and Extend Text Concepts

Salads

3. **RF** Have students plan four luncheon menus, each featuring a different type of salad. Have them include recipes with each menu.
4. **ER** Set up a display of salad greens, such as iceberg lettuce, spinach, watercress, Belgian endive, escarole, red leaf lettuce, romaine, and curly endive. Have students compare the appearance, texture, and flavor of each type of salad green on a *Food Product Evaluation Sheet* (TRB).
5. **EX** Place a piece of leaf lettuce on each of two plates. Place one plate in the refrigerator and leave the other on a table or counter. After one hour, have students compare the two samples and explain how their observations relate to the preparation of salads.
6. **RT** Demonstrate for students how to clean a head of iceberg lettuce following the directions

given in Illustration 20-2 of the text. Then demonstrate how to clean and prepare other types of salad greens for use.

7. **EX** *Salad Recipes,* recipe master 20-1, TRB. Have students use the recipe master and additional recipes, as desired, to plan a salad lab. Have each lab group complete a *Market Order Sheet* (TRB) and a *Time-Work Schedule* (TRB).

8. **EX** *Salad Dressing Recipes,* recipe master 20-2, TRB. Have students use the recipe master to prepare basic salad dressings and variations of basic dressings to serve with the salad lab planned in strategy 7. Students should add ingredients for the dressings to their *Market Order Sheet* (TRB). They should include preparation steps for the dressings on their *Time-Work Schedule* (TRB). After preparing their recipes and sampling their salad and salad dressing products, have each lab group complete a *Lab Evaluation Sheet* (TRB).

9. **RF** *Salads,* Activity A, SAG. Students are to complete exercises about salads as described on the worksheet.

Casseroles

10. **RT** *Casserole Ingredients,* color transparency CT-20, TRB. Use the transparency to illustrate the five basic components used in casseroles.

11. **RF** *Casserole Preparation Guide,* Activity B, SAG. Students are to complete a chart with examples of casserole ingredients and then answer the questions that follow.

12. **EX** *Casserole Recipes,* recipe master 20-3, TRB. Have students use the recipe master and additional recipes, as desired, to plan a casserole lab. Have each lab group complete a *Market Order Sheet* (TRB) and a *Time-Work Schedule* (TRB). After preparing their recipe and sampling their casserole product, have each group complete a *Lab Evaluation Sheet* (TRB).

Stock Soups

13. **ER** Guest speaker. Have a soup cook or pantry chef speak to your class about how he or she creates and prepares the dishes in which he or she specializes.

14. **ER** Have students prepare chicken stock. Have them use the stock to prepare vegetable soup or bouillon.

15. **ER** Have students prepare a beef stock.

Have them add vegetables and pasta to one portion of the stock to make soup. Have them clarify the remaining portion and prepare beef consommé.

16. **RF** *Stock Soups,* Activity C, SAG. Students are to match stock soup terms with their definitions. Then they are to identify the correct order of steps for preparing bouillon.

17. **EX** *Stock Soup Recipes,* recipe master 20-4, TRB. Have students use the recipe master and additional recipes, as desired, to plan a stock soup lab. Have each lab group complete a *Market Order Sheet* (TRB) and a *Time-Work Schedule* (TRB). After preparing their recipe and sampling their soup product, have each group complete a *Lab Evaluation Sheet* (TRB).

Herbs and Spices

18. **ER** Select four herbs, four spices, and two blends. Place a sample of each in a small dish. Blindfold students, one at a time, and ask them to try to identify the substances in each dish by the smell.

19. **ER** Have students look through gourmet cookbooks and magazines. Ask them to note any unusual herbs and spices required for the recipes. Have students investigate where they can obtain these seasonings. Then have them prepare one of the recipes and evaluate the flavor created by the seasoning.

20. **RF** *Herbs, Spices, and Blends,* Activity D, SAG. Students are to complete a chart by listing all the seasonings available in the foods laboratory and identifying whether each seasoning is an herb, a spice, or a blend. Then they are to give examples of foods in which each would be used.

21. **EX** *Seasoning Cooked Food,* food science master 20-5, TRB. Have lab groups complete the experiment as directed on the master. Students will be conducting a blind comparison to determine the optimum time to add whole and ground seasonings to food during cooking.

Chapter Review

22. **RT** *Chapter 20 Study Sheet,* reproducible master 20-6, TRB. Have students complete the statements as they read text pages 328-336.

23. **RF** *Tic Tac Toe,* Software, diskette for Part Three. Have students play the chapter

review game according to the instructions that appear on the screen.

Above and Beyond

24. **EX** Place one of the following labels on each of four small bags: *protein food, vegetable, starchy food,* and *product.* Place a number of small cards in each bag, each giving an example appropriate for the label on the bag. For example, cards in the protein food bag might be labeled *chicken, ground beef,* or *tuna.* Cards in the product bag should be labeled *salad, casserole,* or *soup.* Have each student draw a card from each bag, record what is listed on the card, and then return the card to the bag. Have each student create the type of dish he or she drew from the product bag using the foods drawn from the other three bags as ingredients in the dish. Students should write a recipe for their dish and give it a name. Then they should write a description of the dish that could be used on a menu.

25. **ER** Have students contact the placement office at a culinary institute to find out where some of their graduates have been employed as salad makers or soup cooks. Ask students to share their findings in class.

Answer Key

Text

Review What You Have Read, page 337
1. protein salads, pasta salads, vegetable salads, fruit salads, gelatin salads
2. D; because it contains enzymes that prevent gelatin from setting
3. base, body, dressing
4. (List four:) iceberg lettuce, romaine, Boston bibb, watercress, spinach, escarole, endive, leaf lettuce
5. to prevent bruising
6. French, mayonnaise, cooked
7. (List four. Student response. See pages 329-331 in the text.)
8. protein food, vegetable, starch, sauce, topping (Examples are student response.)
9. A soup stock is seasoned liquid made from meats, poultry, fish, and vegetables. Ingredients are placed in a large pan, covered with cold water, and cooked slowly for

several hours at a simmering temperature. After cooking, the fat is skimmed from the surface, and the stock is strained.
10. Bouillon is clear broth made from stock. Consommé is clear, rich-flavored soup made from stock. Consommé is simmered longer than bouillon.
11. (List three of each. Student response. See page 335 in the text.)
12. Ground spices should be added to food toward the end of cooking. Whole spices should be added to food at the beginning of cooking.

Student Activity Guide

Salads, Activity A, page 97
1. Greens should be washed before they are used to remove soil and pesticide residues.
2. Cutting salad greens with a knife can cause bruising.
3. B
4. C
5. A
6. (Student response. Answers should be based on information from the section, "Kinds of Salads," on page 328 of the text.)
7. (Student response.)

Casserole Preparation Guide, Activity B, page 98
1. because casserole ingredients need to be precooked
2. by putting casseroles in a greased dish
3. by loosely placing a piece of aluminum foil over the top of the casserole

Stock Soups, Activity C, page 99
1. E
2. B
3. F
4. C
5. A
6. D
Steps for preparing bouillon should be numbered in this order: 6, 9, 3, 4, 1, 10, 7, 5, 8, 2.

Herbs, Spices, and Blends, Activity D, page 100
1. Herbs are the leaves of plants usually grown in temperate climates. Spices are the dried roots, stems, and seeds of plants grown mainly in the tropics. Blends are combinations of ground herbs and spices.
2. Always store herbs, spices, and blends in a cool, dry place away from light. Keep the containers tightly closed.

Teacher's Resources

Chapter 20 Test

1. C
2. B
3. A
4. C
5. B
6. C
7. A
8. C
9. C
10. B
11. F
12. T
13. T
14. F
15. F
16. T
17. F
18. F
19. F
20. T
21. A
22. B
23. A
24. D
25. D

26. In one type of protein salad, the protein foods are cut into small pieces and combined with a dressing. In the other type of protein salad, the protein foods are cut into strips or slices and attractively arranged on a plate with cold vegetables or fruits.

27. Quickly dip the mold into warm water or cover it with a warm, damp cloth for a few seconds. Then invert the loosened salad onto a serving plate.

28. (Student response. See pages 332-333 of the text.)

29. A stock can be clarified by adding a slightly beaten egg white and a few pieces of eggshell to the boiling, strained stock. As the egg proteins coagulate, they trap any solid materials.

30. A bouquet garni is a small cheesecloth bag filled with whole herbs and spices. It is added to food during cooking for flavor and allows the herbs and spices to easily be removed once their flavors are released.

Salads, Casseroles, and Soups

Name _____

Date _____ Period _____ Score _____

Chapter 20 Test

Matching: Match the following definitions and examples with the appropriate terms. (You may use each term more than once.)

_____ 1. A dried root, stem, or seed of a plant grown main-ly in the tropics.

_____ 2. A leaf of a plant usually grown in a temperate climate.

_____ 3. A combination of seasonings.

_____ 4. Ginger.

_____ 5. Basil.

_____ 6. Allspice.

_____ 7. Poultry seasoning.

_____ 8. Cinnamon.

_____ 9. Pepper.

_____ 10. Mint.

A. blend
B. herb
C. spice

True/False: Circle *T* if the statement is true or *F* if the statement is false.

T   F   11. Protein salads are usually served as accompaniments.

T   F   12. Vegetable salads are small and light.

T   F   13. Salad greens can be prepared a few hours before serving without losing important vitamins and minerals.

T   F   14. Salad greens should be cut to prevent bruising.

T   F   15. Mayonnaise is a temporary emulsion because it is not cooked.

T   F   16. Leftovers make good casserole ingredients because all the meat, poultry, and fish used in casseroles should be precooked.

T   F   17. Most casseroles must be served immediately after being removed from the oven.

T   F   18. To be rich and flavorful, stocks must be cooked quickly.

T   F   19. The stock that results from browned meat is called consommé.

T   F   20. Dried herbs should be used in cooking unless a recipe specifies otherwise.

Multiple Choice: Choose the best response. Write the letter in the space provided.

_____ 21. Which of the following is *not* considered a vegetable salad?
   A. Chef salad.
   B. Coleslaw.
   C. Three bean salad.
   D. Tossed salad.

(Continued)

Name _____

_____ 22. The main part of a salad is called the _____.
    A. base
    B. body
    C. dressing
    D. garnish

_____ 23. The type of salad dressing thickened with a food starch is _____.
    A. cooked salad dressing
    B. French dressing
    C. mayonnaise
    D. All of the above.

_____ 24. Most casseroles are a combination of _____.
    A. foods prepared in a single dish
    B. ground beef, carrots, rice, and condensed soup
    C. a protein food, a vegetable, a starch, and a sauce
    D. A and C above.

_____ 25. Which of the following is *not* a stock-based soup?
    A. Beef consommé.
    B. Beef with barley soup.
    C. Chicken vegetable soup.
    D. Corn chowder.

Essay Questions: Provide complete responses to the following questions or statements.

26. Describe the two different types of protein salads.
27. Describe how to unmold a gelatin salad.
28. Give two tips for putting a casserole together.
29. How can a stock be clarified?
30. What is a bouquet garni and how is it used?

Cereal Products

Objectives

After studying this chapter, students will be able to
- list a variety of cereal products.
- describe how heat and liquids affect starches.
- prepare cooked breakfast cereals, rice, and pasta.

Bulletin Board

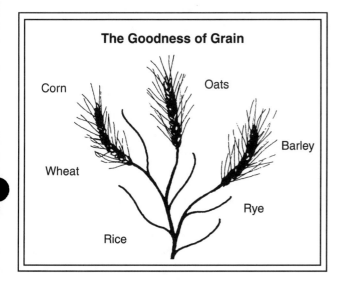

The Goodness of Grain

Corn
Oats
Barley
Wheat
Rye
Rice

Title: "The Goodness of Grain"

Sketch a large stalk of grain in the center of the bulletin board. Place labels around the stalk identifying the six grains most commonly used as food—corn, wheat, rice, oats, barley, and rye.

Teaching Materials

Text, pages 339-350
Student Activity Guide
    A. *Grains and Grain Products*
    B. *Breakfast Cereal Comparison*
    C. *Starch and Cereal Cookery*

Teacher's Resource Binder
    Grain Structure, transparency master 21-1
    Effects of Dry Heat on Starch, food science master 21-2
    Cereal Recipes, recipe master 21-3
    Chapter 21 Study Sheet, reproducible master 21-4
    Chapter 21 Test

Software, diskette for Part Three
    The Matching Game, chapter review game

Introductory Activities

1. Mount samples of the six grains most commonly used as foods—corn, wheat, rice, oats, barley, and rye—on a display poster. See how many of the grains students are able to identify and have them give an example of a food product containing each type of grain.
2. Have students brainstorm a list of cereal products. Write their responses on the chalkboard.

Strategies to Reteach, Reinforce, Enrich, and Extend Text Concepts

Types of Cereal Products

3. **RT** *Grain Structure,* transparency master 21-1, TRB. Use the master to show students the different parts of a kernel of grain. Emphasize the nutritional qualities of each part.
4. **ER** Field trip. Take your class on a tour of a grain mill so they can see how grains are ground into flour.
5. **EX** *Breakfast Cereal Comparison,* Activity B, SAG. Students are to record and compare nutrition information from their choice of two ready-to-eat breakfast cereals.
6. **ER** Have students set up a display on the different types of flour. Have them prepare a baked product from each type of flour to include in the display.
7. **RF** Bring in examples of the variety of pasta shapes and sizes that are available on the market. See how many of them students are able to identify.
8. **RT** Display for students the different types of rice that are available. Display each product with its package so students will recognize the various products when they shop.
9. **ER** Divide the class into eight lab groups. Assign each group to prepare one of the

following foods: cornbread, fried hominy, cooked hominy grits, cherry sauce thickened with cornstarch, beef barley soup, bulgur pilaf, fruit cup sprinkled with wheat germ, and cooked farina. Display the prepared products on an evaluation table. Have students sample the products and comment on their appearance, texture, and taste.

10. **ER** Divide the class into four groups. Assign each group one of the following categories of cereal products: breakfast foods, flours, pastas, and rices. Have each group visit a grocery store and make a list of as many products as they can find that belong in their assigned category. Have them also note the price of each product. (Be sure students check canned and frozen products as well as dried products.) Have each group make a poster showing a price graph of all the products they found.

Selecting and Storing Cereal Products

11. **RF** Ask students to discuss storage guidelines for the various types of cereal products.
12. **RF** *Grains and Grain Products,* Activity A, SAG. Students are to complete exercises about grains and grain products.

Cooking Starches

13. **RT** Demonstrate for students the preparation of a browned flour gravy. As you demonstrate, explain what happened to the starch granules and describe how they were affected by heat.
14. **EX** *Effects of Dry Heat on Starch,* food science master 21-2, TRB. Have lab groups complete the experiment as directed on the master. Students will be evaluating the effects of dry heat on starch by comparing sauces made with browned and unbrowned flour.
15. **EX** Divide the class into six lab groups. Have each group prepare a cooked starch paste using one of the following: cornstarch, potato starch, rice starch, wheat flour, arrowroot starch, and minute tapioca. To do this, each group will add 1 cup (250 mL) cold water to 2 tablespoons (30 mL) starch. (Minute tapioca should be soaked 5 minutes before cooking.) Heat quickly to maximum gelatinization temperature. Hold at this temperature one minute, stirring constantly but gently. Pour paste into custard cups. Unmold or pour cooled starch pastes onto small,

white, ceramic plates. Place the plates on an observation table. Then have students compare clarity, viscosity, and gel structure of each sample and record their observations.

16. **RF** Have students observe syneresis by cutting in half one of the cooled starch paste samples made in strategy 15.
17. **ER** Prepare a flour-thickened pudding, a cornstarch pudding, and a tapioca pudding. Have students compare the starch granules from each under a microscope and sketch what they observe. Then have them write a brief description of their observations.
18. **EX** Have students brainstorm a list of starch-thickened products. Write their responses on the chalkboard.
19. **EX** Working in lab groups, have students stir ½ cup (125 mL) boiling water into each of the following: 1 tablespoon (15 mL) flour; 1 tablespoon (15 mL) flour mixed with 3 tablespoons (45 mL) sugar; 1 tablespoon (15 mL) flour mixed with 1 tablespoon (15 mL) melted fat; and 1 tablespoon (15 mL) flour mixed with 1 tablespoon (15 mL) cold water. Have students record and explain their observations.

Cooking Cereal Products

20. **RF** Have students explain the principles of cereal cookery.
21. **ER** Divide the class into five lab groups. Have each group prepare two of the following: regular oatmeal, quick-cooking oatmeal, farina, yellow cornmeal, cream of rye, cream of rice, hominy, hominy grits, bulgur, and barley. Have students place cooked products on an evaluation table, labeling each product with the amount of cooking time required to prepare it. Have students sample all products, recording the appearance, texture (consistency), flavor, and cooking time of each on a *Food Product Evaluation Sheet* (TRB).
22. **ER** Divide the class into five lab groups. Have each group prepare one of the following: white rice, parboiled rice, instant rice, brown rice, and wild rice. Have students place their cooked samples on an evaluation table. Beside each cooked sample, place a small uncooked sample. Have groups label their cooked products with the water/rice ratio and total cooking time. Have students sample all products and compare them in terms of water/rice ratio, total cooking time, appearance, flavor, and degree of swelling.

Then have them summarize their observations in a brief written report.

23. **EX** *Cereal Recipes,* recipe master 21-3, TRB. Have students use the recipe master and additional recipes, as desired, to plan a cereal lab. Have each lab group complete a *Market Order Sheet* (TRB) and a *Time-Work Schedule* (TRB). After preparing their recipe and sampling their cereal product, have each group complete a *Lab Evaluation Sheet* (TRB).

24. **RF** *Starch and Cereal Cookery,* Activity C, SAG. Students are to complete the worksheet by identifying true and false statements.

Chapter Review

25. **RT** *Chapter 21 Study Sheet,* reproducible master 21-4, TRB. Have students complete the statements as they read text pages 340-348.
26. **RF** *The Matching Game,* Software, diskette for Part Three. Have students play the chapter review game according to the instructions that appear on the screen.

Above and Beyond

27. **ER** Have students investigate the use of grain in another culture. Have them find out what grains are used and how they are prepared and served. Have them prepare visual aids to submit with a written report or to use in giving an oral report.

Answer Key

Text

Review What You Have Read, page 350
1. (List four:) corn, wheat, rice, oats, barley, rye
2. The bran is the outer protective covering of the kernel and is a good source of vitamins and fiber. The endosperm makes up the largest part of the kernel and contains most of the starch and protein. The germ is the smallest part of the kernel and is rich in vitamins, protein, and fat.
3. Whole grain cereals contain all three parts of the kernel. Refined cereals have had the bran and germ removed during processing.
4. (List three:) pastas, cornmeal, hominy, corn-starch, pearl barley, bulgur wheat, wheat germ, farina
5. true
6. D
7. gelatinization
8. coating with fat, combining with sugar, mixing with a cold liquid to form a paste
9. gravies, sauces, puddings
10. true
11. false
12. by continuing to cook them for a short time after gelatinization is complete
13. by adding 1 tablespoon (15 mL) of cooking oil to the water in which the pasta is cooked
14. false

Student Activity Guide

Grains and Grain Products, Activity A, page 101
1. A. endosperm: contains most of the starch and protein of the kernel and holds the food supply that the plant uses to grow
   B. bran: the outer protective covering of the kernel, which is a good source of vitamins and fiber
   C. germ: contains the parts needed to produce a new plant and is rich in vitamins, proteins, and fat

2. wheat	10. J
3. corn	11. H
4. barley	12. E
5. oats	13. K
6. rice	14. G
7. rye	15. D
8. A	16. B
9. C	17. F

Starch and Cereal Cookery, Activity C, page 104

1. F	11. T
2. F	12. T
3. F	13. T
4. F	14. F
5. T	15. T
6. T	16. F
7. F	17. T
8. T	18. F
9. T	19. F
10. T	20. T

Teacher's Resources

Chapter 21 Test

1. B	14. F
2. F	15. T
3. K	16. F
4. A	17. F
5. G	18. F
6. I	19. F
7. H	20. T
8. C	21. C
9. D	22. A
10. E	23. C
11. T	24. B
12. T	25. D
13. T	

26. corn, wheat, rice, oats, barley, and rye
27. During cooking, the starch granules in the cereal absorb water and swell. As they swell, the cereal becomes thicker until it reaches the point of maximum thickness (gelatinization).
28. temperature, time, agitation, and mixing method
29. the size of the cereal particles and whether the bran layer is present
30. Cereal products are less likely to stick and burn when prepared in a microwave oven. Cereal products can be prepared and served in the same dish when cooked in a microwave oven, which saves time on cleanup.

Cereal Products

Name _____

Date _____ Period _____ Score _____

Chapter 21 Test

Matching: Match each of the following cereal products with its description.

_____ 1. Flour made from soft wheat.

_____ 2. Flour treated to blend easily with liquids.

_____ 3. Flour that contains the bran, germ, and endosperm.

_____ 4. Rice that has had the hull removed but contains the bran, germ, and endosperm.

_____ 5. Rice that is dry and fluffy when cooked.

_____ 6. Rice that can be prepared in minutes.

_____ 7. Macaroni, noodles, and spaghetti.

_____ 8. Ground white or yellow corn.

_____ 9. Refined starch obtained from the endosperm of corn.

_____ 10. Wheat product used as a thickener and a cooked breakfast cereal.

A. brown rice
B. cake flour
C. cornmeal
D. cornstarch
E. farina
F. instant flour
G. long grain rice
H. pasta
I. precooked rice
J. self-rising flour
K. whole wheat flour

True/False: Circle *T* if the statement is true or *F* if the statement is false.

T F 11. Refined cereals are cereal grains that have had the bran and germ removed during processing.

T F 12. Converted rice tends to cost more than long grain rice.

T F 13. Grain products should be stored tightly covered.

T F 14. Starch is affected by moist heat but not by dry heat.

T F 15. Heat and moisture are needed for gelatinization to take place.

T F 16. When gelatinization occurs, a starch mixture should be removed from the heat.

T F 17. Flour-thickened mixtures are translucent.

T F 18. As a general rule, use three times as much water as rice when preparing white rice.

T F 19. Adding 1 teaspoon (5 mL) of salt to the cooking water can help keep pasta from sticking together.

T F 20. Cereal products should be covered for microwave cooking.

Multiple Choice: Choose the best response. Write the letter in the space provided.

_____ 21. The largest part of a kernel of grain is the _____.
   A. bran
   B. cereal
   C. endosperm
   D. germ

(Continued)

Name _____

_____ 22. Cereal products that have had nutrients added to them during processing are called _____.
      A. enriched cereal products
      B. refined cereal products
      C. whole grain cereal products
      D. None of the above.

_____ 23. Which of the following techniques should *not* be used to separate starch granules?
      A. Coating the starch granules with fat.
      B. Combining the starch with sugar.
      C. Mixing the starch with boiling water to form a paste.
      D. Mixing the starch with cold water to form a paste.

_____ 24. Which of the following would probably *not* be used to thicken a cherry sauce?
      A. Cornstarch.
      B. Flour.
      C. Tapioca.
      D. All of the above.

_____ 25. Rice may be cooked _____.
      A. in a double boiler
      B. in the oven
      C. over direct heat
      D. Any of the above.

Essay Questions: Provide complete responses to the following questions or statements.

26. Which six grains are used most often for food?
27. Describe what happens when cereals are cooked.
28. List the four factors that must be controlled when cooking starch-thickened mixtures.
29. What two factors determine the amount of cooking water needed to prepare cereals?
30. What are two advantages of preparing cereal products in a microwave oven?

Breads

Objectives

After studying this chapter, students will be able to
■ describe how to select and store baked goods.
■ explain the function of ingredients in baked products.
■ prepare quick breads and yeast breads.

Bulletin Board

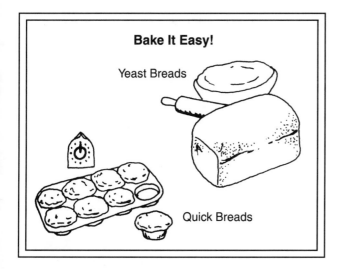

Title: "Bake It Easy!"
Use drawings or cutouts to illustrate one or more quick bread products and one or more yeast bread products. Label each product and post recipes, if desired.

Teaching Materials

Text, pages 351-368
Student Activity Guide
    A. *Functions of Ingredients*
    B. *Adjusting Recipes*
    C. *Characteristics of Quick Breads*
    D. *Yeast Breads*

Teacher's Resource Binder
    The Effects of Baking Powder in Biscuits, food science master 22-1
    Quick Bread Recipes, recipe master 22-2
    Yeast Bread Recipes, recipe master 22-3
    Chapter 22 Study Sheet, reproducible master 22-4

Leavening Agents and Gases, color transparency CT-22
    Chapter 22 Test
Software, diskette for Part Three
    Bingo, chapter review game

Introductory Activities

1. Have students look up the words *bread* and *dough* in a dictionary. Ask them how they think the slang meanings for these two words came about.
2. Nearly every culture in the world has some type of bread as a staple of the diet. Have students name as many breads of other cultures as they can.

Strategies to Reteach, Reinforce, Enrich, and Extend Text Concepts

Selecting and Storing Baked Products

3. **ER** Allow students to sample homemade crescent rolls, bakery crescent rolls, brown-and-serve crescent rolls, and refrigerated crescent rolls. Have them evaluate the appearance, flavor, texture, and cost per dozen on a *Food Product Evaluation Sheet* (TRB).
4. **ER** Have students list all the breads sold at a local grocery store in order by cost, beginning with the least expensive. Have them share their findings in class. Use this information as the basis for a discussion of factors affecting bread costs.
5. **EX** Wrap each of three slices of homemade white bread tightly in plastic wrap. Place one slice in the freezer, another slice in the refrigerator, and leave the third slice sitting on a counter. Have students examine the slices after 3, 5, 7, and 10 days, recording their observations each time. Then have them summarize their observations in a few paragraphs on bread storage.

Ingredients for Baked Products

6. **RF** Have students name the two proteins

found in wheat flour and explain their role in the preparation of bread products.

7. **RF**   Have students explain how bread flour, all-purpose flour, and cake flour differ.

8. **RT**   *Leavening Agents and Gases,* color transparency CT-22, TRB. Use the transparency to illustrate the three basic gases—air, steam, and carbon dioxide—that cause baked products to rise. Explain how each of the different leavening gases might be incorporated into baked products.

9. **RF**   *Functions of Ingredients,* Activity A, SAG. Students are to list at least one function in the preparation of baked products for each ingredient pictured on the worksheet.

10. **RF**   *Adjusting Recipes,* Activity B, SAG. Students are to adjust the ingredients in a biscuit recipe to reflect minimum proportions. Then they are to calculate the calorie, fat, and sodium savings per biscuit that would result from these adjustments.

Quick Breads

11. **ER**   Guest speaker. Invite a baker to speak to your class about how quick breads and yeast breads are prepared in quantities for the retail market.

12. **RF**   Have students name and describe the three basic mixing methods used for quick breads and list the products for which each is used.

13. **RF**   Have students define the term *quick bread* and list as many different quick breads as they can.

14. **RF**   Ask students to describe the difference between pour batters, drop batters, and doughs.

15. **RF**   Ask students to explain why quick breads should not be overmixed.

16. **RF**   *Characteristics of Quick Breads,* Activity C, SAG. Students are to answer questions about the characteristics of quick breads.

17. **EX**   *The Effects of Baking Powder in Biscuits,* food science master 22-1, TRB. Have lab groups complete the experiment as directed on the master. Students will be evaluating the effects of using too little and too much baking powder in dropped biscuits.

18. **EX**   *Quick Bread Recipes,* recipe master 22-2, TRB. Have students use the recipe master to plan a quick bread lab. Have each lab group complete a *Market Order Sheet* (TRB) and a *Time-Work Schedule* (TRB). After preparing

and sampling their quick bread product, have each group complete a *Lab Evaluation Sheet* (TRB).

19. **EX**   Have students plan a puff paste lab. Instruct half of the lab groups to shape their puff paste into cream puffs. Have the other groups shape their paste into eclairs. Have each group choose a different sweet or protein-based filling to serve with their puff paste product. Have each lab group complete a *Market Order Sheet* (TRB) and a *Time-Work Schedule* (TRB). Have students evaluate their cream puffs and eclairs according to the criteria given in the text. Then have each group complete a *Lab Evaluation Sheet* (TRB).

Yeast Breads

20. **ER**   Have students use a microscope to watch yeast grow. Have them explain how yeast differs from other leavening agents.

21. **RF**   Have students explain the function of each of the following ingredients in yeast breads: yeast, flour, salt, sugar, and liquid.

22. **RT**   Demonstrate for students how to mix yeast bread dough using the straight-dough, fast mixing, sponge, and batter methods.

23. **RT**   Demonstrate for students the correct way to knead yeast dough.

24. **RF**   *Yeast Breads,* Activity D, SAG. Students are to complete exercises dealing with yeast breads.

25. **EX**   Working in lab groups, have students prepare two loaves of the same basic white bread, but have them eliminate the salt in one of the loaves. After the loaves have cooled, have students compare the appearance, flavor, and texture on a *Food Product Evaluation Sheet* (TRB). Have them describe how the salt-free dough felt during kneading and explain why it felt this way.

26. **EX**   Prepare a yeast bread recipe that will yield two loaves. After kneading, divide the dough in half. Shape and bake one half immediately. Allow the other half to rise as the recipe directs. After the second loaf has cooled, have students compare it with the first loaf. Have them use their observations as the basis for a discussion of the importance of fermentation.

27. **EX**   *Yeast Bread Recipes,* recipe master 22-3, TRB. Have students use the recipe master to plan a yeast bread lab. Have each group complete a *Market Order Sheet* (TRB) and a

Time-Work Schedule (TRB). After preparing and sampling their yeast bread products have each group complete a *Lab Evaluation Sheet* (TRB).

28. **ER** Have students prepare a basic yeast roll dough and experiment with different roll shapes.

29. **ER** Field trip. Take the class to a bakery so students can watch bakery products being produced in large quantities.

Chapter Review

30. **RT** *Chapter 22 Study Sheet,* reproducible master 22-4, TRB. Have students complete the statements as they read text pages 352-366.

31. **RF** *Bingo,* Software, diskette for Part Three. Have students play the chapter review game according to the instructions that appear on the screen.

Above and Beyond

32. **EX** Have your class plan and prepare a buffet brunch for the faculty featuring quick breads and yeast breads. Have them prepare muffins, biscuits, popovers, and coffee cakes. Have them also prepare a sweet yeast dough and use it to prepare sweet rolls and coffee rings. After the brunch, hold a class discussion to evaluate the outcome of the project. Have students identify strengths and weaknesses in their lab work, in the food products, and in the presentation of the meal. Have them write an article about the event for the local paper.

33. **ER** Have students prepare two loaves from the same basic bread recipe, one traditionally and the other in an automatic bread machine. Have students compare the flavor, texture, and appearance on a *Food Product Evaluation Sheet* (TRB).

Answer Key

Text

Review What You Have Read, page 368

1. Quick breads contain leavening agents other than yeast and can be prepared in a short amount of time. Yeast breads use yeast as a leavening agent and require more time to prepare. (Examples are student response.)

2. flour, leavening agents, liquid, fat, eggs, sugar, salt (For functions, see pages 354-356 in the text.)

3. gliadin, glutenin
4. Proteins found in cake flour produce gluten that is too weak to support the structure of bread.
5. air, steam, carbon dioxide
6. true
7. popovers, cream puffs
8. D
9. A, C, D, B
10. fast rising yeast
11. (List three:) kind of yeast, amount of yeast, temperature of the room, kind of flour
12. Gently push two fingers into the dough. If an indentation remains, the dough has risen enough.
13. oven spring
14. true

Student Activity Guide

Adjusting Recipes, Activity B, page 106
Light 'n Healthy Biscuits
  2 cups flour
     (omit sugar)
 2½ teaspoons baking powder
  ½ teaspoon salt
  ¼ cup shortening
  ¾ cup skim milk

These proportions would result in a total savings of 232 calories, 23 g of fat, and 1195 mg of sodium. This is equivalent to a savings of approximately 19 calories, 2 g of fat, and 100 mg of sodium per biscuit.

Characteristics of Quick Breads, Activity C page 107

1. (List two:) Dropped biscuits have a higher proportion of milk than rolled biscuits. Rolled biscuits are cut with a biscuit cutter; dropped biscuits are dropped from a spoon. Rolled biscuits are baked on an ungreased baking sheet; dropped biscuits are baked on a greased baking sheet.

2. A high-quality rolled biscuit has an even shape with a smooth and level top and straight sides. The crust is an even brown. The interior is white to creamy white. The crumb is moist and fluffy and peels off in layers.

3. A. U   F. H
   B. U   G. H
   C. U   H. H
   D. O   I. O
   E. O   J. H

4. A hot oven is used for the first part of the baking period to allow steam to expand the

walls of the popovers. A lower temperature is used during the second part of the baking period to prevent overbrowning before the interior has set.

5. A popover that has not been baked long enough will collapse when it is taken from the oven. The exterior will be soft instead of crisp, and the interior will be doughy.

6. If the cream puffs have not set, the steam can condense and cause them to collapse.

7. The evaporation of too much liquid occasionally causes cream puffs to ooze fat during baking. This might occur when the water and fat are heated together, or when the puff paste is cooked.

Yeast Breads, Activity D, page 108

1. With the fingers, fold the dough in the half toward the body. Push against the dough with the heels of your hands, and turn the dough one-quarter turn. This folding, pushing, and turning continues until the dough is smooth and elastic.

2. Bread is kneaded to develop the gluten.

3. A, C, F, H

4. (Student response.)

Teacher's Resources

Chapter 22 Test

1. B	15. T
2. E	16. T
3. H	17. F
4. G	18. C
5. D	19. A
6. A	20. B
7. F	21. C
8. T	22. A
9. F	23. A
10. F	24. A
11. T	25. D
12. T	26. D
13. T	27. C
14. F	

28. Pour batters have a large amount of liquid and a small amount of flour. Drop batters have a higher proportion of flour and soft doughs have an even higher proportion of flour.

29. A high-quality rolled biscuit has an even shape with a smooth, level top and straight sides. The crust has an even brown color. When broken open, the interior is white to creamy white. The crumb is moist and fluffy and peels off in layers.

30. Microwave cooking lacks the dry heat popovers and cream puffs need for crust formation.

31. Temperatures that are too hot will kill the yeast cells. Temperatures that are too cool will slow down yeast activity and may stop it altogether.

32. Fermentation is the step in yeast bread production when the yeast cells act upon the sugars in the dough to produce carbon dioxide and alcohol. The carbon dioxide makes the bread rise.

Breads

Name _____

Date _____ Period _____ Score _____

Chapter 22 Test

Matching: Match the following ingredients with their functions in quick breads and yeast breads.

_____ 1. Serves as a tenderizing agent.

_____ 2. Produce gases that make baked products rise.

_____ 3. Helps crusts brown.

_____ 4. Regulates the action of yeast.

_____ 5. Gives structure to baked products.

_____ 6. Add color and flavor and contribute to structure.

_____ 7. Hydrate the protein and starch in flour.

A. eggs
B. fat
C. flavorings
D. flours
E. leavening agents
F. liquids
G. salt
H. sugar

True/False: Circle *T* if the statement is true or *F* if the statement is false.

T F 8. Breads with fruits and nuts usually cost more than plain white or wheat bread.

T F 9. Cake flour forms gluten that is strong enough to support the structure of yeast breads and quick breads.

T F 10. Double-acting baking powder releases most of its carbon dioxide as soon as it is moistened.

T F 11. Eggs and fats are considered to be liquid ingredients in baked products.

T F 12. In the muffin method, the liquid ingredients are added to the dry ingredients all at once.

T F 13. Overdeveloped gluten can cause quick breads to be compact and tough.

T F 14. Cream puff failures are usually caused by overbaking.

T F 15. In yeast dough, most of the gluten is developed by kneading.

T F 16. Carbon dioxide causes yeast bread dough to rise.

T F 17. Bread baked in a microwave oven is microwaved on high power until it is almost done.

Multiple Choice: Choose the best response. Write the letter in the space provided.

_____ 18. Which of the following is *not* a quick bread?
A. Biscuit.
B. Cream puff.
C. English muffin.
D. Waffle.

_____ 19. Which of the following flours would be most suitable for the preparation of muffins?
A. All-purpose flour.
B. Bread flour.
C. Cake flour.
D. Pastry flour.

(Continued)

Name _____

_____ 20. Which leavening gas is the result of chemical reactions that occur between ingredients in baked products?
   A. Air.
   B. Carbon dioxide.
   C. Steam.
   D. All of the above.

_____ 21. Tunnels often are found in _____.
   A. overmixed biscuits
   B. undermixed biscuits
   C. overmixed muffins
   D. undermixed muffins

_____ 22. Sometimes cream puffs will ooze fat during baking. This is caused by _____.
   A. evaporation of too much liquid
   B. too much fat
   C. too much liquid
   D. using the wrong kind of fat

_____ 23. Less flour is used when a yeast dough is mixed by the _____.
   A. batter method
   B. fast mixing method
   C. sponge method
   D. straight-dough method

_____ 24. If a loaf of yeast bread has large, overexpanded cells, the dough was _____.
   A. allowed to rise for too long a time
   B. baked at too high a temperature
   C. kneaded too much
   D. not kneaded long enough

_____ 25. Refrigerator yeast bread doughs usually contain extra _____.
   A. salt
   B. sugar
   C. yeast
   D. All of the above.

_____ 26. Fermentation takes place in a yeast dough when the yeast acts upon the _____.
   A. milk
   B. salt
   C. starch granules in the flour
   D. sugar

_____ 27. The sudden dramatic rise of a yeast dough that takes place during the first few minutes of baking is called _____.
   A. fermentation
   B. lightening
   C. oven spring
   D. sponge formation

Essay Questions: Provide complete responses to the following questions or statements.

28. Explain the difference between pour batters, drop batters, and soft doughs.
29. Describe a high-quality rolled biscuit.
30. Why don't popovers and cream puffs microwave well?
31. Why is temperature so crucial when liquid is added to yeast?
32. What is fermentation in yeast bread production?

Cakes, Cookies, Pies, and Candies

Objectives

After studying this chapter, students will be able to
- discuss gluten development and the interaction of ingredients as they apply to cakes, cookies, and pies.
- prepare shortened and unshortened cakes, six types of cookies, and pastry.
- prepare crystalline and noncrystalline candies.

Bulletin Board

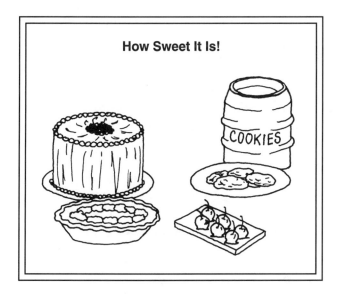

How Sweet It Is!

Title: "How Sweet It Is!"

Use cutouts, drawings, or magazine pictures to illustrate cakes, cookies, pies, and candies.

Teaching Materials

Text, pages 369-386
Student Activity Guide
    A. *Kinds of Cakes*
    B. *Preparation of Cakes*
    C. *Cookies*
    D. *Pie Filling*
    E. *Pastry Preparation*
    F. *Candy*

Teacher's Resource Binder
    Minimum Ingredient Proportions in Baked Goods, reproducible master 23-1
    Cake Recipes, recipe master 23-2

    Cake Decorating Accessories, transparency master 23-3
    Ingredient Proportions in Cookies, food science master 23-4
    Cookie Recipes, recipe master 23-5
    Pie Recipes, recipe master 23-6
    Candy Recipes, recipe master 23-7
    Chapter 23 Study Sheet, reproducible master 23-8
    Chapter 23 Test

Software, diskette for Part Three
    Reverse Thinking, chapter review game

Introductory Activities

1. Divide the chalkboard into four columns headed *Cakes, Cookies, Pies,* and *Candies.* Ask students to name their favorite sweets in each category. List responses under the appropriate headings.
2. Have students use Appendix B (Nutritive Values of Foods) on pages 617-634 of the text to evaluate the caloric content and nutritive value of a variety of cakes, cookies, pies, and candies.
3. Guest speaker. Invite a pastry chef to speak to your class about the desserts he or she creates and prepares.

Strategies to Reteach, Reinforce, Enrich, and Extend Text Concepts

Cakes

4. **RF** Have students name the three basic types of cakes and list the major ingredients in each. Then have them explain the function of each ingredient.
5. **EX** Prepare two shortened cakes. Use all-purpose flour in one of the cakes and cake flour in the other. Have students compare and evaluate appearance, texture, and flavor.
6. **RT** *Minimum Ingredient Proportions in Baked Goods,* reproducible master 23-1, TRB. Go over the handout with students. Explain how students can use it to reduce fat, sugar, and sodium in foods prepared from traditional

recipes. Encourage students to post the handout in their kitchen at home for future reference.

7. **RF** *Kinds of Cakes,* Activity A, SAG. Students are to complete exercises about cakes.

8. **EX**   Prepare three shortened cakes using the recipe in the text. Prepare one recipe as directed. Increase the amount of flour by $2/3$ cup (150 mL) in the second recipe. Decrease the amount of sugar by ½ cup (125 mL) in the third recipe. After the cakes have cooled, have students evaluate them and explain their observations.

9. **RF**   Prepare batter for a two-layer shortened cake. After beating the ingredients for the appropriate amount of time, pour half of the batter into a 9-inch (23 cm) cake pan and bake. Continue beating the remainder of the batter several more minutes. Pour batter into another 9-inch (23 cm) cake pan and bake. Cut each layer in half and have students compare the texture, volume, and exterior. Ask them to summarize their observations in a paragraph explaining why overmixing should be avoided.

10. **EX**   Prepare three shortened cakes using the recipe in the text. Pour the batter of the first cake into two 8-inch (20 cm) pans. Pour the second batter into three 8-inch (20 cm) pans. Pour the third batter into four 8-inch (20 cm) pans. Bake all pans at 350°F (180°C) for 30 to 35 minutes. After cakes have cooled, have students compare volume, texture, and appearance and explain their observations.

11. **RT**   On the chalkboard, draw diagrams showing students how one, two, three, and four cake pans should be arranged in an oven for even heat circulation.

12. **RF**   *Preparation of Cakes,* Activity B, SAG. Students are to explain various principles and techniques used in preparing cakes.

13. **ER**   Divide the class into four lab groups. Assign one of the following cake preparations to each group: an angel food cake from scratch, an angel food cake from a mix, a sponge cake, and a chiffon cake. Have students place the cooled cakes on an evaluation table. Then have them compare the cakes in terms of appearance, volume, grain (cell wall size and uniformity), tenderness, and flavor.

14. **EX**   *Cake Recipes,* recipe master 23-2, TRB. Have students use the recipe master to plan a cake lab. Have each group choose a different frosting or filling for their cake. Each group should complete a *Market Order Sheet* (TRB) and a *Time-Work Schedule* (TRB). After preparing, filling and/or frosting, and sampling their cake, have each group complete a *Lab Evaluation Sheet* (TRB).

15. **RT**   *Cake Decorating Accessories,* transparency master 23-3, TRB. Use the transparency as you explain to students how the various decorating tips and accessories are used to decorate cakes.

16. **ER**   Guest speaker. Invite a professional cake decorator to come to your class and demonstrate cake decorating techniques. Your class can supply the shortened cakes that the speaker will decorate. You may wish to videotape this presentation to show to other classes.

17. **ER**   Have students prepare a cooked frosting and an uncooked frosting. Ask them to compare preparation, spreadability, appearance, and flavor of the two types of frosting.

18. **ER**   Have students prepare cut-up cakes in the shapes of a variety of animals and objects. Arrange to deliver the cakes to a class at a preschool or kindergarten.

19. **ER**   Have students use a decorators' tube and several decorating tips to practice making a variety of flowers and trims.

Cookies

20. **ER**   Assign each lab group a different dropped cookie recipe. Have each group prepare two batches of their assigned recipe. Groups should make one batch according to traditional ingredient proportions. They should make the second batch according to minimum ingredient proportions. Have groups sample and compare the two versions of their recipe.

21. **RT**   Demonstrate for students how crisp cookies and soft cookies should be stored.

22. **RF**   *Cookies,* Activity C, SAG. Students are to identify the basic group to which each of the types of cookies listed on the worksheet belongs. Then they are to identify whether various statements about cookies are true.

23. **ER**   Have students prepare a recipe for refrigerator cookies. Have them bake half the cookies and store them in the freezer. Have

them wrap the other half of the cookie dough and place it in the freezer unbaked. At the end of the school term, thaw the frozen dough and bake the cookies. Thaw the frozen cookies. Have students compare the products.

24. **ER** Divide the class into four lab groups. Assign one of the following chocolate chip cookie preparations to each group: made from scratch, made from a cookie mix, made from a cake mix, and made from commercially refrigerated dough. Have students compare these cookies with at least two brands of commercially prepared chocolate chip cookies. Have them compare appearance, flavor, texture, and cost on a *Food Product Evaluation Sheet* (TRB).

25. **EX** *Ingredient Proportions in Cookies,* food science master 23-4, TRB. Have lab groups complete the experiment as directed on the master. Students will be evaluating the effect of fat and sugar proportions on the crispness of dropped cookies.

26. **EX** *Cookie Recipes,* recipe master 23-5, TRB. Have students use the recipe master and additional recipes to plan a cookie lab. Additional recipes should be chosen so that at least one example is prepared from each of the six basic groups of cookies. Have each group complete a *Market Order Sheet* (TRB) and a *Time-Work Schedule* (TRB). Place all the cookies on a sample table. Then have each group complete a *Lab Evaluation Sheet* (TRB).

Pies

27. **RF** *Pie Filling,* Activity D, SAG. Students are to supply requested information about different kinds of pies.

28. **RF** Have students find recipes for at least three products (other than pies) that are made with pastry.

29. **RF** Have students list the four basic ingredients used to prepare pastry and explain the function of each.

30. **RF** *Pastry Preparation,* Activity E, SAG. Students are to answer questions about pastry preparation.

31. **EX** Using the pastry recipe in the text, prepare pastry for a single-crust pie. Prepare the same recipe again, this time decreasing the shortening by ¼ cup (50 mL). Roll both samples and bake them in a 425°F (220°C) oven until lightly browned. Then have students compare the appearance, tenderness, and flakiness of the two samples and explain their observations.

32. **ER** Have students practice preparing lattice tops, a variety of cut-out tops, and decorative edges used for pastries.

33. **ER** Have students prepare a double-crust cherry pie from scratch. Also have them bake a double-crust frozen cherry pie. Then have them evaluate the appearance, flavor, flakiness, and tenderness of the pastry as well as the eating quality and appearance of the filling of each pie.

34. **EX** *Pie Recipes,* recipe master 23-6, TRB. Have the students use the recipe master and additional recipes to plan a pie lab. Additional recipes should be chosen so that at least one example is prepared from each of the four basic groups of pies. Have each lab group complete a *Market Order Sheet* (TRB) and a *Time-Work Schedule* (TRB). Place the finished pies on an evaluation table. Have students evaluate the appearance, flakiness, and tenderness of the pastry as well as the eating quality and appearance of the filling of each pie. Then have each lab group complete a *Lab Evaluation Sheet* (TRB).

Candy

35. **ER** Field trip. Take your class to a candy shop where students can see different types of candies being made. Have them observe how ingredients are combined and cooked. After the trip, discuss with the class the important candy making principles they observed.

36. **RF** Have students define the terms *crystalline candy* and *noncrystalline candy*. Then have them find recipes for each type of candy.

37. **RT** Demonstrate for students how to use a candy thermometer and how to use the cold water method to test candy when you do not have a candy thermometer.

38. **RF** Have students find recipes for candies cooked to the soft ball, hard ball, soft crack, and hard crack stages.

39. **RF** *Candy,* Activity F, SAG. Students are to complete exercises about the preparation of candy.

40. **ER** Working in lab groups, have students prepare chocolate fudge, white fudge, and penuche. Have them compare appearance, texture, and flavor of the candies on a *Food Product Evaluation Sheet* (TRB).

41. **ER**   Working in lab groups, have students prepare butterscotch, peanut brittle, and English toffee. After the candies have cooled, have students compare the appearance, texture, and flavor on a *Food Product Evaluation Sheet* (TRB). Also have students list the interfering agents used in each candy.

42. **ER**   Have students compare the ease of melting chocolate, caramels, or marshmallows on top of a range with melting these candies in a microwave oven.

43. **EX**   *Candy Recipes,* recipe master 23-7, TRB. Have students use the recipe master and additional recipes, as desired, to plan a candy lab. Have each group complete a *Market Order Sheet* (TRB) and a *Time-Work Schedule* (TRB). After preparing and sampling their candy products, have each group complete a *Lab Evaluation Sheet* (TRB).

Chapter Review

44. **RT**   Make a class desserts and sweets cookbook. Have each student contribute a favorite recipe for cake, cookies, pie, or candy.

45. **RT**   *Chapter 23 Study Sheet,* reproducible master 23-8, TRB. Have students complete the statements as they read text pages 370-385.

46. **RF**   *Reverse Thinking,* Software, diskette for Part Three. Have students play the chapter review game according to the instructions that appear on the screen.

Above and Beyond

47. **EX**   Have each student create a variation of one of the following basic recipes: white or yellow layer cake, sugar cookies, vanilla cream pie, or chocolate fudge. Have students give their variation a name and submit a written explanation of how the recipe would be altered. (Students may want to refer to some standard cookbooks for ideas about how a variation might alter a recipe.) Students should prepare a sample of their creation. If desired, samples may be judged for appearance, texture, flavor, and creativity and awards may be given to those creations receiving the highest ratings.

48. **EX**   Have students prepare two batches of sugar cookies, one with part of the sugar replaced with artificial sweetener. Have students compare the flavor, texture, and appearance on a *Food Product Evaluation Sheet* (TRB).

49. **EX**   Have students plan a bake sale as a fund-raiser. Have them prepare a variety of cakes, cookies, pies, and candies to sell. Students should consider prices of similar commercial products and their time and ingredient costs when pricing their products. Following the sale, discuss whether students were able to charge an adequate profit margin to make this a worthwhile way of raising money.

Answer Key

Text

Review What You Have Read, page 386
1. Cakes are classified as shortened and unshortened. Chiffon cake has characteristics of both types.
2. flour, sugar, eggs, liquid, salt, fat, leavening agent (For functions, see pages 370-372 in the text.)
3. makes egg whites whiter, makes the cake grain finer, stabilizes the egg white proteins which increases the volume of the baked cake
4. (List three:) spices, extracts, fruits, nuts, poppy seeds, coconut
5. conventional method, quick mix method
6. If the pans are too small, the batter will overflow. If the pans are too large, the cake will be too flat and it may become dry. A cake baked in pans that are the right size will have a gently rounded top. Pans should be arranged in the oven so they do not touch each other or the sides of the oven. Air should circulate freely around them.
7. false
8. false
9. rolled, dropped, bar, pressed, molded, refrigerator; Brownies are bar cookies.
10. Cookies baked on a shiny cookie sheet have light, delicately browned crusts. Those baked on dark cookie sheets have dark bottoms.
11. flour, fat, salt, water
12. tender, flaky
13. (List two:) too much liquid, too little fat, too much flour, dough overmixed, rolling pin used too vigorously
14. Add cocoa or instant coffee to the flour when making pastry. Brush the pastry with a mixture of molasses and egg yolk.

15. Crystalline candy is smooth and creamy. Noncrystalline candy may be chewy or brittle.

Student Activity Guide

Kinds of Cakes, Activity A, page 109
1. A, C, E, F, G
2. Pound cakes contain no chemical leaveners. They are more compact than other shortened cakes, and they have a closer grain.
3. A, B, C, E
4. Sponge cakes contain the whole egg rather than just the egg white.
5. A, B, C
6. H
7. D
8. E
9. C
10. A
11. G
12. B
13. F

Preparation of Cakes, Activity B, page 110
1. A cake made with too much flour is compact and dry. A cake made with too little flour is coarse, and it may fall.
2. Overmixing will cause the gluten to overdevelop and the cake will be tough.
3. If the pans are too small, the batter will overflow. If the pans are too large, the cake will be too flat and may be dry.
4. Angel food and sponge cake batters must cling to the sides of the pan during baking.
5. Cakes baked for too long may be dry.
6. This will allow the heat to circulate freely, and will prevent hot spots and uneven baking.
7. If the toothpick comes out clean or the cake springs back when touched, the cake is done.
8. This makes it easier to remove the cake from the pan.
9. Round or ring-shaped pans give the most even cooking in a microwave oven.
10. This will allow the egg whites to achieve maximum volume when they are beaten.
11. This breaks down large air pockets and seals the batter against the sides of the pan and tube.
12. If the cracks feel dry and no imprint remains, the cake is done.
13. This prevents a loss of volume during cooling.

Cookies, Activity C, page 111
1. E
2. A
3. D
4. A
5. C
6. B
7. C
8. B
9. F
10. F
11. T
12. T
13. F
14. T
15. T
16. F
17. T
18. F
19. F
20. F
21. F
22. T

Pie Filling, Activity D, page 112
1. A fruit pie is typically a two-crust pie with a filling made from canned, frozen, dried, or fresh fruit or commercially prepared pie filling.
2. A cream pie is typically a one-crust pie with a filling made from a cornstarch-thickened pudding mixture.
3. A custard pie is typically a one-crust pie filled with a custard made from milk, eggs, and sugar.
4. A chiffon pie is typically a one-crust pie filled with a light, airy mixture containing gelatin and beaten egg whites.
5. A high-quality pie has a tender, flaky, crisp crust. It should be evenly browned and the filling should have a pleasing flavor and texture.
6. (Student response.)

Pastry Preparation, Activity E, page 113
1. A, C, F, H, I, K, M, N, P, Q, R
2. The bottom and sides of the crust are not pricked.
3. A second crust is placed on top of a filled pie. The edges are sealed and fluted together. Several small slits are made in the top crust to allow steam to escape during baking.
4. The crust would be microwaved in six to seven minutes. Special techniques would also need to be used if you desire a crust that appears to be browned.

Candy, Activity F, page 114
1. C
2. NC
3. NC
4. C
5. NC
6. C
7. B
8. C
9. NC
10. NC
11. B
12. B
13. B
14. C
15. NC

188

16. A sugar syrup is a heated mixture of sugar and liquid that is the basis of all cooked candies.
17. High-quality fudge tastes smooth and creamy because it contains small sugar crystals. It has a deep brown color and a satiny sheen.
18. High-quality peanut brittle has a golden color and looks foamy.
19. These candies are less likely to stick and burn in a microwave oven than on a conventional range.
20. Both crystalline and noncrystalline candies can be successfully prepared in a microwave oven.

Teacher's Resources

Chapter 23 Test

1. D		14. F
2. E		15. F
3. B		16. T
4. F		17. C
5. G		18. B
6. A		19. B
7. T		20. C
8. T		21. A
9. T		22. B
10. F		23. B
11. F		24. D
12. T		25. B
13. T		26. D

27. In the quick mix method, the fat and part of the liquid are added to the sifted dry ingredients and beaten. The remaining liquid and unbeaten eggs are added last. In the conventional method, the fat and sugar are creamed together. The eggs are added, followed by the dry and liquid ingredients, which are added alternately, beginning and ending with the dry ingredients.
28. Crisp cookies should be stored in a container with a loose-fitting cover. Soft cookies should be stored in a container with a tight-fitting cover. The two types of cookies never should be stored together.
29. Pastry should be handled as little and as gently as possible to avoid overdeveloping the gluten and toughening the pastry.
30. A high-quality pie should have pastry that is tender, flaky, and crisp. It should be lightly and evenly browned, and the filling should have a pleasing flavor and be neither too runny nor too firm.
31. to produce small, fine crystals that will give the finished candy a creamy texture

Cakes, Cookies, Pies, and Candies

Name _____

Date _____ Period _____ Score _____

Chapter 23 Test

Matching: Match each of the following kinds of cookies with the basic group of cookies to which it belongs.

_____ 1. Crescents.

_____ 2. Spritz.

_____ 3. Chocolate chip.

_____ 4. Pinwheels.

_____ 5. Gingerbread figures.

_____ 6. Brownies.

A. bar cookies

B. dropped cookies

C. formed cookies

D. molded cookies

E. pressed cookies

F. refrigerator cookies

G. rolled cookies

True/False: Circle *T* if the statement is true or *F* if the statement is false.

T F   7. Unshortened cakes contain no fat.

T F   8. Fat tenderizes the gluten in cakes.

T F   9. Cream of tartar is used in angel food cakes to stabilize the egg white proteins, improve the color of the egg whites, and make the cake grain finer.

T F   10. Cake pans for unshortened cakes should be greased and floured.

T F   11. Molded cookies are made from a soft dough that is dropped from a spoon onto a cookie sheet.

T F   12. Many cookies can be frozen in both baked and unbaked form.

T F   13. The four basic kinds of pies are fruit, cream, custard, and chiffon.

T F   14. Oil-based pastry is tender and flaky.

T F   15. Fudge, fondant, and divinity are noncrystalline candies.

T F   16. High-quality fudge has small sugar crystals.

Multiple Choice: Choose the best response. Write the letter in the space provided.

_____ 17. Which of the following fats is *not* used in cakes?
   A. Butter.
   B. Hydrogenated vegetable shortening.
   C. Lard.
   D. Margarine.

_____ 18. Which of the following ingredients gives cakes structure?
   A. Butter.
   B. Flour.
   C. Milk.
   D. Sugar.

_____ 19. Which of the following can make a cake tough?
   A. Too little liquid.
   B. Too many eggs.
   C. Too much fat.
   D. Too much flour.

(Continued)

Name _____

_____ 20. A shortened cake that contains no chemical leavener is a _____.
A. butter cake
B. chiffon cake
C. pound cake
D. sponge cake

_____ 21. What type of pan should be used for cookies with light, delicate crusts?
A. Bright, shiny pans.
B. Dark pans.
C. Pans with high sides.
D. All of the above.

_____ 22. Cookies that contain beaten egg whites, such as macaroons, meringues, and kisses, are mixed _____.
A. by the biscuit method
B. like angel food and sponge cakes
C. using the conventional mixing method used for cakes
D. using the quick mix method

_____ 23. Crumbly pastry usually is the result of _____.
A. too little fat
B. too much fat
C. too much flour
D. too much water

_____ 24. Tough pastry usually is caused by _____.
A. overmixing the dough when adding liquid
B. rolling pastry too vigorously
C. too much liquid
D. All of the above.

_____ 25. All the following are crystalline candies *except* _____.
A. caramels
B. fudge
C. peanut brittle
D. toffee

_____ 26. Which of the following substances is *not* an interfering agent used in candy making?
A. Butter.
B. Corn syrup.
C. Heavy cream.
D. Sugar.

Essay Questions: Provide complete responses to the following questions or statements.

27. How does the quick mix, or one-bowl, method differ from the conventional method used to mix cakes?
28. How should cookies be stored?
29. How should pastry be handled?
30. Describe a high-quality pie.
31. Why must fudge be vigorously beaten after it has cooled to lukewarm?

Parties, Picnics, and Dining Out

Objectives

After studying this chapter, students will be able to
- plan a party.
- prepare party foods and beverages.
- safely prepare and pack food for outdoor meals.
- follow etiquette rules when dining out.

Bulletin Board

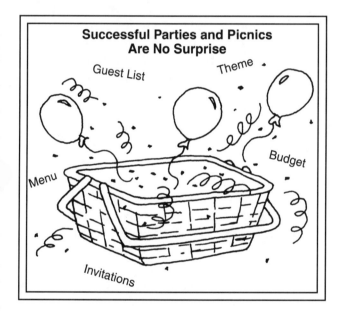

Successful Parties and Picnics Are No Surprise

Guest List

Theme

Menu

Budget

Invitations

Title: "Successful Parties and Picnics Are No Surprise"

Use cutouts or a drawing to show a large picnic basket with party balloons, streamers, and confetti coming out of it. Interspersed with the party trimmings should be words, such as *menu, invitations, budget, guest list,* etc., that emphasize key concepts in the chapter.

Teaching Materials

Text, pages 387-404
Student Activity Guide
- A. *Planning a Party*
- B. *Table Manners*
- C. *Food and Beverages for Parties*
- D. *Entertaining Outdoors*
- E. *Dining Out*

Teacher's Resource Binder
- *Food for Parties,* recipe master 24-1
- *The Effect of Water Temperature on Tea,* food science master 24-2
- *Beverage Recipes,* recipe master 24-3
- *Picnic Food,* recipe master 24-4
- *The Cost of Dining Out,* transparency master 24-5
- *Chapter 24 Study Sheet,* reproducible master 24-6
- Chapter 24 Test
Software, diskette for Part Three
- *The Matching Game,* chapter review game

Introductory Activities

1. Ask students what they think makes a party fun. Then ask them what makes a party boring.
2. Ask students to explain what they feel is the most difficult part of giving a party or planning a picnic. Focus on their responses when covering chapter material.

Strategies to Reteach, Reinforce, Enrich, and Extend Text Concepts

Planning a Party

3. **EX** Have the class brainstorm a list of party themes. Discuss how the themes could be carried out.
4. **EX** Have each student plan a menu for one of the parties listed in strategy 3. Have students set up time-work schedules for their menus.
5. **RF** Ask students to discuss what factors should be considered when planning a guest list for a party.
6. **EX** Have students role-play making introductions at a party.
7. **EX** Have the class brainstorm a list of activities that could be used to "break the ice" at parties.
8. **RF** Ask one student to give a responsibility of a party host. Then ask another student to state why that responsibility is important. Repeat this activity with different students around the room.

9. **RF**   Have students list the responsibilities of a party guest. Then have them discuss the difference between being a good guest and being a poor guest.
10. **RF**   Have students make a list of etiquette guidelines for dining in a friend's home.
11. **EX**   *Planning a Party,* Activity A, SAG. Students are to complete the party planning activities outlined on the worksheets.
12. **RF**   *Table Manners,* Activity B, SAG. Students are to provide appropriate solutions to etiquette problems described on the worksheet.
13. **ER**   Guest speaker. Invite a caterer to speak to your class about how parties are professionally planned and carried out.

Food for Parties

14. **RF**   Ask students what factors should be considered when choosing food to serve at a party.
15. **RF**   Have students find recipes for party appetizers that can be cooked in a microwave oven.
16. **EX**   *Food for Parties,* recipe master 24-1, TRB. Have students use the recipe master and additional recipes found in strategy 15 to plan a party food lab. Have each lab group complete a *Market Order Sheet* (TRB) and a *Time-Work Schedule* (TRB). Have groups share their foods with the class. Then have each group complete a *Lab Evaluation Sheet* (TRB).

Beverages for Parties

17. **ER**   Working in lab groups, have students prepare iced coffee and a variety of flavored coffees. Ask students when these coffee beverages would be most appropriate.
18. **EX**   Brew fine, medium, and coarse grind coffee each in a drip coffeemaker. Have students compare the color, flavor, body, and aroma of the three brews. Use their observations as the basis for a discussion of choosing the right grind for the brewing method.
19. **ER**   Have students compare the appearance of several varieties of tea leaves. Then have them prepare and sample the teas and compare color, aroma, and flavor.
20. **EX**   *The Effect of Water Temperature on Tea,* food science master 24-2, TRB. Have lab groups complete the experiment as directed on the master. Students will be analyzing the effect of water temperature on the extraction of flavoring substances from tea leaves.

21. **ER**   Have students prepare iced tea by first brewing hot tea. Then have them prepare "sun tea" by placing eight tea bags in a one-gallon jar filled with water and leaving it in the sun for several hours until the tea has reached the desired strength. Have students compare the two chilled beverages and identify the one they prefer. Have them give reasons for their choice.
22. **EX**   Divide the class into five lab groups. Assign one of the following hot chocolate or cocoa preparations to each group: made with natural process cocoa, made with Dutch process cocoa, made with unsweetened chocolate, made with powdered chocolate mix, and made with chocolate syrup. Have students use fluid, fresh milk for all preparations. Place the prepared beverages on an evaluation table. Have students compare the appearance, flavor, body, and color of the beverages on a *Food Product Evaluation Sheet* (TRB). Also have students note the amount of chocolate or cocoa that settles out into the cup for each sample.
23. **RF**   Have students find a variety of punch recipes that would be refreshing party beverages.
24. **EX**   *Beverage Recipes,* recipe master 24-3, TRB. Have students use the recipe master and additional recipes found in strategy 23 to plan a beverage lab. Have each lab group complete a *Market Order Sheet* (TRB) and a *Time-Work Schedule* (TRB). Have groups share their beverages with the class. Then have each group complete a *Lab Evaluation Sheet* (TRB).
25. **RF**   *Food and Beverages for Parties,* Activity C, SAG. Students are to complete exercises about food and beverages for parties.

Outdoor Entertaining

26. **ER**   Guest speaker. Invite someone from your local park district to speak to your class about safe and courteous picnicking guidelines.
27. **EX**   Have students plan menus that would be suitable for each of the following types of picnics: a bicycle picnic for four people; a weekday, noon-hour picnic for two in a city park; a tailgate picnic for four before a football game; and an all-day picnic for a group of 25.
28. **ER**   Have students prepare short oral reports on the selection, cost, use, or care of a barbecue grill.
29. **ER**   Have students plan a barbecue display

for a school bulletin board or showcase. Have them include pictures and descriptions of barbecue equipment along with lists of safety precautions.

30. **ER** Have students prepare two-page written reports on campfire cooking. Have them include descriptions of cooking equipment suitable for use at campfires as well as a list of foods that can be carried long distances without spoilage.
31. **RT** Discuss with the class safety precautions that should be followed when cooking and eating outdoors.
32. **ER** Have students investigate different types of equipment available for transporting hot and cold foods.
33. **EX** *Picnic Food,* recipe master 24-4, TRB. Have lab groups prepare a variety of foods, including fruits, vegetables, and breads, to serve with the entrees on the recipe master. Have each lab group complete a *Market Order Sheet* (TRB) and a *Time-Work Schedule* (TRB). After students have prepared and sampled the picnic foods, have each lab group complete a *Lab Evaluation Sheet* (TRB).
34. **RF** *Entertaining Outdoors,* Activity D, SAG. Students are to complete the worksheet by writing a picnic menu, identifying safe barbecuing techniques, and listing staple items that belong in a picnic basket.

Dining Out

35. **ER** Field trip. Take your class to visit a restaurant during nonbusiness hours. Ask restaurant personnel about reservations, dress codes, methods of payment, and tipping.
36. **EX** Have students debate the pros and cons of eating out versus eating at home. Include such factors as time, energy, cost, family size, cooking skills, and enjoyment.
37. **RT** *The Cost of Dining Out,* transparency master 24-5, TRB. Use the transparency to illustrate for students how the cost of eating out compares with the cost of preparing meals at home. Note that the home-cooked meal cost includes labor costs for shopping, preparing, and cleanup.
38. **RT** Discuss with students appropriate attire for different types of restaurants.
39. **EX** Have students role-play ordering from a menu at a restaurant.
40. **RT** Discuss with students how etiquette guidelines for dining in a friend's home

resemble etiquette guidelines for dining in a restaurant.
41. **RF** Give students some mock restaurant bills and have them practice determining how much money should be given for tips.
42. **RF** On the chalkboard, list each type of restaurant discussed in the chapter. Define each type, then have students cite the advantages and disadvantages of dining in each type. Ask students what factors determine which type of restaurant they choose.
43. **RF** *Dining Out,* Activity E, SAG. Students are to complete a chart describing the atmosphere, menu items, price range, and popular characteristics of various types of restaurants in their area.

Chapter Review

44. **RT** *Chapter 24 Study Sheet,* reproducible master 24-6, TRB. Have students complete the statements as they read text pages 388-402.
45. **RF** *The Matching Game,* Software, diskette for Part Three. Have students play the chapter review game according to the instructions that appear on the screen.

Above and Beyond

46. **EX** Have your class plan a school dance or party or a class picnic. Have them determine a budget; publicize the event; sell tickets; plan, purchase, and prepare the food; and set up and serve at the event. You may want to make this project a cooperative effort. Art classes could be responsible for designing posters, business classes could be responsible for doing the budgeting and bookkeeping, etc. After the event, discuss the outcome with your students. Ask them to identify strengths and weaknesses.
47. **ER** Have students contact a hotel or resort facility to find out what types of special events are held for guests. Students should also ask what member of the staff is responsible for planning these events. Have students share their findings in class.

Answer Key

Text

Review What You Have Read, page 404
 1. date, time, place

2. budget, cooking skills, time schedule, equipment available
3. (List three. Student response. See pages 389-390 in the text.)
4. (List five. Student response. See pages 390-391 in the text.)
5. true
6. Bulk containers allow consumers to buy just as much coffee as they want. Vacuum-sealed packages help coffee stay fresh longer.
7. C
8. starch cookery principles, milk cookery principles
9. Freeze fruit juices in ice cube trays to make ice cubes that will not dilute drinks.
10. (List four:) place grill in the open, keep all flammable materials away from the fire, wear tight-fitting clothes, tie hair back away from the face, never use gasoline or kerosene to start the fire, never pour more lighter fluid on coals after they have been lighted, keep water handy for flare-ups
11. false
12. a la carte
13. $2.00.
14. A. almondine
    B. marengo
    C. a la mode
    D. Florentine

Student Activity Guide

Table Manners, Activity B, page 117
1. Open the napkin to a comfortable size and place it on your lap.
2. Tear a slice of bread into two parts and then in two again. Butter only one-fourth of a slice at a time.
3. Keep the hand you are not eating with in your lap while eating.
4. Remove it from your mouth with your fingers as inconspicuously as possible.
5. Ask for it to be passed to you.
6. Eating utensils are used in the order in which they have been placed on the table—from the outside toward the plate.
7. Do not use the utensil anymore. The host should get you another one.
8. Use your handkerchief, quietly excuse yourself, and leave the table.
9. Leave it without comment.

10. Place your knife on the rim of the plate with the sharp edge pointing toward the center. Place the fork parallel to the knife.

Food and Beverages for Parties, Activity C, page 118
(Appetizer descriptions are student response.)
1. T
2. HC
3. CD
4. C
5. C
6. HC
7. T
8. C
9. CD
10. HC

Entertaining Outdoors, Activity D, page 119
(Menu is student response.)
(The following items should be checked as safe barbecuing techniques:) 1, 4, 5, 7, 8
(Items for picnic basket are student response.)

Teacher's Resources

Chapter 24 Test
1. C
2. D
3. A
4. B
5. E
6. I
7. H
8. G
9. K
10. F
11. T
12. F
13. T
14. F
15. T
16. T
17. F
18. T
19. T
20. T
21. F
22. T
23. D
24. C
25. C
26. A
27. D
28. A
29. B
30. B
31. available space, cooking equipment, cooking skills (Students may justify other responses.)
32. (Student response. See pages 390-391 in the text.)
33. The starch granules must be separated (starch cookery principles), and low temperatures must be used to heat the beverage to prevent scorching (milk cookery principles).
34. Coals in a barbecue grill are ready to cook food when they are covered with a gray ash.
35. Quietly call the problem to your waiter's attention. Avoid making a scene and disturbing other diners. If the waiter is unwilling or unable to correct the problem, ask to speak to the manager.

Parties, Picnics, and Dining Out

Name _____

Date _____ Period _____ Score _____

Chapter 24 Test

Matching: Match the following terms and identifying phrases.

_____ 1. Several varieties of coffee beans mixed together.

_____ 2. A compound found in products like coffee, tea, and chocolate that acts as a stimulant.

_____ 3. Menu in which each food item is individually priced.

_____ 4. A small, light food served at the beginning of a meal to stimulate the appetite.

_____ 5. A term describing coffee or tea from which a stimulating compound has been removed.

_____ 6. Type of menu in which one price is given for an entire meal.

_____ 7. An abbreviation used on invitations, which means, "Please respond."

_____ 8. An arrangement made with a restaurant to hold a table for a given date and time.

_____ 9. Money left for a waiter for service rendered.

_____ 10. Rules set by society to guide social behavior.

A. a la carte

B. appetizer

C. blend

D. caffeine

E. decaffeinated

F. etiquette

G. reservation

H. RSVP

I. table d'hôte

J. tea

K. tip

True/False: Circle *T* if the statement is true or *F* if the statement is false.

T   F   11. A formal party always requires a written invitation.

T   F   12. The best party menus include unique, new recipes that the party giver has been waiting to try.

T   F   13. A younger guest should be introduced to an older guest by giving the older person's name first.

T   F   14. A diner should begin eating as soon as food is placed in front of him or her.

T   F   15. Seeds, pits, and fish bones should be removed from the mouth with the fingers.

T   F   16. Placing appetizers with cracker bases on paper towels helps absorb excess moisture during microwaving.

T   F   17. Coffee should be allowed to sit for a while before serving so the flavors have a chance to intensify.

T   F   18. Iced tea is prepared by first making hot tea.

T   F   19. An ice ring will keep punch cold longer than ice cubes.

T   F   20. The type of food served at a picnic depends partly on the cooking facilities available at the picnic site.

T   F   21. Charcoal lighter fluid and gasoline are equally safe for starting a fire in a barbecue.

T   F   22. When a restaurant check is brought in a folder, the waiter will take the payment and bring the change.

(Continued)

Name _____

Multiple Choice: Choose the best response. Write the letter in the space provided.

_____ 23. When planning a party menu, you should consider _____.
    A. the theme of your party
    B. your time schedule
    C. special dietary needs of your guests
    D. All of the above.

_____ 24. Which of the following appetizers should be microwaved at a lower setting?
    A. Chicken wings with honey mustard glaze.
    B. Cocktail sausages with barbecue sauce.
    C. Hot sour cream dip with green onions.
    D. Toasted nuts with herb seasoning.

_____ 25. Which coffee grind should be used in a drip coffeemaker?
    A. Coarse grind.
    B. Fine grind.
    C. Medium grind.
    D. Regular grind.

_____ 26. The type of tea made from fully fermented tea leaves is _____.
    A black tea
    B. green tea
    C. herbal tea
    D. oolong tea

_____ 27. The part of a barbecue grill on which food is cooked is called the _____.
    A. bowl
    B. briquettes
    C. fire box
    D. grate

_____ 28. In what order are foods in restaurants generally served?
    A. Appetizer, salad, entree, and dessert.
    B. Appetizer, entree, soup, and dessert.
    C. Salad, appetizer, entree, and dessert.
    D. Soup, salad, appetizer, and dessert.

_____ 29. What would be an appropriate tip for average service on a $12.00 restaurant bill?
    A. $1.00.
    B. $1.80.
    C. $2.50.
    D. None of the above amounts is appropriate.

_____ 30. Which type of restaurant generally has a rather limited menu?
    A. Family restaurant.
    B. Fast-food restaurant.
    C. Formal restaurant.
    D. Specialty restaurant.

Essay Questions: Provide complete responses to the following questions or statements.

31. What factors should be taken into consideration when planning a guest list?
32. Describe three responsibilities of a well-mannered party guest.
33. When preparing chocolate or cocoa beverages, what cooking principles must be followed?
34. How can you tell when the coals in a barbecue grill are ready to cook food?
35. What should you do if the food you are served in a restaurant has not been prepared as you ordered it?

Preserving Foods

Objectives

After studying this chapter, students will be able to
- explain principles of food preservation.
- discuss techniques for home canning and making jellied products.
- describe procedures for freezing and drying foods.
- identify methods of commercial food preservation.

Bulletin Board

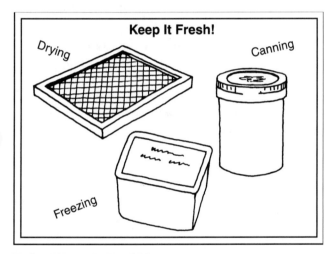

Title: "Keep It Fresh!"

Use cutouts or drawings to illustrate the three basic methods of home food preservation—canning, freezing, and drying.

Teaching Materials

Text, pages 405-423
Student Activity Guide
   A. *Microorganisms and Enzymes*
   B. *Home Canning*
   C. *Jellied Products Crossword*
   D. *Freezing*
   E. *Drying*
   F. *Storage Life of Foods*

Teacher's Resource Binder
   Preserving Food, transparency master 25-1
   Mold Growth, food science master 25-2
   Preparing Fruits for Freezing, reproducible master 25-3

Preparing Vegetables for Freezing, reproducible master 25-4
   Preparing Fruits for Drying, reproducible master 25-5
   Preparing Vegetables for Drying, reproducible master 25-6
   Microwaving Fruit Leather, reproducible master 25-7
   Chapter 25 Study Sheet, reproducible master 25-8
   Chapter 25 Test
Software, diskette for Part Three
   Bingo, chapter review game

Introductory Activities

1. *Preserving Food,* transparency master 25-1, TRB. Use the master to introduce students to the three main methods of home food preservation—canning, freezing, and drying. Explain the basic principles of each method.
2. Discuss with students how people in earlier times used root cellars and springhouses to store foods for long periods of time. Ask students to evaluate the effectiveness of those storage methods compared to methods used today.

Strategies to Reteach, Reinforce, Enrich, and Extend Text Concepts

Food Spoilage

3. **RF** Have students divide a sheet of paper vertically into two columns. In one column, have them list the good effects microorganisms can have. In the other column, have them list the bad effects they can have.
4. **RF** *Microorganisms and Enzymes,* Activity A, SAG. Students are to identify whether the phrases on the worksheet describe microorganisms or enzymes. Then they are to answer the questions that follow.
5. **EX** *Mold Growth,* food science master 25-2, TRB. Have lab groups complete the experiment as directed on the master. Students will

be analyzing conditions that promote and inhibit mold growth on food.

Canning Foods

6. **RF**   Have students discuss the various reasons people choose to do home canning.
7. **RT**   Display approved canning jars and closures for students to examine.
8. **ER**   Guest speaker. Invite a county extension agent to speak to your class about safe home canning methods.
9. **RF**   Ask students to explain the difference between the raw pack and hot pack methods of filling canning jars. Then have them describe the function of leaving headspace in filled jars.
10. **ER**   Have students write two paragraphs describing the two methods of home canning.
11. **ER**   Have students use the boiling water canning method to can fresh fruit.
12. **RF**   Have students draw a picture of a pressure canner. Have them label the following parts of the canner and describe the function of each: petcock, safety valve, gasket, and pressure gauge.
13. **ER**   Have students locate an authorized agency in your area that provides a gauge testing service. If possible, have them ask for a demonstration.
14. **ER**   Have students pressure can a fresh, low-acid vegetable.
15. **RT**   Demonstrate for students how to test the seals on canning jars.
16. **ER**   Have students design a brochure about the safe use of home-canned foods. The brochure should describe how to check for spoilage, what types of spoilage to be aware of, what to do with spoiled foods, and how to prepare foods that appear to be wholesome.
17. **RF**   *Home Canning*, Activity B, SAG. Students are to complete exercises about home canning.

Making Jellied Products

18. **RF**   Have students list and describe the functions of the four basic ingredients needed to make jelly.
19. **ER**   Working in lab groups, have students prepare jelly, preserves, marmalade, jam, and conserves and process them in a boiling water canner. Later in the term, have them evaluate the color, flavor, and texture of each product on a *Food Product Evaluation Sheet* (TRB).

20. **ER**   Have students prepare an uncooked jam and a cooked jam made with the same fruit. Have them compare the two products in terms of flavor, texture, and appearance using a *Food Product Evaluation Sheet* (TRB).
21. **RF**   *Jellied Products Crossword*, Activity C, SAG. Students are to complete a crossword puzzle using terms related to jellied products.

Freezing Foods

22. **RT**   *Preparing Fruits for Freezing*, reproducible master 25-3, TRB. Distribute the handout as you discuss with students how to prepare various fruits for freezing.
23. **ER**   Have students freeze strawberries using the dry pack, sugar pack, and syrup pack methods. At the end of the school term, thaw the fruits. Have students compare the appearance, flavor, color, and texture of the three products on a *Food Product Evaluation Sheet* (TRB). Ask students to specify which product they prefer and state why.
24. **RT**   *Preparing Vegetables for Freezing*, reproducible master 25-4, TRB. Distribute the handout as you discuss with students how to prepare various vegetables for freezing.
25. **EX**   Have students clean 1 pound (450 g) of green beans. Have them steam blanch half of the beans and leave the other half unblanched. Freeze beans in separate freezer containers, labeling each. At the end of the school term, thaw the beans and cook them. Have students compare the appearance, flavor, color, and texture of the two groups of beans on a *Food Product Evaluation Sheet* (TRB). Ask students to specify which product they prefer and state why.
26. **EX**   Freeze a gelatin dessert, a vanilla cornstarch pudding, and an egg salad sandwich. Thaw the products a week later. Have students analyze them and explain why these foods should not be frozen.
27. **RF**   *Freezing*, Activity D, SAG. Students are to complete statements about freezing food and then arrange circled letters to spell a term related to freezing food.

Drying Foods

28. **ER**   Have students visit a supermarket and make a list of all the dried food products that are available. Have them be sure to look for dried mixes and convenience items as well as fruits and vegetables.

29. **RT** *Preparing Fruits for Drying,* reproducible master 25-5, TRB. Distribute the handout as you discuss with students how to prepare various fruits for drying.
30. **RT** *Preparing Vegetables for Drying,* reproducible master 25-6, TRB. Distribute the handout as you discuss with students how to prepare various vegetables for drying.
31. **ER** *Microwaving Fruit Leather,* reproducible master 25-7, TRB. Have students follow the directions on the duplicating master to prepare a fruit leather in a microwave oven.
32. **RF** *Drying,* Activity E, SAG. Students are to place the steps for drying fruits and vegetables in the proper order. Then they are to answer the questions that follow.

Commercial Food Preservation

33. **ER** Have students investigate how foods for which irradiation has been approved are being preserved, if not by irradiation. Have them share their findings in class.
34. **ER** Have students prepare an oral report with visual aids on one of the commercial preservation methods discussed in the chapter. Reports should include information about the types of foods with which the method is used and how it affects the cost of products.
35. **RF** Have students design a game they can play to help them remember how long various foods can be stored in a refrigerator, in a freezer, or on a shelf.
36. **RF** *Storage Life of Foods,* Activity F, SAG. Students are to give the storage life for various frozen, refrigerated, and shelf-stored foods.

Chapter Review

37. **RT** *Chapter 25 Study Sheet,* reproducible master 25-8, TRB. Have students complete the statements as they read text pages 406-422.
38. **RF** *Bingo,* Software, diskette for Part Three. Have students play the chapter review game according to the instructions that appear on the screen.

Above and Beyond

39. **ER** Have students investigate the costs of home canning equipment and supplies. Assuming they grew produce at a negligible cost, have them determine how much canning they would need to do to realize a return on their investment in canning equipment over the cost of purchasing canned goods in a grocery store. Then have them interview someone who does home canning about why he or she chooses to do it. Students should compile the information from their cost analysis and their interview into a three-page report on the topic "Motivation for Home Canning in Today's Society."
40. **ER** Have students prepare a dinner. Then have them compare the cost, including labor and ingredients, of the homemade dinner with a comparable commercial frozen dinner. Also have them compare the two dinners in terms of appearance and flavor. Students should summarize their comparison in a three-page written report.
41. **ER** Have students build a home food dryer and use it to dry several food items. Have them compare these items in terms of cost, appearance, and flavor with commercially dried products. Students should summarize their comparison in a three-page written report.

Answer Key

Text

Review What You Have Read, page 423
1. true
2. food, moisture, favorable temperatures
3. two-piece vacuum caps comprised of a metal screw band and a flat metal lid with sealing compound on one side
4. headspace
5. pressure canning
6. (List three:) freezing temperatures, dampness, heat, light
7. (List five:) bulging lids; leaking jars; spurting liquid; off odor; mold; gas bubbles; unusually soft food; looks spoiled, foams, or has an off odor during heating
8. fruit juice, pectin, acid, sugar
9. marmalade
10. Quick-freezing produces very small ice crystals. Slow-freezing causes large ice crystals to form that damage the cell structure of food and change the texture.
11. dry pack, sugar pack, syrup pack
12. (List five:) lettuce, salad greens, custards, gelatin products, meringues, sour cream,

hard-cooked egg white, sandwiches containing salad dressing or mayonnaise
13. sun drying, oven drying
14. A

Student Activity Guide

Microorganisms and Enzymes, Activity A, page 121

1. M		6. E	
2. E		7. E	
3. M		8. M	
4. M		9. M	
5. E		10. E	

11. Freezing temperatures prevent microorganisms from growing and retard the action of enzymes.
12. High temperatures destroy microorganisms and enzymes.
13. Drying removes the moisture needed for growth.
14. Vegetables and some fruits can be blanched. Other fruits can be treated with sulfur dioxide or sulfites.

Home Canning, Activity B, page 122

1. A	10. A	
2. B	11. F	
3. A	12. T	
4. B	13. T	
5. B	14. T	
6. B	15. T	
7. B	16. T	
8. A	17. T	
9. B	18. F	

Jellied Products Crossword, Activity C, page 123

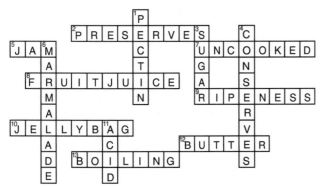

Freezing, Activity D, page 124
1. quick-frozen
2. ice crystals
3. freezer
4. freezer burn
5. containers
6. underripe

7. ascorbic
8. head
9. enzymatic browning
10. blanched
11. serving
12. vapor
Circled letters: I, S, E, R, T, P, R, E, A, N, V, O
Freezing is one method of food PRESERVATION.
13. Fruits have the best flavor if served with a few ice crystals remaining.
14. Meat, poultry, and fish should be allowed to thaw overnight in a refrigerator or using the defrost setting on a microwave oven.
15. If food is partially thawed but still firm, it can be refrozen. If food is fully thawed, it should not be refrozen.

Drying, Activity E, page 125

1. I	7. G	
2. L	8. E	
3. D	9. A	
4. B	10. F	
5. J	11. H	
6. C	12. K	

13. Microorganisms that cause food spoilage need moisture to grow. Drying removes moisture, thus stopping the growth of microorganisms.
14. (List five:) Milk, eggs, coffee, fruit drinks, dessert mixes, salad dressing mixes, fruits, vegetables, and complete meals are all examples of commercially dried food products.
15. Dried foods are popular with campers, hikers, and backpackers because they are lightweight and take up less space than their reconstituted counterparts.
16. You can use a salt solution made by dissolving 3 to 6 tablespoons (45 to 90 mL) salt in one gallon (4L) of water.
17. Trays with screen bottoms allow foods to dry faster than cookie sheets because they allow air to circulate around the food.
18. Oven drying can be done in a food dehydrator or a conventional oven.
19. Soak dried vegetables in water for 1¼ to 2 hours. Cook vegetables in the same water used for soaking.
20. Dried fruits and vegetables can be stored on a shelf for up to one year.

Storage Life of Foods, Activity F, page 126
1. 6 to 12 months
2. 2 to 3 months
3. 3 to 4 months
4. 9 to 12 months

5. 3 months
6. 2 months
7. 2 months
8. 6 to 9 months
9. 3 to 6 months
10. 6 to 8 months
11. 5 to 7 days
12. 2 to 4 days
13. 4 to 8 weeks
14. 1 to 2 days
15. varies according to type
16. 2 to 4 days
17. 1 to 2 days
18. varies according to type
19. 6 months
20. 1 year
21. 1 year
22. 1 year
23. 1 year
24. 4 weeks
25. 1 year

Teacher's Resources

Chapter 25 Test

1. A		14. T
2. K		15. F
3. E		16. F
4. I		17. T
5. B		18. F
6. J		19. T
7. C		20. T
8. D		21. C
9. G		22. B
10. F		23. C
11. F		24. B
12. F		25. A
13. T		26. C

27. Press the center of the lid. Make sure it is concave and does not flex up and down. Then remove the screw band and make sure you cannot lift the lid off with your fingertips.
28. Dispose of it so that neither humans nor animals can eat it. Use a food waste disposer, or burn it.
29. Fully ripe fruit can be used and the cooking time is shortened. Using commercial pectin also allows more jelly to be made from the same amount of fruit.
30. Containers used in freezing must be moisture- and vapor-resistant to avoid dehydration. Containers made of aluminum, glass, plastic-coated paper, and plastic all are suitable.
31. The principle behind drying food is the removal of moisture. Microorganisms that cause food spoilage need moisture to grow.

Preserving Foods

Name _____

Date _____ Period _____ Score _____

Chapter 25 Test

Matching: Match the following terms and identifying phrases.

_____ 1. A food additive that prevents color and flavor loss.

_____ 2. Antidarkening treatment used on some fruits before drying.

_____ 3. Method of commercial food preservation in which water vapor is removed from frozen foods.

_____ 4. Process of subjecting foods to extremely low temperatures for a short time.

_____ 5. Commercial packaging method in which a food and its packaging material are sterilized separately.

_____ 6. Commercial packaging method in which food is sealed in a foil pouch.

_____ 7. To scald or parboil in water or steam.

_____ 8. A complex protein that is produced by living cells and causes specific chemical reactions.

_____ 9. A microscopic living substance.

_____ 10. Space between the food and the closure of a canning jar.

A. ascorbic acid
B. aseptic packaging
C. blanch
D. enzyme
E. freeze-drying
F. headspace
G. microorganism
H. mold
I. quick-freezing
J. retort packaging
K. sulfuring

True/False: Circle *T* if the statement is true or *F* if the statement is false.

T F 11. If a canning jar has a small chip, it still can be used.

T F 12. A boiling water canner is used to can low-acid foods such as green beans and meats.

T F 13. The safety valve on a pressure canner helps prevent explosions.

T F 14. Sugar helps preserve jelly.

T F 15. Marmalades often contain raisins and nuts.

T F 16. Gelatin products freeze well.

T F 17. For best flavor, frozen fruits should be served with a few ice crystals remaining.

T F 18. Meats, poultry, and fish should always be thawed before cooking.

T F 19. Vegetables must be dried completely to prevent spoilage, but fruits may contain some moisture.

T F 20. Most dried vegetables need to be soaked before cooking.

(Continued)

Name _____

Multiple Choice: Choose the best response. Write the letter in the space provided.

_____ 21. Freezing temperatures _____.
A. destroy enzymes
B. destroy microorganisms
C. prevent microorganisms from growing
D. retard the action of bacteria and mold

_____ 22. Which of the following pieces of canning equipment *cannot* be reused?
A. Glass canning jar.
B. Metal lid with sealing compound.
C. Metal screw band.
D. Pressure canner.

_____ 23. Which of the following ingredients helps jelly become firm?
A. Fruit juice.
B. Pectin.
C. Sugar.
D. All of the above.

_____ 24. Which of the following is *not* a packing method used for freezing fruit?
A. Dry pack.
B. Raw pack.
C. Sugar pack.
D. Syrup pack.

_____ 25. Before drying, vegetables should be _____.
A. blanched
B. sulfured
C. treated with a salt solution
D. None of the above.

_____ 26. Which type of commercial food preservation exposes food to low level doses of gamma rays, electron beams, or X rays?
A. Aseptic packaging.
B. Freeze-drying.
C. Irradiation.
D. Retort packaging.

Essay Questions: Provide complete responses to the following questions or statements.

27. Describe how to test the seals of canning jars.
28. What is the appropriate way to dispose of home-canned food suspected of contamination?
29. What are the advantages of adding commercial pectin when making jelly?
30. Describe the characteristics of a suitable freezing container.
31. Explain the principle behind drying food as a method of preservation.

Regional Cuisine of the United States

Objectives

After studying this chapter, students will be able to
- trace the development of cuisine of the United States.
- prepare foods that are representative of the seven main regions of the United States and identify their origins.

Bulletin Board

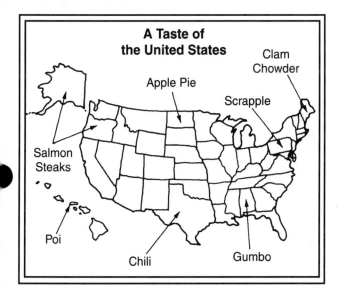

A Taste of the United States

- Clam Chowder
- Apple Pie
- Scrapple
- Salmon Steaks
- Poi
- Chili
- Gumbo

Title: "A Taste of the United States"

Place a map of the United States on the bulletin board. Around the map, place cards with labels or pictures of foods from the various regions. Punch a hole in each card and attach a small piece of yarn that is long enough to reach the map. As you cover chapter material, or as a student self-check, have students attach the free end of the yarn to the proper region on the map.

Teaching Materials

Text, pages 427-459
Student Activity Guide
- A. *Cultural Influences on Food*
- B. *U.S. Regions Maze*
- C. *Regional Foods Match*

Teacher's Resource Binder
   Nutrition Around the World, reproducible master 26-1
   Regions of the United States, transparency master 26-2
   New England Recipes, recipe master 26-3
   Mid-Atlantic Recipes, recipe master 26-4
   Southern Recipes, recipe master 26-5
   Midwestern Recipes, recipe master 26-6
   Southwestern Recipes, recipe master 26-7
   Pacific Coast Recipes, recipe master 26-8
   Hawaiian Recipes, recipe master 26-9
   Chapter 26 Study Sheet, reproducible master 26-10
   Map of the World, color transparency CT-26
   Chapter 26 Test
Software, diskette for Part Four
   Tic Tac Toe, chapter review game

Introductory Activities

1. *Map of the World,* color transparency CT-26, TRB. Use the transparency to introduce students to the geographic locations of the regions they will be studying. Be sure to point out the relationship of each region to the United States.
2. *Nutrition Around the World,* reproducible master 26-1, TRB. Use the handout as you discuss the various groups of people who have influenced cuisine in the United States. Discuss the contributions various groups have made to nutrition as well as variety. Encourage students to keep the handout available for reference as you study Chapters 27-31 in the text.
3. *Regions of the United States,* transparency master 26-2, TRB. Use the master to introduce students to the seven regions of the United States they will be focusing on in this chapter.
4. Go around the room asking students which states they have visited. Place pins on the map on the bulletin board to indicate their responses. Ask students what, if any, regional foods they

sampled when traveling in different areas of the country.

Strategies to Reteach, Reinforce, Enrich, and Extend Text Concepts

A Historical Overview

5. **RF** Ask the class to list and discuss reasons why Europeans left their homes and came to the United States.
6. **ER** Have students research the food customs of Native Americans and write a two-page report summarizing their findings.
7. **ER** Field trip. Take your class to a historical museum where they can see exhibits on foods and cooking utensils used by the Native Americans and early American settlers.
8. **RF** Invite students to share their heritage with other class members. Discuss the various nationalities that your students represent. Ask what cultural dishes they serve in their home.
9. **ER** Have students prepare a Thanksgiving dinner similar to the first one prepared by the early colonists. Discuss with students which foods the colonists introduced and which were native.

New England

10. **ER** Ask students to prepare short oral reports describing some of the obstacles that were overcome by the early settlers in New England.
11. **RF** Have students make a list of foods typical of New England colonists. Have them underline those foods that people still associate with the New England states today.
12. **ER** Have students plan and prepare a New England breakfast.
13. **EX** *New England Recipes,* recipe master 26-3, TRB. Have students use the recipe master to plan a New England dinner. Have each lab group prepare a different dish. Ask each group to complete a *Market Order Sheet* (TRB) and a *Time-Work Schedule* (TRB). After preparing their recipe, have each group share their dish with the rest of the class. Then have each group complete a *Lab Evaluation Sheet* (TRB).

Mid-Atlantic

14. **ER** Have students research the food customs of the Pennsylvania Dutch and present their findings in a two-page written report.
15. **RF** Have students make a list of seven sweets and seven sours that might be served as part of a typical Pennsylvania Dutch meal.
16. **RT** Discuss with students the development of the "melting pot" found in the Mid-Atlantic states.
17. **RF** Have students write menus that exemplify the ethnic feeling typical of many Mid-Atlantic cities.
18. **EX** *Mid-Atlantic Recipes,* recipe master 26-4, TRB. Have students use the recipe master to plan a typical Mid-Atlantic dinner. Have each lab group prepare a different dish. Ask each group to complete a *Market Order Sheet* (TRB) and a *Time-Work Schedule* (TRB). After preparing their recipe, have each group share their dish with the rest of the class. Then have each group complete a *Lab Evaluation Sheet* (TRB).

South

19. **RT** Discuss with students the origin of the expression, "Southern hospitality."
20. **ER** Divide the class into small study groups. Assign each group an important agricultural product of the South. Have the groups research where and how their assigned product is grown and how it is used. Ask each group to present their findings to the rest of the class in a brief oral report.
21. **ER** Divide the class into three groups. Have each group research one of the following types of Southern cooking: soul, Creole, or Cajun. Have each group prepare visual aids and sample menus to illustrate their findings. Then ask one member of each group to participate in a panel presentation.
22. **ER** Have students find out all they can about the history, people, and food customs of New Orleans before planning and preparing an authentic Creole brunch.
23. **RF** Have students write a menu for a Southern buffet that includes Creole specialties, soul food specialties, Cajun specialties, and other Southern favorites.

24. **EX** *Southern Recipes,* recipe master 26-5, TRB. Have students use the recipe master to plan a typical Southern dinner. Have each lab group prepare a different dish. Ask each group to complete a *Market Order Sheet* (TRB) and a *Time-Work Schedule* (TRB). After preparing their recipe, have each group share their dish with the rest of the class. Then have each group complete a *Lab Evaluation Sheet* (TRB).

Midwest

25. **RT** Discuss with the class the development of the potluck dinner.
26. **RF** Have students write a menu for a Midwest farm breakfast typical of the early 1900s.
27. **ER** Have each student investigate one of the agricultural products produced in the Midwest. Have students discuss the production of their chosen product in a one-page report.
28. **ER** Arrange for students to attend a county fair to watch the judging of homemade food products.
29. **EX** *Midwestern Recipes,* recipe master 26-6, TRB. Have students use the recipe master to plan a typical Midwestern dinner. Have each lab group prepare a different dish. Ask each group to complete a *Market Order Sheet* (TRB) and a *Time-Work Schedule* (TRB). After preparing their recipe, have each group share their dish with the rest of the class. Then have each group complete a *Lab Evaluation Sheet* (TRB).

West and Southwest

30. **ER** Have students trace the development of Southwestern cooking, including the contributions made by the Spanish, the Mexicans, and Native Americans. Have them summarize their findings in a short oral report.
31. **ER** Have students research the life of cowboys and write a two-page report. Then have them write a menu for a meal that cowboys of the early 1900s might have eaten on the trail.
32. **RF** Prepare several types of wild game for students to sample.
33. **EX** *Southwestern Recipes,* recipe master 26-7, TRB. Have students use the recipe master to plan a typical Southwestern dinner. Have each lab group prepare a different dish. Ask

each group to complete a *Market Order Sheet* (TRB) and a *Time-Work Schedule* (TRB). After preparing their recipe, have each group share their dish with the rest of the class. Then have each group complete a *Lab Evaluation Sheet* (TRB).

Pacific Coast

34. **ER** Have students use the library resources to write a three-page report on the diversity of the Pacific states.
35. **RF** Have students obtain recipes for at least four dishes that developed in California.
36. **ER** Have students find a variety of recipes for sourdough products. Prepare a sourdough starter and then have lab groups each prepare a different sourdough product.
37. **ER** Have students write menus for a Pacific coast buffet. Have them include specialties of each Pacific state and foods representative of the various ethnic groups that populate the region.
38. **EX** *Pacific Coast Recipes,* recipe master 26-8, TRB. Have students use the recipe master to plan a typical Pacific Coast dinner. Have each lab group prepare a different dish. Ask each group to complete a *Market Order Sheet* (TRB) and a *Time-Work Schedule* (TRB). After preparing their recipe, have each group share their dish with the rest of the class. Then have each group complete a *Lab Evaluation Sheet* (TRB).

Hawaiian Islands

39. **RF** Have students prepare a time line illustrating important dates in Hawaii's history.
40. **ER** Guest speaker. Invite someone who has recently visited Hawaii to speak to your class about the Hawaiian people, their customs, and their foods. Invite the speaker to bring slides, movies, or videotapes to illustrate the discussion.
41. **EX** Have students brainstorm a list of fresh fruits, vegetables, and seafood that are products of Hawaii.
42. **EX** *Hawaiian Recipes,* recipe master 26-9, TRB. Have students use the recipe master to plan a traditional Hawaiian luau. Have each lab group prepare a different dish. Ask each group to complete a *Market Order Sheet* (TRB) and a *Time-Work Schedule* (TRB). Have students decorate the classroom appropriately and plan musical entertainment. Have each

group prepare their recipe and share their dish with the rest of the class. Then have each group complete a *Lab Evaluation Sheet* (TRB).

Chapter Review

43. **RF** *Cultural Influences on Food*, Activity A, SAG. Students are to answer questions regarding food customs in a chosen region of the United States.
44. **RF** *U.S. Regions Maze*, Activity B, SAG. Students are to complete statements with terms related to food customs in the United States. Then they are to find and circle the terms in a maze.
45. **RF** *Regional Foods Match*, Activity C, SAG. Students are to match the regions of the United States with foods typical of each region. Then they are to list the groups of people that influenced the cuisine in each region.
46. **RT** *Chapter 26 Study Sheet*, reproducible master 26-10, TRB. Have students complete the statements as they read text pages 428-455.
47. **RF** *Tic Tac Toe*, Software, diskette for Part Four. Have students play the chapter review game according to the instructions that appear on the screen.

Above and Beyond

48. **ER** Have students investigate how the Native Americans contributed to the success of the first American colonists. Then have them plan and prepare a meal that would have been typical of one of the tribes that assisted the early settlers.

Answer Key

Text

Review What You Have Read, page 459
1. (List three:) to escape debtors' prisons, to find religious freedom, to escape famine and/or disease, to work as forced laborers, to find fame and fortune
2. by drying and salting
3. (List three. Student response. See pages 434-435 in the text.)
4. (List two:) soul food, Creole cuisine, Cajun cuisine

5. (List six:) corn, wheat, soybeans, beef, pork, lamb, poultry, fish, dairy products, fruits, vegetables
6. Spanish, Mexicans, Native Americans, cowboys
7. false
8. The prospectors mixed together flour, water, and salt and then exposed the mixture to air to absorb yeast plants. They used the dough as a leavening agent to make a variety of baked products. They kept a small amount of the dough after each baking to serve as a starter for the next batch.
9. (Student response. See pages 454-455 in the text.)
10. (Student response. See page 455 in the text.)
11. G, A, F, E, D, C, B

Student Activity Guide

U.S. Regions Maze, Activity B, pages 128-129
1. Native
2. British
3. immigrants
4. clam chowder
5. maple
6. Dutch
7. shoofly
8. soul food
9. okra
10. yams
11. Creole
12. filé
13. gumbo
14. jambalaya
15. Cajun
16. breadbasket
17. potluck
18. game
19. longhorn
20. Pacific Coast
21. sourdough
22. muumuu
23. tourism
24. luau
25. imu

Regional Foods Match, Activity C, page 130
1. I, L, R
2. G, N, T
3. B, M, O
4. H, P, Q
5. A, D, U
6. C, E, S
7. F, J, K

New England: English

Mid-Atlantic: Dutch, Germans, Swedes, English

South: French, English, Irish, Scots, Spaniards, African slaves, Native Americans

Midwest: Scandinavians, Germans, Irish, French, Italians, Greeks, Poles, Spaniards

West and Southwest: Native Americans, Mexicans, Spaniards, cowboys

Pacific Coast: Chinese, Japanese, Koreans, Polynesians, Mexicans

Hawaiian Islands: Polynesians, Europeans, Chinese, Japanese

Teacher's Resources

Chapter 26 Test

1. J		16. F	
2. I		17. F	
3. E		18. T	
4. G		19. F	
5. K		20. T	
6. B		21. C	
7. A		22. A	
8. F		23. D	
9. H		24. B	
10. D		25. A	
11. F		26. D	
12. F		27. A	
13. T		28. C	
14. T		29. A	
15. T		30. C	

31. The Native Americans taught the colonists how to hunt; fish; and plant corn, squash, and beans.

32. The Pennsylvania Dutch were a group of German immigrants who settled in the southeast section of Pennsylvania. (Characteristics of foods are student response. See pages 434-435 in the text.)

33. Rich soil, good climate, and advanced farming techniques have made the Midwest one of the world's most agriculturally productive regions. Corn, wheat, and soybeans grow in large enough quantities to be exported to many parts of the world.

34. Chinese, Japanese, Koreans, Polynesians, Mexicans, Spanish, and prospectors

35. The tropical climate of the islands make the production of many fresh fruits and vegetables possible year-round. Many of the fruits, such as pineapples, mangoes, coconuts, and papayas, are important to Hawaiian cooking. Because water surrounds Hawaii, fishing is an important industry. Hawaiian cooking uses fish and shellfish of all types. Cuttlefish, squid, convict fish, bone fish, crabs, and opihi (a clamlike mollusk) are especially popular.

Regional Cuisine of the United States

Name _____

Date _____ **Period** _____ **Score** _____

Chapter 26 Test

Matching: Match the following terms and identifying phrases.

_____ 1. A dough containing active yeast plants that is used as a leavening agent.

_____ 2. A cuisine that combines food customs of African slaves with food customs of Native Americans and European sharecroppers.

_____ 3. A traditional Creole dish that is a mixture of rice; seasonings; and shellfish, poultry, and/or sausage.

_____ 4. A pod-shaped vegetable brought to the United States from Africa.

_____ 5. A dark orange tuber with moist flesh.

_____ 6. A flavoring and thickening agent made from sassafras leaves.

_____ 7. The hearty fare of rural Southern Louisiana that reflects the foods and cooking methods of the Acadians, French, Native Americans, Africans, and Spanish.

_____ 8. An elaborate outdoor feast that is popular in the Hawaiian Islands.

_____ 9. A shared meal to which each person or family brings food for the whole group to eat.

_____ 10. A pit lined with hot rocks used to roast a whole, young pig.

A. Cajun cuisine
B. filé
C. gumbo
D. imu
E. jambalaya
F. luau
G. okra
H. potluck
I. soul food
J. sourdough
K. yam

True/False: Circle *T* if the statement is true or *F* if the statement is false.

T   F   11. Food customs in the United States began with the first English colonists.

T   F   12. The people of New England have always been known for their elaborate meals.

T   F   13. Succotash is a mixture of corn and lima beans.

T   F   14. Heavy German foods were the basis of the Pennsylvania Dutch diet.

T   F   15. Fresh fish and homegrown fruits and vegetables were staple foods in the diets of early settlers in the mid-Atlantic region.

T   F   16. Mobile, Alabama is the home of Creole cuisine.

T   F   17. Traditional Cajun dishes include beignets, café au lait, café brulot, and pralines.

T   F   18. The buffet and potluck dinner developed in the Midwest.

T   F   19. Pork plays an important part in Western cooking.

T   F   20. Caribou sausage and reindeer steak are Alaskan specialties.

(Continued)

Name _____

Multiple Choice: Choose the best response. Write the letter in the space provided.

_____ 21. Which of the following foods is *not* typical of New England?
    A. Blueberry grunt.
    B. Clam chowder.
    C. Shoofly pie.
    D. Succotash.

_____ 22. Red-flannel hash obtains its bright color from _____.
    A. beets
    B. red cabbage
    C. sour cherries
    D. tomatoes

_____ 23. Which of the following foods is a Pennsylvania Dutch specialty?
    A. Cranberry catsup.
    B. Pralines.
    C. Sopapillas.
    D. Sticky buns.

_____ 24. Which of the following foods is *not* representative of soul cooking?
    A. Chitterlings.
    B. Jambalaya.
    C. Pone.
    D. Sweet potato pie.

_____ 25. Which of the following is *not* an ingredient in Creole cooking?
    A. Cracklin' corn bread.
    B. Filé.
    C. Rice.
    D. Seafood.

_____ 26. Tamales, chili, and barbecued beef are typical of the _____.
    A. Midwest
    B. Pacific Coast
    C. South
    D. Southwest

_____ 27. Which of the following is a dessert?
    A. Sopapillas.
    B. Tacos.
    C. Tamales.
    D. Tostadas.

_____ 28. Dungeness crabs, butter clams, and Columbia River salmon are specialties of _____.
    A. the mid-Atlantic states
    B. New England
    C. the Pacific Coast
    D. the South

_____ 29. Which of the following ingredients was *not* used by the prospectors to make their sourdough starter?
    A. Active dry yeast.
    B. Flour.
    C. Salt.
    D. Water.

(Continued)

Name _____

_____   30. Poi is made from _____.
        A. cassava
        B. corn
        C. taro
        D. wheat

Essay Questions: Provide complete responses to the following questions or statements.

31. How were the Native Americans instrumental in assuring the success of the first colonial settlements?
32. Explain who the Pennsylvania Dutch were and describe three characteristics of their foods.
33. Why is the Midwest sometimes called the "breadbasket" of the nation?
34. What groups of people influenced the cuisine of the Pacific Coast?
35. What foods are popular in Hawaii as a result of the climate and geography?

Latin America

Objectives

After studying this chapter, students will be able to
■ identify the geographic, climatic, and cultural factors that have influenced the food customs of Mexico and the South American countries.
■ prepare foods native to Latin America.

Bulletin Board

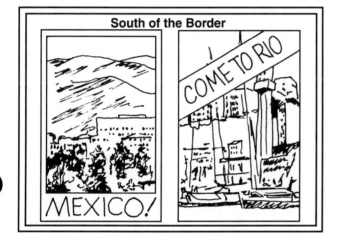

Title: "South of the Border"

Contact a travel agency for travel posters and brochures on Latin American countries. Arrange these in an attractive display on the bulletin board.

Teaching Materials

Text, pages 461-480
Student Activity Guide
    A. *Mexican Cuisine*
    B. *Latin America Maze*
    C. *South American Culture and Cuisine*
Teacher's Resource Binder
    Map of Latin America, transparency master 27-1
    Mexican Recipes, recipe master 27-2
    South American Recipes, recipe master 27-3
    Chapter 27 Study Sheet, reproducible master 27-4
    Chapter 27 Test
Software, diskette for Part Four
    The Matching Game, chapter review game

Introductory Activities

1. *Map of Latin America,* transparency master 27-1, TRB. Use the master to introduce students to the geographic areas they will be studying in this chapter and to illustrate the relationship of one country to another.
2. Ask students to describe Latin American foods with which they are familiar. Ask students to note how many new Latin American foods they are introduced to as they study the chapter.

Strategies to Reteach, Reinforce, Enrich, and Extend Text Concepts

Mexican Geography and Culture

3. **ER** Guest speaker. Invite someone who has recently visited Mexico to speak to your class about the Mexican people, their customs, and their foods. Invite the speaker to bring slides, movies, or videotapes to illustrate the discussion.
4. **ER** Have students use the research materials available in your school library to write a three-page report explaining how climate and geography have affected the development of Mexican cuisine.
5. **RT** Discuss with students how the Aztecs and the Spaniards contributed to Mexican cuisine.

Mexican Cuisine

6. **ER** Field trip. Tour a local supermarket so students can see what Mexican foods are sold there. Be sure they check the canned and packaged food sections as well as the produce counter and frozen food case. Ask them what Mexican dishes they would be able to make from the ingredients available.
7. **RF** Have students use Mexican cookbooks to make a list of Mexican dishes made with corn.
8. **ER** Using the recipe in the text, have students

prepare tortillas from scratch. (If a tortilla press and a comal are not available, have students use a rolling pin and a lightly greased skillet.)

9. **ER** Working in lab groups, have students use the tortillas prepared in strategy 8 to make tacos, tostadas, enchiladas, quesadillas, and burritos.

10. **RT** Demonstrate for students how hot peppers should be cleaned and how peppers can be skinned.

11. **RF** *Mexican Cuisine,* Activity A, SAG. Students are to identify whether the Aztecs or the Spanish contributed various foods important to Mexican cuisine. Then they are to answer several questions.

12. **EX** *Mexican Recipes,* recipe master 27-2, TRB. Have students use the recipe master to plan a typical Mexican dinner. Have each group prepare a different dish. Ask each group to complete a *Market Order Sheet* (TRB) and a *Time-Work Schedule* (TRB). After preparing their recipe, have groups share their dish with the rest of the class. Then have each group complete a *Lab Evaluation Sheet* (TRB).

South American Geography and Culture

13. **ER** Guest speaker. Invite a Native South American to visit your class and talk about the customs of his or her home.

14. **ER** Have students use research materials available in your school library to write a three-page report about the factors that have enabled each South American country to develop independently, thus preserving a unique culture.

15. **ER** Have students research the history of the Inca and write a two-page report summarizing their findings.

South American Cuisine

16. **RF** Have each student write a menu typical of the South American country of his or her choice.

17. **RF** *South American Culture and Cuisine,* Activity C, SAG. Students are to match foods with the South American country with which the foods are associated and provide brief descriptions.

18. **EX** *South American Recipes,* recipe master 27-3, TRB. Have students use the recipe master to plan a typical South American dinner. Have each lab group prepare a different dish.

Ask each group to complete a *Market Order Sheet* (TRB) and a *Time-Work Schedule* (TRB). After preparing their recipe, have groups share their dish with the rest of the class. Then have each group complete a *Lab Evaluation Sheet* (TRB).

Chapter Review

19. **RF** *Latin America Maze,* Activity B, SAG. Students are to complete statements with terms related to Latin America. Then they are to find and circle the terms in a maze.

20. **RT** *Chapter 27 Study Sheet,* reproducible master 27-4, TRB. Have students complete the statements as they read text pages 462-475.

21. **RF** *The Matching Game,* Software, diskette for Part Four. Have students play the chapter review game according to the instructions that appear on the screen.

Above and Beyond

22. **ER** Have each student choose one Latin American country that particularly interests him or her. Have students research the climate, geography, culture, and food customs of the country they have chosen. Have them prepare visual aids to use as they share their findings with the rest of the class in an oral presentation.

Answer Key

Text

Review What You Have Read, page 480
1. (Student response. See page 463 in the text.)
2. (Name four contributions of each:) Aztecs—chocolate, vanilla, corn, peppers, peanuts, tomatoes, avocados, squash, beans, sweet potatoes, pineapples, papayas
   Spaniards—oil, wine, cinnamon, cloves, rice, wheat, peaches, apricots, beef, chicken.
3. A tortilla is flat, unleavened bread made from cornmeal and water. The dough is shaped into a thin pancake in a tortilla press. Then it is cooked on a lightly greased griddle called a *comal.* (For descriptions of three foods made from the tortilla, see page 465 in the text.)
4. The peppers used in Mexican cooking are red and green. Red peppers are used dried except for ripe bell peppers and pimientos. Green peppers are used fresh.
5. false

6. The mole used to prepare the traditional turkey mole is made from a variety of chilies, almonds, raisins, garlic, sesame seeds, onions, tomatoes, cinnamon, cloves, coriander seeds, and anise seeds that are finely chopped and added to chicken stock. Unsweetened chocolate is added just before serving.
7. comida; appetizer, soup, small dish of stew, main course, tortillas or bread, beans, dessert, coffee
8. arepa
9. papa (potato); freeze-drying
10. A
11. Native South American, Portuguese, African
12. false

Student Activity Guide

Mexican Cuisine, Activity A, page 131

1. A	9. S
2. S	10. A
3. S	11. A
4. A	12. S
5. S	13. S
6. A	14. S
7. A	15. A
8. A	16. A

17. A. corn
    B. beans
    C. peppers (Dishes are student response. See page 465 in the text.)
18. (List three of each:) vegetables—zucchini, artichokes, white potatoes, spinach, chard, lettuce, beets, cauliflower, carrots, huazontle, jicama, nopole, chayotes
    fruits—avocados, bananas, pineapples, guavas, papayas, prickly pears (Dish is student response. See pages 465-466 in the text.)
19. (Student response. See page 467 in the text.)
20. (Student response. See page 467 in the text.)

Latin American Maze, Activity B, pages 132-133

1. Mexico	14. tamales
2. Spanish	15. rice
3. oil	16. abara
4. Mestizos	17. bananas
5. beans	18. Aztecs
6. peppers	19. comida
7. guacamole	20. tortilla
8. Pampas	21. taco
9. empanadas	22. manioc
10. Chileans	23. molinillo
11. cassava	24. Inca
12. plantains	25. flan
13. coffee	

South American Culture and Cuisine, Activity C, page 134

A. Venezuela, arepa
B. Colombia, ajiaco
C. Ecuador, bananas
D. Peru, papa
E. Chile, pastel de choclo
F. Argentina, chimichurri
G. Brazil, dendé oil
(Descriptions are student response and should reflect information on text pages 473-475.)

Teacher's Resources

Chapter 27 Test

1. K		16. T	
2. H		17. F	
3. D		18. T	
4. I		19. T	
5. J		20. F	
6. B		21. B	
7. A		22. B	
8. C		23. A	
9. F		24. A	
10. G		25. A	
11. T		26. A	
12. T		27. A	
13. T		28. C	
14. F		29. C	
15. T		30. C	

31. (Describe three. Student response. See page 465 in the text.)
32. Mexican families with an ample income often eat four meals a day. Desayuno is a substantial breakfast. The main meal of the day, comida, is served in the middle of the day. Merienda is a light snack served around five or six o'clock. Supper, cena, may be served between eight and ten o'clock.

```
S A N A N A B A A S N B O U T Y P W E A
O R O D A P S A D A N A P M E J Q F N E
Z E T E U T Z Y Y I T O R T I L L A M J
I B O N I S O W U Q D T I V I E V C A C
T A M A L E S R C H I L E A N S J Z N X
S I D P P G U A C A M O L E E Y T Y I M
E U P C L M D E A U E B O J S E A E O U
M N A R L A A H U D X B R Y C X C A C S
O Y V Q A P N E Z E I I E S L I O W L A
L A A P H B H T S G C Y M B R W I U I P
I S S E O M R E A R O O E H I X L R V M
N N S P K D Q B F I H S M E I A R A B A
I R A P M T E T A F N M S I F F O G O P
L N C E Y A T E T G A S L A D F Q E N R
L N S R N R G H L U L L X U Z A O T W K
O F H S I N A P S V F U H A G P A C N I
```

33. Both bananas and plantains are boiled, fried, baked, and added to soups and stews. Plantains, thinly sliced and fried until crisp, are a popular snack. Banana leaves are used to wrap hallacas, Venezuela's national dish, which is a cornmeal dough filled with other foods.

34. The Inca freeze-dried potatoes by alternately exposing them to the cold night air and the warm sunshine high up in the Andes mountains. As the potatoes repeatedly froze and thawed, moisture evaporated. Soon the potatoes became hard as stone but very lightweight. The Inca could then store the potatoes indefinitely.

35. The Portuguese brought Africans to Brazil to work in the sugar fields. African cooks were the first to use dendé oil, red pepper, bananas, and coconut in Brazilian dishes.

Latin America

Name _____

Date _____ Period _____ Score _____

Chapter 27 Test

Matching: Match the following terms and identifying phrases.

_____ 1. A flat, unleavened bread made from cornmeal and water.

_____ 2. Refried beans.

_____ 3. Hot peppers.

_____ 4. A complex sauce used in Mexican cuisine.

_____ 5. A green, starchy fruit that has a bland flavor and looks much like a large banana.

_____ 6. A starchy root plant eaten as a side dish and used in flour form in cooking and baking.

_____ 7. A corn pancake that is a traditional Venezuelan bread.

_____ 8. A marinated raw fish dish.

_____ 9. An Argentine appetizer.

_____ 10. Brazil's national dish, which is made with meat and black beans.

A. arepa
B. cassava
C. ceviche
D. chilies
E. dendé oil
F. empanada
G. feijoada completa
H. frijoles refritos
I. mole
J. plantain
K. tortilla

True/False: Circle *T* if the statement is true or *F* if the statement is false.

T F 11. The Aztecs ate some of their foods raw, but cooked many others.

T F 12. The Spanish introduced peaches, rice, beef, and wheat to Mexico.

T F 13. Sauces often are used in Mexican cooking.

T F 14. Mexicans eat their main meal of the day around six o'clock in the evening.

T F 15. Most food customs in South America have developed on a regional basis because of the geographic isolation of the different areas.

T F 16. The Pampas are rich lands located in Argentina and Uruguay where large herds of cattle and sheep are raised.

T F 17. Ají is a seasoning made from banana leaves.

T F 18. Colombia is an important coffee-producing country.

T F 19. Potatoes are a staple food in Peru.

T F 20. Dendé oil gives Brazilian dishes a brilliant green color.

(Continued)

Name _____

Multiple Choice: Choose the best response. Write the letter in the space provided.

_____ 21. Which of the following is Mexico's most important crop?
   A. Citrus fruits.
   B. Corn.
   C. Sugarcane.
   D. Wheat.

_____ 22. Which of the following foods was *not* contributed to Mexican cuisine by the Aztecs?
   A. Chocolate.
   B. Oil.
   C. Squash.
   D. Tomatoes.

_____ 23. In Mexico, tortillas are cooked on a _____.
   A. comal
   B. desayuno
   C. molinillo
   D. tortilla press

_____ 24. Tortillas wrapped around a meat or bean filling are called _____.
   A. burritos
   B. enchiladas
   C. tacos
   D. tostadas

_____ 25. Guacamole is a popular spread made from mashed _____.
   A. avocados
   B bananas
   C. huazontle
   D. plantains

_____ 26. A molinillo is used to _____.
   A beat chocolate into a frothy foam before serving
   B. chop chilies
   C. cook paella
   D. grind corn for tortillas

_____ 27. Which of the following is a Colombian soup made with potatoes, chicken, corn, and cassava?
   A. Ajiaco.
   B. Humitas.
   C. Papa.
   D. Vatapa.

_____ 28. The cuisine of Peru reflects traditions of the _____.
   A. Aztecs and Africans
   B. French and English
   C. Inca and Spanish
   D. Portuguese and Dutch

_____ 29. Porotos granados, pastel de choclo, and chupe de marisco are specialties of _____.
   A. Argentina
   B. Brazil
   C. Chile
   D. Venezuela

(Continued)

Name _____

_____ 30. Which of the following is *not* a staple food in Brazil?
     A. Beans.
     B. Manioc.
     C. Potatoes.
     D. Rice.

Essay Questions: Provide complete responses to the following questions or statements.

31. Describe three Mexican dishes made from tortillas.
32. Describe Mexican meal patterns.
33. How do Venezuelans use bananas and plantains?
34. How did the Inca preserve their potato crop?
35. How did Africans come to be in Brazil and what influence did they have on Brazilian cuisine?

Europe

Objectives

After studying this chapter, students will be able to
■ describe the food customs of the British Isles, France, Germany, and the Scandinavian countries.
■ explain how and why these customs have evolved.
■ recognize and prepare foods native to each of these countries.

Bulletin Board

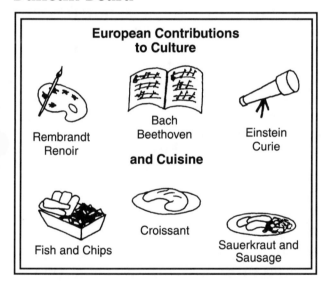

Title: "European Contributions to Culture and Cuisine"

Use the words of the title to divide the bulletin board into upper and lower halves, as shown. In the top half, place pictures or drawings of an artist's palette, sheet music, and a telescope or microscope. With each of these illustrations, list the names of several European artists, composers, and scientists, respectively. In the bottom half of the bulletin board, place pictures or drawings of classic European foods labeled with their name.

Teaching Materials

Text, pages 481-522
Student Activity Guide
　A. *British Food and Customs*
　B. *France Crossword*
　C. *Foods of Germany*
　D. *Influences on Scandinavian Cuisine*
　E. *Cuisine Travel Guide*

Teacher's Resource Binder
　British Recipes, recipe master 28-1
　French Recipes, recipe master 28-2
　German Recipes, recipe master 28-3
　Scandinavian Recipes, recipe master 28-4
　Chapter 28 Study Sheet, reproducible master 28-5
　A Size Comparison, color transparency CT-28
　Chapter 28 Test

Software, diskette for Part Four
　Reverse Thinking, chapter review game

Introductory Activities

1. *A Size Comparison,* color transparency CT-28, TRB. Use the transparency to show students the size of the European countries they will be studying compared to the United States.
2. Go around the room asking each student to name a famous European, the accomplishment for which he or she is known, and his or her country of origin. Use student responses as the basis for a discussion of European contributions to Western civilization.
3. Guest speaker. Invite someone who has visited Europe to come to your class and talk about his or her experiences.

Strategies to Reteach, Reinforce, Enrich, and Extend Text Concepts

The British Isles

4. **RT** Discuss with students the important geographic features of the British Isles.
5. **ER** Have students research the history of the English monarchy and summarize their findings in a two-page report.
6. **ER** Ask students to identify major cities of the British Isles. Have students investigate how these cities evolved into major centers of business and industry.

England

7. **RF** Have students use a map of England to locate the places where such native foods as Cheddar cheese originated.

8. **ER** Have students use library resources to write a dinner menu for a meal that might have been served to members of the English court at the time of Henry VIII.

9. **RF** Have the class compare the cuisine of England with the cuisine of the United States. Discuss similarities and differences.

10. **ER** Have each student research an English holiday he or she thinks is especially interesting. Have students share their findings with the class in a brief oral report.

11. **EX** Discuss the custom of tea in the British Isles. Have the class plan and prepare a tea for faculty members and classmates. Students should be sure their menu includes foods from each of the countries in the British Isles.

12. **RF** Have students find recipes for each of the following types of English puddings: sweet, protein-based, and summer.

Scotland

13. **ER** Have each student research the history of one of the Scottish clans. Have students summarize their findings in a two-page report.

14. **ER** Have each student find a fabric swatch or draw a sample of the tartan representing the clan he or she researched in strategy 13. Each student should summarize information about his or her chosen clan on a large index card and create a class display with the tartans.

15. **ER** Working in lab groups, have students prepare a variety of Scottish baked goods.

Ireland

16. **RT** Share the story of St. Patrick with your class. Ask students how, or if, they celebrate St. Patrick's Day.

17. **RF** Have students prepare a time line noting important dates in Irish history for the last three centuries. Ask students to identify factors that have led to the current political situation in Ireland.

18. **RF** Have students find recipes for a variety of Irish potato dishes.

19. **ER** Working in lab groups, have students prepare some of the Irish potato recipes they found in strategy 18.

20. **ER** Have students prepare a traditional Irish breakfast including Irish soda bread.

Wales

21. **ER** Have students research the political relationship between England and Wales. Have them summarize their findings in a two-page report.

22. **ER** Have students find recipes for Welsh crempog, bara ceirch, and bara brith. Have them prepare and serve these items as part of a typical Welsh tea.

23. **EX** *British Recipes,* recipe master 28-1, TRB. Have students use the recipe master to plan a dinner including specialties from each of the countries of the British Isles. Have each lab group prepare a different dish. Ask each group to complete a *Market Order Sheet* (TRB) and a *Time-Work Schedule* (TRB). After preparing their recipe, have each group share their dish with the rest of the class. Then have each group complete a *Lab Evaluation Sheet* (TRB).

24. **RF** *British Food and Customs,* Activity A, SAG. Students are to identify the countries indicated on the map of the British Isles. Then they are to identify the British country with which each of the listed phrases about food and customs is most closely associated.

France

25. **RF** Have students locate major cities and geographic features on a map of France.

26. **RF** Discuss with students the differences between haute cuisine, provincial cuisine, and nouvelle cuisine. Then have them use French cookbooks to write a menu that would be typical of each class.

27. **ER** Working in lab groups, have students prepare the following French sauces: béchamel, velouté, hollandaise, demi-glace, and vinaigrette.

28. **EX** Have students plan and prepare an hors d'oeuvres buffet including both hot and cold hors d'oeuvres.

29. **ER** Working in lab groups, have students prepare a variety of French breads, including brioche, croissants, and traditional long loaves of crusty French bread.

30. **RF** Allow students to sample a variety of French cheeses.

31. **EX** Have students plan and prepare a French dessert buffet including such items as

soufflés, éclairs, baba au rhum, and dessert crêpes.

32. **EX** *French Recipes,* recipe master 28-2, TRB. Have students use the recipe master to plan a typical French dinner. Have each lab group prepare a different recipe. Ask each group to complete a *Market Order Sheet* (TRB) and a *Time-Work Schedule* (TRB). After preparing their recipe, have each group share their dish with the rest of the class. Then have each group complete a *Lab Evaluation Sheet* (TRB).

33. **RF** *France Crossword,* Activity B, SAG. Students are to complete a crossword puzzle with terms relating to French culture and cuisine.

Germany

34. **ER** Have each student investigate the production and economic importance of one of Germany's primary industrial or agricultural products. Then have students share their findings in a brief oral report.

35. **ER** Have students visit the meat department of a supermarket and make a list of all the sausages with German origins. Have students compare lists.

36. **ER** Guest speaker. Invite a butcher to your class to talk about German sausages.

37. **ER** Have students use a basic yeast dough to practice making the German picture breads called gebildbrote.

38. **EX** Have students plan and prepare a German dessert buffet including such items as stollen, lebkuchen, schnecken, and Schwarzwälder Kirschtorte.

39. **RF** Have each student choose one geographic region in Germany and write a menu that might be found in a local restaurant.

40. **EX** *German Recipes,* recipe master 28-3, TRB. Have students use the recipe master to plan a typical German dinner. Have each lab group prepare a different recipe. Ask each group to complete a *Market Order Sheet* (TRB) and a *Time-Work Schedule* (TRB). After preparing their recipe, have each group share their dish with the rest of the class. Then have each group complete a *Lab Evaluation Sheet* (TRB).

41. **RF** *Foods of Germany,* Activity C, SAG. Students are to complete statements about German foods by filling in blanks with words listed on the worksheet.

Scandinavia

42. **ER** Have students visit an import shop or department store or do library research to learn more about Scandinavian design in furniture, glassware, or ceramics. Have each student prepare visual aids to use in giving an oral report on his or her findings.

43. **RT** Discuss with the class the role climate and geography have played in the development of food customs in Sweden, Norway, and Finland.

44. **ER** Have students visit a supermarket to see how many Danish dairy products are available in your area.

45. **ER** Working in lab groups, have students prepare a variety of smørrebrød.

46. **RF** Have students write a menu for a Norwegian breakfast that might precede a day of skiing.

47. **EX** Have students plan and prepare a Norwegian dessert buffet including such items as sour cream waffles, kringla, krumkaker, and rosettes.

48. **EX** Have students brainstorm a list of 30 or more foods that might be included in an authentic Swedish smörgåsbord.

49. **ER** Have students research Scandinavian Christmas traditions and summarize their findings in a three-page report.

50. **EX** *Scandinavian Recipes,* recipe master 28-4, TRB. Have students use the recipe master to plan a dinner including specialties from each of the Scandinavian countries. Have each lab group prepare a different recipe. Ask each group to complete a *Market Order Sheet* (TRB) and a *Time-Work Schedule* (TRB). After preparing their recipe, have each group share their dish with the rest of the class. Then have each group complete a *Lab Evaluation Sheet* (TRB).

51. **RF** *Influences on Scandinavian Cuisine,* Activity D, SAG. Students are to answer questions about Scandinavian climate, geography, and cuisine.

Chapter Review

52. **ER** *Cuisine Travel Guide,* Activity E, SAG. Students are to use the worksheet to prepare a travel brochure emphasizing the cuisine of one of the European countries discussed in the chapter.

53. **RT** *Chapter 28 Study Sheet,* reproducible master 28-5, TRB. Have students complete the statements as they read text pages 482-517.
54. **RF** *Reverse Thinking,* Software, diskette for Part Four. Have students play the chapter review game according to the instructions that appear on the screen.

Above and Beyond

55. **ER**   Have students research the origins of the people of one of the European countries discussed in this chapter. Have them investigate where the founding groups came from, what skills and knowledge they brought with them, and what factors were important in the development of their food customs. Have students prepare visual aids to use in an oral presentation to share their findings with the rest of the class.

Answer Key

Text

Review What You Have Read, page 522
1. meat, cheese, bread, ale (Puddings and pies were added later.)
2. eggs, bacon, fried bread served with marmalade, tea (In some parts of the country, the following foods might be added: fruits, fruit juices, main dish pies, ham, smoked fish, and oatmeal porridge.)
3. *Tea* can be defined as a beverage or as a light meal served throughout the British Isles.
4. false
5. potatoes
6. (Student response. See page 494 in the text.)
7. (Student response. See pages 494 and 496 in the text.)
8. false
9. (List three:) ratatouille, aioli, bouillabaisse, leg of lamb, grilled fish, chicken
10. (Describe three. Student response. See page 506 in the text.)
11. false
12. Traditionally, Germans who could afford to do so ate five meals. The two "extra" meals were a second breakfast and an afternoon coffee.
13. (List two:) Danish blue cheese with raw egg yolk, sliced roast pork garnished with dried fruit, smoked salmon and scrambled eggs garnished with chives

14. (Describe three. Student response. See page 515 in the text.)
15. herring dishes; cold fish, meats, and salads; hot meats, eggs, or fish; breads; cheeses; and desserts
16. true

Student Activity Guide

British Food and Customs, Activity A, page 135

1. A. Scotland
   B. England
   C. Wales
   D. Ireland
2. A
3. B
4. B
5. C
6. C
7. D
8. A
9. A
10. B
11. C
12. B
13. D
14. D
15. D
16. A
17. C
18. A
19. B
20. C
21. C
22. D
23. A
24. B
25. D

France Crossword, Activity B, page 136

```
                              ¹M
                  ²G          A        ³H
                ⁴P R O V I N C I A L          ⁵T
                  A           U        U       R
                  P           F        T       U
                  E           A    ⁶H E ⁷R B S  F
        ⁸S N A I L S          C        O       F
                              T    ⁹N O U V E L L E
    ¹⁰C                ¹¹Q     U        X       E
    ¹²H O R S D O E U V R E S          S
    E                  I      I
    E                  C      N
    S                  H      G
    E                  E
```

Foods of Germany, Activity C, page 137

1. bratwurst
2. spätzle
3. hasenpfeffer
4. preiselbeeren
5. Westphalian ham
6. lebkuchen
7. kasseler rippenspeer
8. sauerkraut
9. braunschweiger
10. schnitzel
11. stollen
12. pumpernickel
13. sauerbraten

14. strudel
15. kartoffelpuffer
16. gebildbrote
17. salzkartoffeln
18. eintopf

Influences on Scandinavian Cuisine, Activity D, page 138

1. A. Winters in Norway, Sweden, and Finland are long and severe. Summers are short and cool.
   B. The growing season in Norway, Sweden, and Finland is short so agricultural production is limited.
   C. Careful preservation of food is important in Norway, Sweden, and Finland. Pickled, dried, and salted foods are common.
2. A. The geography of Norway, Sweden, and Finland is rugged. Norway has a mountainous coast. Much of northern Sweden is covered by forests. Finland is stony and rough with many lakes and marshy areas.
   B. Only a small percentage of the land in Norway, Sweden, and Finland can be farmed.
3. The climate in Denmark is mild with plenty of rainfall. The winters are warmer than they are in the other Scandinavian countries.
4. The land in Denmark is less rugged. Forests fringe the eastern shore and hills cut through the central part of the country.
5. Denmark has a longer growing season than the other Scandinavian countries and about 75 percent of the land can be farmed.
6. Fishing is an important industry to all four Scandinavian countries.
7. Pigs, cows, and chickens are Denmark's main agricultural products.
8. Grain and livestock are the main agricultural products of Norway, Sweden, and Finland. Norway also produces large quantities of potatoes.
9. Danish food is richer than that of the other Scandinavian countries due to the use of large quantities of butter, cream, cheese, and eggs. Fish is not as popular in Denmark as in the other countries. Danes eat more pork and chicken.
10. (Examples and descriptions of typical Scandinavian dishes are student response. Answers should be based on information from the section, "Scandinavian Cuisine," found on pages 513-517 of the text.)

Teacher's Resources

Chapter 28 Test

1.	F	20.	F
2.	G	21.	F
3.	B	22.	T
4.	A	23.	F
5.	E	24.	T
6.	C	25.	F
7.	P	26.	T
8.	D	27.	T
9.	K	28.	B
10.	H	29.	A
11.	L	30.	A
12.	N	31.	D
13.	O	32.	D
14.	M	33.	A
15.	J	34.	C
16.	F	35.	D
17.	F	36.	A
18.	T	37.	C
19.	T		

38. (Student response. See pages 483-484 in the text.)
39. Tea is served throughout the day as a beverage. Tea is also a light meal served in the afternoon or evening. This meal may be a snack including cookies or cake, or it may include sandwiches, sausages, cheeses, and breads.
40. haute cuisine, provincial cuisine, nouvelle cuisine (Descriptions are student response. See page 494 in the text.)
41. (Student response. See page 507 in the text.)
42. Geography has made food production difficult. Human isolation has caused cuisine to develop on a regional basis. Climate has caused much effort to be put into food preservation.

Europe

Name _____

Date _____ Period _____ Score _____

Chapter 28 Test

Matching: Match the following terms and identifying phrases.

_____ 1. Battered, deep-fried fish fillets served with a British version of French fries.

_____ 2. A Scottish dish made from a sheep's stomach stuffed with a pudding made from oatmeal and the sheep's organs.

_____ 3. An Irish dish made with mashed potatoes mixed with chopped scallions, shredded cooked cabbage, and melted butter.

_____ 4. A type of mussel common along the coast of Wales.

_____ 5. A mixture of fresh chives, parsley, tarragon, and chervil used to flavor many French soups and stews.

_____ 6. A flaky, buttery yeast roll shaped into a crescent.

_____ 7. A rare type of fungi that grow underground near oak trees and are used in many French recipes.

_____ 8. A snail eaten as food.

_____ 9. A custard tart served in many variations as an appetizer and a main dish.

_____ 10. German potato pancakes.

_____ 11. Fermented or pickled cabbage.

_____ 12. Small dumplings made from wheat flour, which are a popular German side dish.

_____ 13. A German dessert made with paper-thin layers of pastry filled with fruit.

_____ 14. Danish open-faced sandwiches usually made with thin, sour rye bread spread thickly with butter.

_____ 15. Dried cod that have been soaked in a lye solution before cooking.

A. cockles
B. colcannon
C. croissant
D. escargot
E. fines herbes
F. fish and chips
G. haggis
H. kartoffelpuffer
I. lingonberry
J. lutefisk
K. quiche
L. sauerkraut
M. smørrebrød
N. spätzle
O. strudel
P. truffles

True/False: Circle *T* if the statement is true or *F* if the statement is false.

T   F   16. Steamed puddings are a Welsh specialty.

T   F   17. Crumpets are an English dessert similar to cream puffs.

T   F   18. Oats, a staple food in Scotland, are used to make haggis.

T   F   19. Potatoes have been a staple food in Ireland for centuries.

(Continued)

Name _____

T   F   20. Provincial cuisine was developed by chefs employed by the French nobility.

T   F   21. Hors d'oeuvres are small bowls of soup served before the main course.

T   F   22. In France, bread is served at every meal.

T   F   23. Crêpes are pastry shells filled with custard and fruit.

T   F   24. Of all meats, pork is served most often in Germany.

T   F   25. Lebkuchen is a snail-shaped coffee cake served throughout Germany.

T   F   26. Danish foods are the richest of all Scandinavian foods.

T   F   27. Weinerbrød are layers of buttery pastry filled with fruit or custard and sprinkled with sugar or nuts.

Multiple Choice: Choose the best response. Write the letter in the space provided.

_____   28. Which of the following English dishes is *not* made with leftovers?
A. Bubble and squeak.
B. Fish and chips.
C. Shepherd's pie.
D. Toad in the hole.

_____   29. Which of the following is *not* an Irish potato dish?
A. Barmbrack.
B. Boxty.
C. Champ.
D. Colcannon.

_____   30. When milk is added to a roux, the mixture is called a _____.
A. béchamel sauce
B. demi-glace sauce
C. hollandaise sauce
D. velouté sauce

_____   31. In France, a green salad usually is served _____.
A. after the soup course
B. before the main course
C. with the main course
D. after the main course but before dessert

_____   32. Ratatouille, aioli, and bouillabaisse are specialties of _____.
A. Alsace
B. Brittany
C. Languedoc
D. Provence

_____   33. Which of the following foods is popular in both Germany and Scandinavia?
A. Herring.
B. Ostkaka.
C. Pumpernickel bread.
D. Sauerkraut.

_____   34. Which of the following desserts contains a liqueur made from cherries?
A. Pflaumenkuchen.
B. Schnecken.
C. Schwarzwälder Kirschtorte.
D. Stollen.

(Continued)

Name _____

_____ 35. In Germany, spätzle are served as a(n) _____.
   A. appetizer
   B. breakfast cereal
   C. dessert
   D. side dish

_____ 36. Danes often serve their smørrebrød with chilled glasses of _____.
   A. aquavit
   B. cranberry liqueur
   C. dark beer
   D. vodka

_____ 37. Lutefisk, lefse, and kringla are specialties of _____.
   A. Denmark
   B. Finland
   C. Norway
   D. Sweden

Essay Questions: Provide complete responses to the following questions or statements.

38. What are three contributions the Germanic invaders made to British cuisine?
39. How is tea served in the British Isles?
40. Name and describe the three classes of French cooking.
41. Briefly describe the five meals that may be served throughout the day in Germany. Give examples of foods that may be served at each meal.
42. List and describe the three major factors that have influenced Scandinavian cuisine.

Mediterranean Countries

Objectives

After studying this chapter, students will be able to
- describe the food customs of Spain, Italy, and Greece.
- discuss how climate, geography, and culture have influenced these customs.
- recognize and prepare foods that are native to each of these countries.

Bulletin Board

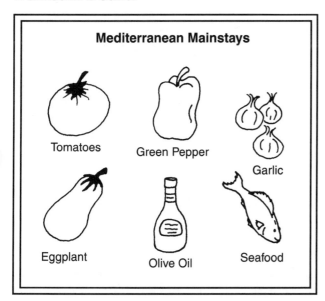

Mediterranean Mainstays

Tomatoes
Green Pepper
Garlic
Eggplant
Olive Oil
Seafood

Title: "Mediterranean Mainstays"
Use pictures, drawings, or cutouts to illustrate some of the foods that are typical of Spanish, Italian, and Greek cuisines. Such foods might include tomatoes, green peppers, eggplant, seafood, garlic, and olive oil. Label each of the illustrated foods.

Teaching Materials

Text, pages 523-552
Student Activity Guide
   A. *Spanish Culture and Cuisine*
   B. *Italian Foods Identification*
   C. *Italian Culture and Cuisine*
   D. *Greece Maze*
   E. *Mediterranean Climate, Geography, and Cuisine*

Teacher's Resource Binder
   Map of the Mediterranean, transparency master 29-1
   Spanish Recipes, recipe master 29-2
   Italian Recipes, recipe master 29-3
   Greek Recipes, recipe master 29-4
   Chapter 29 Study Sheet, reproducible master 29-5
   Pasta—An Italian Staple Food, color transparency CT-29
   Chapter 29 Test
Software, diskette for Part Four
   Bingo, chapter review game

Introductory Activities

1. *Map of the Mediterranean,* transparency master 29-1, TRB. Use the master to introduce students to the geographic region they will be studying in this chapter and to illustrate the relationship of one country to another.
2. Ask students what Spanish, Italian, and Greek dishes they have tried. Use this indication of students' familiarity with Mediterranean cuisine to emphasize new information as you cover the chapter.

Strategies to Reteach, Reinforce, Enrich, and Extend Text Concepts

Spanish Geography and Culture

3. **RF** Have students use a map to identify major cities and geographic features of Spain.
4. **RT** Discuss with students how geography influenced the development of Spanish food customs.
5. **ER** Guest speaker. Invite a Spanish teacher to come to your class and talk about Spanish customs.
6. **ER** Have students research the Moors and their influence on the development of Spanish cuisine. Have them summarize their findings in a two-page report.

Spanish Cuisine

7. **RF** Have students head a sheet of paper

and write their answers as you read the statement, "Name two Spanish dishes that fall under each of the following categories: tapas, soups, main dishes, accompaniments, and desserts."

8. **RF**   Have students use a Spanish cookbook to find recipes for a variety of tapas (Spanish appetizers).

9. **ER**   Working in lab groups, have students prepare a variety of tapas from the recipes they found in strategy 8. Have them serve the tapas with mock sangria.

10. **EX**   Have each lab group experiment to develop a unique version of gazpacho.

11. **ER**   Assign the preparation of one regional version of paella to each lab group. Serve the paellas buffet-style. Ask students to analyze the major differences that are apparent.

12. **EX**   *Spanish Recipes,* recipe master 29-2, TRB. Have students use the recipe master to plan a dinner including a variety of typical Spanish foods. Have each lab group prepare a different recipe. Ask each group to complete a *Market Order Sheet* (TRB) and a *Time-Work Schedule* (TRB). After preparing their recipe, have each group share their dish with the rest of the class. Then have each group complete a *Lab Evaluation Sheet* (TRB).

13. **RF**   *Spanish Culture and Cuisine,* Activity A, SAG. Students are to match terms and descriptions related to the culture and cuisine of Spain.

Italian Geography and Culture

14. **RF**   Have students trace a map of Italy and outline the locations of Italy's northern, central, and southern regions. In the margins, have students list three characteristics that make each of the regions unique.

15. **ER**   Have students research the history of Italy up to World War II. Have them write a two-page report highlighting the contributions Italians made to Western civilization.

16. **EX**   Divide the class into small study groups. Have each group use library resources to prepare a presentation on a different aspect of the Renaissance in Italy.

Italian Cuisine

17. **ER**   Have each student write a paragraph explaining the following statement: Italian cuisine belongs to the Greeks.

18. **RT**   *Pasta—An Italian Staple Food,* color transparency CT-29, TRB. Use the transparency to illustrate for students some of the many pasta shapes used in Italian cooking. Bring in samples of these pastas to show students.

19. **RF**   Have students use several Italian cookbooks as references to make a collection of recipes featuring pasta.

20. **ER**   Have lab groups prepare several shapes of pastas. Serve the pastas buffet-style with a variety of sauces.

21. **ER**   Field trip. Plan a trip to a food store in an Italian neighborhood or visit a local grocery store. Have students note how many different kinds of pasta and Italian cheeses are sold.

22. **ER**   Allow students to sample a variety of Italian cheeses. (Serve pieces of crusty Italian bread with the cheeses.) Have students make a chart describing the appearance and flavor of each of the cheeses.

23. **EX**   *Italian Recipes,* recipe master 29-3, TRB. Have students use the recipe master to plan a typical Italian dinner. Have each lab group prepare a different recipe. Ask each group to complete a *Market Order Sheet* (TRB) and a *Time-Work Schedule* (TRB). After preparing their recipe, have each group share their dish with the rest of the class. Then have each group complete a *Lab Evaluation Sheet* (TRB).

24. **RF**   *Italian Foods Identification,* Activity B, SAG. Students are to identify Italian foods and answer several questions.

25. **RF**   *Italian Culture and Cuisine,* Activity C, SAG. Students are to determine whether statements about Italian culture and cuisine are true or false.

Greek Geography and Culture

26. **RT**   Discuss with students how the peoples of neighboring countries influenced the development of Greek civilization and vice versa.

27. **EX**   Have students brainstorm a list of accomplishments of the Greeks that benefited Western civilization.

Greek Cuisine

28. **ER**   Have students use research materials available in the school library to prepare a short written report tracing the development of Greek cuisine.

29. **RT**   Demonstrate for students three uses of phyllo. (Be sure to include at least one main dish.)

30. **RF** Have students use Greek cookbooks to find five recipes for lamb dishes. Have them identify common ingredients used in the recipe.
31. **ER** Have each lab group prepare avgolemono and serve it in a different way.
32. **EX** *Greek Recipes,* recipe master 29-4, TRB. Have students use the recipe master to plan a typical Greek dinner. Have each lab group prepare a different recipe. Ask each group to complete a *Market Order Sheet* (TRB) and a *Time-Work Schedule* (TRB). After preparing their recipe, have each group share their dish with the rest of the class. Then have each group complete a *Lab Evaluation Sheet* (TRB).
33. **RF** *Greece Maze,* Activity D, SAG. Students are to complete statements with terms related to Greek culture and cuisine. Then they are to find and circle the terms in a maze.

Chapter Review

34. **RF** *Mediterranean Climate, Geography, and Cuisine,* Activity E, SAG. Students are to complete a chart describing the climate, geography, and cuisine of Spain, Italy, and Greece.
35. **RT** *Chapter 29 Study Sheet,* reproducible master 29-5, TRB. Have students complete the statements as they read text pages 524-548.
36. **RF** *Bingo,* Software, diskette for Part Four. Have students play the chapter review game according to the instructions that appear on the screen.

Above and Beyond

37. **ER** Have each student prepare a map of one of the Mediterranean countries discussed in this chapter. Have students identify major trade centers in the country. Have them draw and label important geographical features. Then have them indicate where key agricultural products are produced. Ask students to submit their map with a written report discussing the relationship between the geographical features, the agricultural products, and the staple ingredients in the cuisine of the country.

Answer Key

Text

Review What You Have Read, page 552
1. Moors brought citrus fruits, peaches, bananas, and figs. They introduced the cultivation of rice and a variety of spices. They planted large almond groves and often used almonds in cooking.
2. tapas
3. In Spain, tortillas are omelets prepared with a variety of fillings and served as a separate course or as an accompaniment. In Mexico, tortillas are flat, unleavened bread made from cornmeal and water and used as the base of many dishes.
4. because Italian cuisine is the source of all other Western cuisines
5. (Describe three. Student response. See pages 536, 538, and 540 in the text.)
6. false
7. antipasto, minestra (soup), main course served with a vegetable or salad (pasta replaces this course if meat is too costly), fruit and cheese (For examples, see page 540 in the text.)
8. (Name three dishes contributed by invading groups:) pasta dishes, kebabs, yogurt, rich pastries, Greek coffee, lamb, beans (Name two native Greek foods:) olives, grapes, seafood
9. C
10. honey

Student Activity Guide

Spanish Culture and Cuisine, Activity A, page 141

1. W	14. O
2. K	15. T
3. P	16. Y
4. I	17. U
5. Z	18. X
6. D	19. A
7. H	20. F
8. N	21. S
9. M	22. Q
10. L	23. B
11. G	24. R
12. V	25. E
13. J	

Italian Foods Identification, Activity B, page 142

1. C	9. P
2. P	10. H
3. P	11. S
4. H	12. S
5. C	13. H
6. S	14. P
7. H	15. C
8. S	16. C

17. P

18. S

19. C

20. H

21. H

22. C

23. S

24. P

25. A. In Northern Italy, pasta bolognese are served. These fat, ribbon-shaped pastas are usually made at home and contain egg. In Southern Italy, pasta naploetania are served. These tubular-shaped pastas are usually produced commercially and do not contain egg.

B. (Student response. See page 538 in the text.)

C. (Student response. See page 540 in the text.)

Italian Culture and Cuisine, Activity C, page 143

1. T
2. T
3. F
4. T
5. T
6. T
7. F
8. T
9. T
10. F
11. F
12. T
13. T
14. T
15. T
16. F
17. T
18. T
19. T
20. F
21. T
22. F
23. T
24. T
25. F

Greece Maze, Activity D, pages 144-145

1. classical
2. city states
3. Sparta
4. ancient
5. Orthodox
6. farmers
7. shipping
8. tavernas
9. ouzo
10. bouzoukia
11. Athens
12. cookbooks
13. kebabs
14. herbs
15. eggplant
16. moussaka
17. lamb
18. seafood
19. squid
20. olives
21. feta
22. honey
23. phyllo
24. baklava
25. mezedhes

Teacher's Resources

Chapter 29 Test

1. D
2. E
3. C
4. G
5. J
6. I
7. A
8. F
9. B
10. H
11. T
12. T
13. F
14. F
15. T
16. F
17. T
18. F
19. T
20. T
21. D
22. A
23. A
24. B
25. A
26. D
27. A
28. C
29. D
30. B

31. The Romans contributed olive oil and garlic. The Moors contributed citrus fruits, peaches, bananas, figs, almonds, a variety of spices, and the cultivation of rice. The colonists in the New World contributed tomatoes, chocolate, potatoes, and sweet and hot peppers.

32. The comida is the main meal of the day in Spain. It is eaten in the middle of the afternoon, around two or three o'clock. A main course of fish, poultry, or meat usually follows salad or soup. A light dessert ends the meal.

33. Catherine de Medici, an Italian, brought her cooks to France when she married the future French king, Henri II. These Italian cooks taught new cooking skills to the French. They also introduced new foods, such as peas, haricot beans, artichokes, and ice cream.

34. because most Italian restaurants in the United States are Neapolitan, and Naples is the heart of Southern Italian cooking

35. Greece is surrounded on three sides by water, thus seafood is a staple of Greek cuisine. Olive trees have deep roots that grow well in Greece's mountainous terrain, thus olives and olive oil are staples of Greek cuisine. Sheep thrive on the short grasses of the more mountainous areas of Greece, therefore, lamb is a staple of Greek cuisine. (Students may justify other responses.)

Mediterranean Countries

Name _____

Date _____ **Period** _____ **Score** _____

Chapter 29 Test

Matching: Match the following terms and identifying phrases.

_____ 1. A fleshy, oval-shaped vegetable with a deep purple skin.

_____ 2. A Spanish soup made with coarsely pureed tomatoes, onions, garlic, and green peppers; olive oil; and vinegar.

_____ 3. A dark sausage with a spicy, smoky flavor.

_____ 4. A variable Spanish rice dish often containing chicken, shrimp, mussels, whitefish, peas, and rice and flavored with saffron, salt, pepper, and pimiento.

_____ 5. A Spanish punch made with red wine, fruit juice, and sparkling water.

_____ 6. An Italian rice dish made with butter, chopped onion, stock or wine, and Parmesan cheese.

_____ 7. An Italian appetizer course.

_____ 8. A popular Italian vegetable soup thick with pasta.

_____ 9. A popular Greek sauce made from a mixture of egg yolks and lemon juice.

_____ 10. A paper-thin pastry made with flour and water used to make many Greek desserts.

A. antipasto
B. avgolemono
C. chorizo
D. eggplant
E. gazpacho
F. minestrone
G. paella
H. phyllo
I. risotto
J. sangria
K. tapas

True/False: Circle *T* if the statement is true or *F* if the statement is false.

T F 11. The Moors planted almond groves in Spain and used almonds in cooking.

T F 12. Many Spanish dishes are a mixture of two or more food flavors.

T F 13. Gazpacho is an avocado-based soup.

T F 14. Italian cooks use few herbs and spices.

T F 15. After pasta, Italy's most important staple food is seafood.

T F 16. Gorgonzola, ricotta, and provolone are examples of ribbon-shaped pastas.

T F 17. Chicken alla cacciatore is a Northern Italian specialty.

T F 18. The meat used most often in Greek dishes is beef.

T F 19. Feta cheese is a slightly salty, white cheese made from goat's milk.

T F 20. Honey sweetens many Greek desserts.

(Continued)

Name _____

Multiple Choice: Choose the best response. Write the letter in the space provided.

_____ 21. Which of the following foods is *not* an important ingredient in Spanish cuisine?
   A. Almonds.
   B. Garlic.
   C. Olive oil.
   D. Potatoes.

_____ 22. Buñeulitos, empanadillas, and banderillas are popular Spanish _____.
   A. appetizers
   B. desserts
   C. main dishes
   D. salads

_____ 23. Which of the following types of poultry is most popular in Spain?
   A. Chicken.
   B. Partridge.
   C. Pheasant.
   D. Pigeon.

_____ 24. Which of the following Italian foods is likely to be served "al dente?"
   A. Gnocchi.
   B. Orecchietta.
   C. Osso buco.
   D. Panettone.

_____ 25. Which of the following cheeses does *not* have Italian origins?
   A. Camembert.
   B. Mozzarella.
   C. Parmesan.
   D. Romano.

_____ 26. In Northern Italy _____.
   A. dairy products are popular
   B. foods are not as heavily spiced as they are in the South
   C. ribbon-shaped pastas are popular
   D. All of the above.

_____ 27. Marinated red peppers, Parma ham, salami, hard-cooked eggs, and stuffed tomatoes are foods used in _____.
   A. antipasto
   B. minestrone
   C. polenta
   D. risotto

_____ 28. Which of the following is served in Greek tavernas?
   A. Bouzoukia.
   B. Malaga.
   C. Retsina.
   D. Sangria.

_____ 29. Which of the following Greek dishes has Italian origins?
   A. Baklava.
   B. Kebabs.
   C. Moussaka.
   D. Pastitisio.

(Continued)

Name _____

_____ 30. Which of the following dishes is *not* made with phyllo?
   A. Baklava.
   B. Diples.
   C. Galat oboureko.
   D. Kopenhai.

Essay Questions: Provide complete responses to the following questions or statements.

31. What did the Romans, Moors, and Spanish colonists in the New World each contribute to the development of Spanish cuisine?
32. Describe the Spanish comida.
33. Why is Italy given credit for laying the foundation for French haute cuisine?
34. Why is Southern Italian cooking the cooking with which most people in the United States are familiar?
35. Give three examples of how the geography of Greece has contributed to certain foods becoming staples of Greek cuisine.

Middle East and Africa
Chapter 30

Objectives

After studying this chapter, students will be able to
- describe the food customs of the Middle East and Africa.
- discuss how climate, geography, and culture have influenced these customs.
- recognize and prepare foods that are native to each of these countries or regions.

Bulletin Board

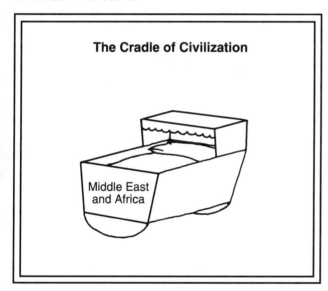

The Cradle of Civilization

Middle East and Africa

Title: "The Cradle of Civilization"

Place a cutout of a large cradle labeled "Middle East and Africa" in the middle of the bulletin board.

Teaching Materials

Text, pages 553-576
Student Activity Guide
- A. *Middle East Match*
- B. *Middle East Regional Cuisine*
- C. *Israeli Culture and Cuisine*
- D. *An African Buffet*

Teacher's Resource Binder
Map of the Middle East and Africa, transparency master 30-1
Middle Eastern Recipes, recipe master 30-2
Israeli Recipes, recipe master 30-3

African Recipes, recipe master 30-4
Chapter 30 Study Sheet, reproducible master 30-5
The Kwanzaa Table, color transparency CT-30
Chapter 30 Test
Software, diskette for Part Four
The Matching Game, chapter review game

Introductory Activities

1. *Map of the Middle East and Africa,* transparency master 30-1, TRB. Use the master to introduce students to the geographic regions they will be studying in this chapter and to illustrate the relationship of one region to another.
2. Have students bring in articles from newspapers and news magazines about current events in the Middle East and Africa. Have them share and discuss their articles with the rest of the class.

Strategies to Reteach, Reinforce, Enrich, and Extend Text Concepts

Middle Eastern Geography and Culture

3. **RF** Have students locate the countries that make up the core of the Middle East on a world map. Have them identify major geographical features.
4. **RT** Discuss with the class some Middle Eastern customs that differ sharply from those of the Western world.
5. **EX** Have students investigate the average annual rainfall of various regions of the Middle East. Ask them to analyze how rainfall affects agricultural production in those regions.
6. **ER** Have students research food customs of the ancient Egyptians and compare them with those of modern Egyptians. Have them present their findings in a short oral report.

Middle Eastern Cuisine

7. **RF** Have students name at least five foods that are served throughout most of the Middle East.

237

8. **RF**   Have students use cookbooks to find Middle Eastern recipes that are made with bulgur.

9. **RT**   Demonstrate for students how to prepare yogurt.

10. **ER**   Have lab groups prepare some of the recipes gathered in strategy 8. Use the yogurt prepared in strategy 9 in recipes calling for yogurt.

11. **ER**   Have each lab group prepare a different Middle Eastern dessert for a dessert buffet.

12. **ER**   Have each student research the food customs of one Middle Eastern country and write a menu for a meal typical of that country.

13. **EX**   *Middle Eastern Recipes,* recipe master 30-2, TRB. Have students use the recipe master to plan a Middle Eastern dinner including foods from several Middle Eastern countries. Have each lab group prepare a different recipe. Ask each group to complete a *Market Order Sheet* (TRB) and a *Time-Work Schedule* (TRB). After preparing their recipe, have each group share their dish with the rest of the class. Then have each group complete a *Lab Evaluation Sheet* (TRB).

14. **RF**   *Middle East Match,* Activity A, SAG. Students are to match descriptions related to the culture and cuisine of the Middle East with the terms they describe.

15. **RF**   *Middle East Regional Cuisine,* Activity B, SAG. Students are to answer questions about similarities and distinctions among the regional cuisines of the Middle East.

Israeli Geography and Culture

16. **ER**   Have students use library resources to find historical accounts of the establishment of the state of Israel. Have them summarize what they have read in a brief written report.

17. **ER**   Have each student conduct research and prepare a presentation on some aspect of life in a kibbutz.

18. **ER**   Divide the class into three groups. Have each group investigate the significance of the city of Jerusalem to one of the following religious groups: Christians, Jews, and Muslims.

19. **ER**   Guest speaker. Invite a rabbi to come to your class and talk about the origin and practice of Jewish customs.

Israeli Cuisine

20. **ER**   Guest speaker. Invite a kosher cook to speak to your class about Jewish dietary laws. Ask the speaker questions about kosher foods and how they are prepared.

21. **ER**   Field trip. Take your class to visit a Jewish delicatessen. Identify the country of origin for as many foods as possible.

22. **RF**   Have students divide a sheet of paper vertically into three columns. Have them head the columns *fleishig foods, milchig foods,* and *pareve foods.* Have students list at least 10 foods that belong in each category.

23. **ER**   Have each student select one Jewish holiday that interests him or her and research the traditions surrounding that holiday. Have students share their findings with the rest of the class.

24. **EX**   *Israeli Recipes,* recipe master 30-3, TRB. Have students use the recipe master to plan a typical Israeli meal. Have each lab group prepare a different recipe. Ask each group to complete a *Market Order Sheet* (TRB) and a *Time-Work Schedule* (TRB). After preparing their recipe, have each group share their dish with the rest of the class. Then have each group complete a *Lab Evaluation Sheet* (TRB).

25. **RF**   *Israeli Culture and Cuisine,* Activity C, SAG. Students are to determine whether statements about the culture and cuisine of Israel are true or false.

African Geography and Culture

26. **RT**   Show students a film about the culture of Africa or an African country. Ask them to pay particular attention to the foods and food customs mentioned in the film.

27. **ER**   Guest speaker. Invite an African student or someone who has recently visited Africa to talk to your class about life in the African countries with which he or she is familiar.

28. **ER**   Have each student research the climate and geography of the African nation of his or her choice. Have students share their findings with the class.

29. **RT**   Discuss with students the colonization of Africa by Europeans and how this European influence has affected the culture and cuisine of Africa.

30. **ER**   Have students investigate the origin and significance of the fast of Ramadan and summarize their findings in a two-page report.

31. **RT**   *The Kwanzaa Table,* color transparency CT-30, TRB. Use this transparency as you

discuss the symbolism of some of the items that appear on a table set for karamu—the Kwanzaa feast held on the next to last night of the weeklong celebration.

32. **ER**   Have students investigate the origin of Kwanzaa and the seven principles on which it is based.

African Cuisine

33. **ER**   Have each student research in detail the food customs of one African country and present his or her findings in a short oral report.

34. **EX**   *African Recipes,* recipe master 30-4, TRB. Have students use the recipe master to plan an African meal including dishes from several African countries. Have each lab group prepare a different recipe. Ask each group to complete a *Market Order Sheet* (TRB) and a *Time-Work Schedule* (TRB). After preparing their recipe, have each group share their dish with the rest of the class. Then have each group complete a *Lab Evaluation Sheet* (TRB).

35. **ER**   *An African Buffet,* Activity D, SAG. Have students research recipes they would serve as part of an African buffet and describe how the buffet would be served.

Chapter Review

36. **RT**   *Chapter 30 Study Sheet,* reproducible master 30-5, TRB. Have students complete the statements as they read text pages 554-572.

37. **RF**   *The Matching Game,* Software, diskette for Part Four. Have students play the chapter review came according to the instructions that appear on the screen.

Above and Beyond

38. **EX**   Have students prepare presentations comparing and contrasting the political, economic, and cultural settings of a Middle Eastern or African country with those of the United States. Students should develop several visual aids to use in giving the presentation.

Answer Key

Text

Review What You Have Read, page 576
1. garlic, lemon, green pepper, eggplant, tomato
2. false
3. (Describe three. Student response. See page 559 in the text.)

4. C
5. Chelo is boiled, buttered rice served with a topping. Polo is similar to pilaf in that all the accompaniments cook with the rice.
6. kibbutzim
7. E, B, C, A, D
8. (List five:) meat, cheese, potato, chicken, chicken liver, kasha
9. cacao
10. During the entire ninth calendar month, Muslims abstain from eating from sunrise to sunset. Meals eaten after sunset are light.
11. Injera is a large, sourdoughlike pancake. It is served with wat, a spicy sauce or stew. The injera is torn into pieces, rolled in the wat, and eaten with the fingers.
12. pillows, folded carpets, or the floor

Student Activity Guide

Middle East Match, Activity A, page 147

1. E, G, H, K, T	9. J
2. I	10. D
3. F	11. O
4. P	12. B
5. L	13. R
6. A	14. C
7. N	15. S
8. M	

Middle East Regional Cuisine, Activity B, page 148
1. Pork is forbidden by religions widely practiced in all Middle Eastern countries.
2. Lamb is the staple meat in the Middle East.
3. Yogurt is a dairy product served throughout the Middle East in a variety of dishes.
4. Wheat and rice are the staple grains in the Middle East.
5. Beans, lentils, and chick-peas are the staple legumes in the Middle East.
6. A. Turkey
   B. Iran
   C. Arab states

7. A	16. A
8. C	17. B
9. C	18. C
10. B	19. A
11. C	20. C
12. B	21. C
13. A	22. A
14. C	23. B
15. A	24. B

Israeli Culture and Cuisine, Activity C, page 149

1. T	14. F
2. T	15. T
3. F	16. T
4. T	17. F
5. F	18. F
6. T	19. F
7. T	20. T
8. T	21. T
9. F	22. T
10. T	23. T
11. T	24. F
12. F	25. T
13. F	

Teacher's Resources

Chapter 30 Test

1. A	15. T
2. H	16. F
3. C	17. F
4. G	18. T
5. D	19. T
6. B	20. F
7. I	21. C
8. F	22. B
9. J	23. D
10. K	24. D
11. F	25. C
12. F	26. A
13. T	27. D
14. F	28. A

29. Yogurt is eaten as a side dish, snack, and dessert. It also is used to make cakes and hot and cold soups. In some parts of the Middle East, yogurt is diluted with water and served as a beverage.

30. Scholars believe that wine, cheese, sherbet, and ice cream were first made by the Persians. The Persians were also the first to extract the essence of roses and to combine exotic herbs and spices with other foods.

31. As Jews have moved back into the present state of Israel, they have brought with them foods from 80 nations. These foods were combined with the area's native Middle Eastern cuisine. In addition, Israeli cooks have developed many totally new dishes based on foods readily available in Israel.

32. (Student response. See pages 564-565 of the text.)

33. African meals are often served on low tables with pillows, folded carpets, or the floor used as seats. The food is usually arranged on one large tray and placed in the center of the table. Each household member takes his or her individual share and foods are usually eaten with the fingers.

Middle East and Africa

Name _____

Date _____ Period _____ Score

Chapter 30 Test

Matching: Match the following terms and identifying phrases.

_____ 1. Grain product made from whole wheat that has been cooked, dried, and partly debranned, and cracked.

_____ 2. Arabian appetizers.

_____ 3. Iran's national dish, which consists of thin slices of marinated, charcoal-broiled lamb served with plain rice accompanied by a pat of butter, a raw egg, and a bowl of sumac.

_____ 4. Meal made from unleavened bread used in Jewish cooking.

_____ 5. A mixture of ground chick-peas, bulgur, and spices that is formed into balls and deep-fried.

_____ 6. A plant that produces beans that are ground into cocoa or made into chocolate.

_____ 7. A flat, round hollow bread.

_____ 8. Ethiopia's main dish, which is a large, sour-doughlike pancake.

_____ 9. A milletlike grain.

_____ 10. A spicy sauce or stew that is part of Ethiopian cuisine.

A. bulgur
B. cacao
C. chelo kebab
D. felafel
E. fleishig foods
F. injera
G. matzo meal
H. mazza
I. pita bread
J. teff
K. wat

True/False: Circle *T* if the statement is true or *F* if the statement is false.

T F 11. The origins of most Middle Eastern dishes can easily be traced to the invading tribe that introduced them into the cuisine.

T F 12. Large herds of swine are raised in the Middle East for food.

T F 13. In the Middle East, olive oil is used in place of butter or lard for cooking.

T F 14. In most of the Middle East, tea is the preferred beverage.

T F 15. Foods prepared according to Jewish dietary laws are called *kosher foods*.

T F 16. Jewish dishes containing both milk and meat are called *pareve dishes*.

T F 17. Blintzes are squares of noodle dough stuffed with a filling made of meat, cheese, potato, or chicken.

T F 18. The French influenced the foods of the North African countries.

T F 19. Ethiopia has a cuisine different from the rest of Africa because it was founded by Christians in an otherwise Muslim continent.

T F 20. Africans cut their food at the table with knives and eat it with forks, just as in the United States.

(Continued)

Name _____

Multiple Choice: Choose the best response. Write the letter in the space provided.

_____ 21. Which of the following is *not* a staple ingredient in Middle Eastern cuisine?
A. eggplant
B. green pepper
C. onion
D. tomato

_____ 22. Most middle Eastern meat dishes are made with _____.
A. beef
B. lamb
C. pork
D. poultry

_____ 23. Which Middle Eastern country is known for halva?
A. Egypt.
B. Iran.
C. Jordan.
D. Turkey.

_____ 24. Which of the following foods is *not* likely to be served in Israel?
A. Challah.
B. Gefilte fish.
C. Kreplach.
D. All of the above are served.

_____ 25. Many Jewish soups are served with _____.
A. blintzes
B. challah
C. knaidlach
D. kugel

_____ 26. Which of the following foods is *not* a pareve food?
A. Blintzes filled with cottage cheese.
B. Eggs.
C. Gefilte fish.
D. Oranges.

_____ 27. A bread found throughout Africa as well as in the Middle East is _____.
A. brik
B. challah
C. kesra
D. pita bread

_____ 28. An African root vegetable that is much like a sweet potato is _____.
A. cassava
B. guava
C. okra
D. papaya

Essay Questions: Provide complete responses to the following questions or statements.

29. How is yogurt used in the Middle East?
30. What contributions to Middle Eastern cuisine were made by the Persians?
31. Why is Israel's cuisine so varied?
32. Give three examples of Jewish dietary laws.
33. How are meals in Africa typically served and eaten?

Asia

Objectives

After studying this chapter, students will be able to
- discuss how climate, geography, and culture have influenced the food customs of Russia, India, China, and Japan.
- recognize and prepare foods that are native to each of the countries.

Bulletin Board

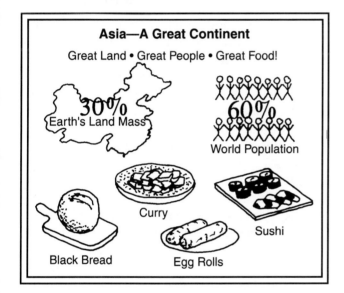

Title: "Asia—A Great Continent"

Play on the various definitions of the word "great" by dividing the bulletin board into three centers of focus—great land, great people, and great food. Use a cutout of the continent labeled to illustrate that Asia represents 30 percent of the earth's land mass. Use drawings of stick people, labeled to illustrate that Asia holds 60 percent of the world population. Then use labeled photos of classic Asian foods to illustrate Asia's interesting and varied cuisine.

Teaching Materials

Text, pages 577-615
Student Activity Guide
   A. *Russian Culture and Cuisine*
   B. *Indian Culture and Cuisine*
   C. *China Match*
   D. *Japan Maze*
   E. *Chinese and Japanese Cuisine*

Teacher's Resource Binder
   Map of Asia, transparency master 31-1
   Russian Recipes, recipe master 31-2
   Indian Recipes, recipe master 31-3
   Chinese Recipes, recipe master 31-4
   Japanese Recipes, recipe master 31-5
   Chapter 31 Study Sheet, reproducible master 31-6
   Using Chopsticks, color transparency CT-31
   Chapter 31 Test

Software, diskette for Part Four
   Hangman, chapter review game

Introductory Activities

1. *Map of Asia,* transparency master 31-1, TRB. Use the master to introduce students to the geographic regions they will be studying in this chapter and to illustrate the relationship of one country to another.
2. Have students brainstorm a list of Russian, Indian, Chinese, and Japanese foods. Use their responses as an indication of topics that you should emphasize when covering the chapter.

Strategies to Reteach, Reinforce, Enrich, and Extend Text Concepts

Russian Geography and Culture

3. **RT**   On a world map, point out for students the boundaries of Russia. Also indicate the dividing line betwen Asia and Europe.
4. **ER**   Have students use resource materials available in your school library to research the food habits of the czars. Have them share their findings with other class members in a short oral report.
5. **ER**   Guest speaker. Invite someone who has recently visited Russia to talk to your class about life in that country.

Russian Cuisine

6. **RF** Have students use the information they gathered in strategy 4 to write a menu for a meal that might have been served by a czar to visiting dignitaries.
7. **ER** Have each student choose one region of Russia that interests him or her and write a menu featuring specialties of that region.
8. **RT** Demonstrate for students how chicken Kiev is prepared. (Bone the chicken breasts as part of the demonstration.)
9. **EX** *Russian Recipes,* recipe master 31-2, TRB. Have students use the recipe master to plan a typical Russian dinner. Have each lab group prepare a different recipe. Ask each group to complete a *Market Order Sheet* (TRB) and a *Time-Work Schedule* (TRB). After preparing their recipe, have each group share their dish with the rest of the class. Then have each group complete a *Lab Evaluation Sheet* (TRB).
10. **RF** *Russian Culture and Cuisine,* Activity A, SAG. Students are to use a provided list of words to complete statements about the culture and cuisine of Russia.

Indian Geography and Culture

11. **RF** Have students use the following statement as the basis for a large group discussion: Religion has played an important role in the development of Indian cuisine.
12. **ER** Have each student use library resources to answer the following question in a one-page essay: How did the British influence Indian food customs?
13. **ER** Have students investigate food shortages in India. Ask them each to write a report summarizing what they learned about efforts to alleviate shortages and prevent shortages in the future.

Indian Cuisine

14. **RT** Demonstrate for students how to prepare ghee.
15. **RF** Have students use Indian cookbooks to compile a group of curry recipes. Ask students to identify how the various recipes differ and what characteristics make them similar.
16. **ER** Working in lab groups, have students prepare the various curry recipes they found in strategy 15.
17. **ER** Working in lab groups, have students prepare several Indian desserts and serve them buffet-style.

18. **RT** Demonstrate for students how to prepare a dry masala, using a mortar and pestle to grind spices.
19. **EX** *Indian Recipes,* recipe master 31-3, TRB. Have students use the recipe master to plan a typical Indian dinner. Have each lab group prepare a different recipe. Ask each group to complete a *Market Order Sheet* (TRB) and a *Time-Work Schedule* (TRB). After preparing their recipe, have each group share their dish with the rest of the class. Then have each group complete a *Lab Evaluation Sheet* (TRB).
20. **RT** *Indian Culture and Cuisine,* Activity B, SAG. Students are to determine whether various statements about Indian culture and cuisine are true or false.

Chinese Geography and Culture

21. **RF** Have students trace maps of China and draw in and label the major cities and geographic features. Then have them explain why much of western and southwestern China is sparsely populated.
22. **ER** Have each student research one of the Chinese dynasties and present his or her findings in a brief oral report to the rest of the class.
23. **ER** Have students write a paper comparing Buddhism, Taoism, and Confucianism.
24. **ER** Have students find articles in newspapers or news magazines about current social issues in the People's Republic of China. Have them share their articles with the rest of the class.

Chinese Cuisine

25. **ER** Field trip. Take the class to have lunch or dinner in a good Chinese restaurant located in your area. If possible, have the chef speak to your class about the ingredients and techniques he or she uses to prepare menu items.
26. **ER** Have students visit a Chinese grocery store or the international food section of a large supermarket. Ask them to make a list of all the Chinese foods that are available.
27. **RF** Using the list of foods compiled in strategy 25 and several Chinese cookbooks, have students make a list of recipes that they could prepare. Help students investigate where to obtain any missing ingredients.
28. **RT** Demonstrate for students how to use a cleaver by preparing vegetables, meats,

poultry, and fish for stir-frying. Use a wok and the foods you cut to prepare a Chinese main dish for students.

29. **ER** Working in lab groups, have students prepare a variety of dim sum. Serve the dim sum with several kinds of Chinese tea.

30. **RT** *Using Chopsticks,* color transparency CT-31, TRB. Use this transparency as you demonstrate how to use chopsticks.

31. **EX** *Chinese Recipes,* recipe master 31-4, TRB. Have students use the recipe master to plan a typical Chinese dinner. Have each lab group prepare a different recipe. Ask each group to complete a *Market Order Sheet* (TRB) and a *Time-Work Schedule* (TRB). After preparing their recipe, have each group share their dish with the rest of the class. Then have each group complete a *Lab Evaluation Sheet* (TRB).

32. **RF** *China Match,* Activity C, SAG. Students are to match terms related to Chinese culture and cuisine with their descriptions.

Japanese Geography and Culture

33. **RT** Discuss with the class the land scarcity and farming difficulties found in Japan.

34. **ER** Have each student use library resources to write a two-page report outlining the major effects the arrival of the first Occidentals had on Japanese culture.

35. **ER** Have students use flowers, rocks, fabric, and other materials to create a small decorative arrangement that would be appropriate in a Japanese home.

Japanese Cuisine

36. **RF** Demonstrate for students the preparation of Japanese tempura and American-style deep-fried, breaded shrimp. Emphasize the differences between the Japanese method of deep-frying and the method used in Western nations. Allow students to sample the products you have prepared. Ask them which product they prefer and why.

37. **RF** Have students use a Japanese cookbook to find recipes using tofu in a variety of ways.

38. **ER** Have students practice preparing attractive garnishes that would be appropriate to serve with various Japanese dishes.

39. **ER** Guest speaker. Invite a Japanese person who is familiar with the tea ceremony to come to your class to talk about the ceremony and its importance to the Japanese people.

40. **EX** *Japanese Recipes,* recipe master 31-5, TRB. Have students use the recipe master to plan a typical Japanese dinner. Have each lab group prepare a different recipe. Ask each group to complete a *Market Order Sheet* (TRB) and a *Time-Work Schedule* (TRB). After preparing their recipe, have each group share their dish with the rest of the class. Then have each group complete a *Lab Evaluation Sheet* (TRB).

41. **RF** *Japan Maze,* Activity D, SAG. Students are to complete statements with terms related to Japanese culture and cuisine. Then they are to find and circle the terms in a maze.

42. **EX** *Chinese and Japanese Cuisine,* Activity E, SAG. Students are to identify phrases that describe Chinese cuisine, Japanese cuisine, or both cuisines. Then they are to analyze similarities and differences between the two cuisines.

Chapter Review

43. **RT** *Chapter 31 Study Sheet,* reproducible master 31-6, TRB. Have students complete the statements as they read text pages 578-612.

44. **RF** *Hangman,* Software, diskette for Part Four. Have students play the chapter review game according to the instructions that appear on the screen.

Above and Beyond

45. **ER** Have students write a survey about Asian geography, climate, culture, cuisine, and current events. Have them conduct the survey throughout the school and the community. Then have them summarize their findings in an article for a local newspaper about local awareness of Asian concerns.

Answer Key

Text

Review What You Have Read, page 615
1. (List four:) broiled meats, sauerkraut, yogurt, kumys, curd cheese, tea drinking
2. bread, kasha, soup
3. (Name and describe two:) charlotte russe—ladyfinger mold with cream filling, fruit tart, kisel—pureed fruit, samsa—sweet walnut fritters, medivnyk—honey cake, paskha—rich cheesecake, kulich—tall, cylindrical yeast cake filled with fruits and nuts

4. In Northern India, foods are rich and heavily seasoned. In Southern India, foods are hotter and not as subtle or refined.
5. ghee
6. B
7. rice
8. (List and define four. Student response. See pages 597-598 in the text.)
9. wok
10. Land is scarce and the teachings of Buddhism forbid the eating of meat.
11. miso—fermented soybean paste, tofu—cus- tardlike cake with a mild flavor, shoyu— Japanese soy sauce that is used as a seasoning
12. (Describe two. Student response. See pages 611-612 in the text.)

Student Activity Guide

Russian Culture and Cuisine, Activity A, page 151

1. czar
2. Bolsheviks
3. samovar
4. kasha
5. zakuska
6. caviar
7. schi
8. borscht
9. ouba
10. shashlik
11. beef stroganov
12. chicken Kiev
13. blini
14. pirozhki
15. koumys
16. kisel
17. paskha
18. kulich

Indian Culture and Cuisine, Activity B, page 152

1. T
2. F
3. T
4. T
5. T
6. F
7. T
8. F
9. F
10. F
11. F
12. F
13. T
14. T
15. T
16. T
17. T
18. F
19. T
20. T
21. T
22. F
23. F
24. T
25. T
26. T
27. T
28. T
29. F
30. T

China Match, Activity C, page 153

1. I
2. K
3. D
4. M
5. O
6. Q
7. C
8. U
9. R
10. B
11. S
12. N
13. L
14. T
15. J
16. A
17. P
18. G
19. H
20. F

Japan Maze, Activity D, pages 154-155

1. sappari
2. typhoon
3. Occidentals
4. dictatorship
5. Buddhism
6. gohan
7. sake
8. soybean
9. tofu
10. shoyu
11. fugu
12. sushi
13. seaweed
14. daikon
15. mandarin
16. tempura
17. teriyaki
18. sukiyaki
19. hibachi
20. green
21. kaiseka
22. oshibori
23. plum
24. nori
25. soaked

Chinese and Japanese Cuisine, Activity E,
page 156

1. B
2. J
3. C
4. B
5. B
6. C
7. J
8. J
9. C
10. B
11. B
12. J
13. C
14. J
15. B
16. B
17. J
18. C
19. (Student response.)
20. (Student response.)
21. (Student response.)

Teacher's Resources

Chapter 31 Test

1. I
2. C
3. N
4. B
5. A
6. M
7. J
8. F
9. G
10. K
11. D
12. E
13. P
14. O
15. L
16. T
17. F
18. F
19. T
20. F
21. T
22. F
23. F
24. F
25. T
26. T
27. T
28. T
29. F
30. T
31. C
32. C
33. A
34. A
35. B
36. A
37. D
38. B
39. A
40. C
41. B
42. A

43. Mongols taught the Slavs how to broil meat and how to make yogurt, sauerkraut, kumys (a mild alcoholic beverage), and curd cheese. They also introduced tea drinking and the samovar.
44. The czars had elaborate banquets and served a variety of European foods. The peasants ate much simpler meals, consisting mainly of bread, kasha, and soup.
45. because many Indians are Hindus and many Hindus are vegetarian
46. Foods are stir-fried by heating a small amount of oil in a wok. The foods with the longest cooking time are added to the wok first. They are quickly stirred over high heat until the vegetables are crisp-tender.
47. (Student response. See page 611 in the text.)

Asia

Name _____

Date _____ **Period** _____ **Score** _____

Chapter 31 Test

Matching: Match the following terms and identifying phrases.

_____ 1. A Russian staple food made of buckwheat or other grains that are fried and then simmered until tender.

_____ 2. The processed, salted eggs of large fish.

_____ 3. Cabbage soup.

_____ 4. Russian beet soup.

_____ 5. A popular Russian meat dish made with tender strips of beef, mushrooms, and a seasoned sour cream sauce.

_____ 6. A rich cheesecake that is a popular Russian dessert.

_____ 7. A tall, cylindrical Russian yeast cake filled with fruits and nuts.

_____ 8. A type of Indian stew.

_____ 9. Indian clarified butter.

_____ 10. A mixture of spices used to make curry.

_____ 11. A flat bread that is common in India.

_____ 12. A thick porridge made from rice or barley often served for breakfast in China.

_____ 13. A mild-flavored, custardlike cake made from soybeans.

_____ 14. A popular Japanese dish made of thinly sliced meat, bean curd, and vegetables cooked in a sauce.

_____ 15. Japanese terms for green teas.

A. beef stroganov
B. borscht
C. caviar
D. chapatis
E. congee
F. curry
G. ghee
H. gohan
I. kasha
J. kulich
K. masala
L. nihon-cha
M. paskha
N. schi
O. sukiyaki
P. tofu

True/False: Circle *T* if the statement is true or *F* if the statement is false.

T   F   16. Russian cuisine has Slavic origins.

T   F   17. A samovar is used to prepare Russian coffee.

T   F   18. Most Russian meals end with zakuska.

T   F   19. Beef has been the traditional meat of Russian cuisine.

T   F   20. Beef is a staple food in the diets of the Hindus.

T   F   21. In Southern India where many people are vegetarians, pulses are an important protein source.

(Continued)

Name _____

T F 22. Vegetable oil is the preferred cooking fat in India.
T F 23. Most Chinese dishes are broiled or baked.
T F 24. Meat is more important to the Chinese diet than fish.
T F 25. Most Chinese soups are meant to be an accompaniment rather than a main dish.
T F 26. Chinese cooks use few dairy products.
T F 27. Tofu, shoyu, and miso all are made from soybeans.
T F 28. A number of Japanese fish dishes are eaten raw.
T F 29. In Japan, beef is of poor quality.
T F 30. Green tea, rather than black tea, is preferred by the Japanese.

Multiple Choice: Choose the best response. Write the letter in the space provided.

_____ 31. Which of the following was *not* a staple food in the Russian peasant's diet?
   A. Bread.
   B. Kasha.
   C. Lamb.
   D. Soup.

_____ 32. Which of the following food probably would *not* appear on a zakuska table?
   A. Caviar.
   B. Pickled herring.
   C. Roast suckling pig.
   D. Salads.

_____ 33. The major ingredient in borscht is _____.
   A. beets
   B. cabbage
   C. fish
   D. potatoes

_____ 34. Which of the following is *not* one of the basic spices used in Indian cooking?
   A. Cinnamon.
   B. Cumin seed.
   C. Fennel seed.
   D. Turmeric.

_____ 35. When meats are braised in yogurt, they have been prepared using the cooking technique known as _____.
   A. chasnidarth
   B. korma
   C. tandoori
   D. vindaloo

_____ 36. Samosas are popular Indian _____.
   A. appetizers
   B. breads
   C. main dishes
   D. vegetable dishes

_____ 37. Wheat flour is used to make _____.
   A. egg roll wrappers
   B. lo mein noodles
   C. wonton wrappers
   D. All of the above.

(Continued)

Name _____

_____ 38. In China, which of the following foods is considered a sign of good luck?
  A. Dim sum.
  B. Eggs.
  C. Lychee nuts.
  D. Red tea.

_____ 39. Which of the following foods is *not* basic to Japanese cuisine?
  A. Meat.
  B. Rice.
  C. Seaweed.
  D. Soybeans.

_____ 40. Which of the following Japanese dishes is prepared by deep-frying?
  A. Beef sukiyaki.
  B. Chicken teriyaki.
  C. Shrimp tempura.
  D. Yakitori.

_____ 41. In Japan, a hibachi is used to _____.
  A. bake foods
  B. grill foods
  C. steam foods
  D. stir-fry foods

_____ 42. The Japanese prefer to end a meal with _____.
  A. fruit
  B. rice cakes
  C. steamed dumplings
  D. sweet pudding or pastry

Essay Questions: Provide complete responses to the following questions or statements.

43. What contributions did the Mongols make to Russian cuisine?
44. How did the diets of the Russian czars and Russian peasants differ?
45. Why are vegetarian dishes prominent in Indian cuisine?
46. How are foods stir-fried?
47. Describe the tradition of the Japanese tea ceremony.